ALSO BY ELLEN SANDBECK

Eat More Dirt: Diverting and Instructive Tips for Growing and Tending an Organic Garden

Slug Bread & Beheaded Thistles: Amusing and Useful Techniques for Nontoxic Housekeeping and Gardening

Organic Housekeeping

IN WHICH THE NONTOXIC AVENGER SHOWS YOU HOW TO
IMPROVE YOUR HEALTH AND THAT OF YOUR FAMILY
WHILE YOU SAVE TIME, MONEY, AND, PERHAPS, YOUR SANITY

Written and Illustrated by

ELLEN SANDBECK

Scribner
NEW YORK   LONDON   TORONTO   SYDNEY

SCRIBNER
1230 Avenue of the Americas
New York, NY 10020

SCRIBNER and design are trademarks of
Macmillan Library Reference USA, Inc., used under license
by Simon & Schuster, the publisher of this work.

DESIGNED BY KYOKO WATANABE

Text set in Goudy

Manufactured in the United States of America

ISBN-13: 978-0-7432-5620-9
ISBN-10: 0-7432-5620-4

This book is dedicated to my husband, Walter.
Wherever I am with him, I am home.

Acknowledgments

This book is the product of a truly collaborative effort involving my friends and family, as well as a few very patient and knowledgeable safety experts, and contains the collective knowledge and experience of a great many people of assorted ages who run the complete housekeeping gamut from neat as a pin to out of control.

I would never have maintained my sanity or finished this book without help from the following well-loved friends and family members:

My wonderful and patient husband and children, Walter, Dmitri, and Addie Sandbeck, who cheerfully endured years of experimentation.

Jean Sramek, who patiently, carefully, and with great good humor read and reread my manuscript and helped me avoid committing horrible errors in print.

The ever patient, encouraging, and brilliant Ann Klefstad, who never refuses a plea for grammatical assistance.

Janis Donnaud, the world's best literary agent, who keeps me going.

My amazing editors, Beth Wareham and Mindy Werner, who whipped the manuscript into shape.

Pat Hamon, for manuscript reading.

Al and Lynda Parella and Charlie Nichol, my chemical consultants.

Philip Cook of the EPA.

Jim Mlodozyniec, lead housing inspector for the city of Duluth, Minnesota.

Captain Marcus Hardin, Hazardous Materials Coordinator for the Duluth Fire Department.

Tim Lundell, Household Hazardous Waste Technician, WLSSD.

The entire staff of the Duluth Public Library.

Housekeeping and lifestyle consultants and technique testers: Traci Eaton, Theresa Koenig, Rebecca Ellenson, Susie Newman, Sarah Benning, Alison Aune, Jenny Bergal, Carolyn Olson, Tim Kaiser, Suzanne Seeley, Terry Johnson, John Bankson, Susan Sjoberg, Cynthia Niemela, and Grace Miller.

Thank you all!

Contents

Organic Housekeeping

Introduction

Ever since I first began landscaping organically in 1980, friends have been asking me for advice about how to solve problems around the home and garden without using chemicals or breaking too much of a sweat; in 1995, after I first self-published *Slug Bread & Beheaded Thistles: Amusing and Useful Techniques for Nontoxic Housekeeping and Gardening*, total strangers began contacting me as well. When asked for housekeeping tips, I always made it clear that I was primarily an organic gardener and that the sole focus of my housekeeping was to keep my family healthy and happy. Period. But a couple of years ago, my focus broadened a bit: A few of my friends were unable to maintain control of their homes and the disorder was making them suffer. I spent many long, chatty days helping them clear out and reclaim their living and storage spaces. The profoundly life-changing effects of these cleaning and organizing sessions made me realize that I wanted to write a book about nontoxic housekeeping.

For several months, my big party joke went something like this: "Guess what the subject of my next book is?" Everyone guessed that I was writing another gardening book. After a well-calculated pause, I would deliver the punch line: "It's about organic housekeeping!" Incredulous and hysterical laughter generally erupted. The joke worked so well because I am one of the least domestic people I know. I prefer to spend as little time as possible doing housework: I would rather dig a ditch than iron a shirt. But on the other hand, my family is extremely healthy; I am quite knowledgeable about managing living systems, controlling pest organisms, and preventing disease; no one has ever gotten sick from my cooking or cleaning; and although both my husband and I had allergies when we were children, our offspring have no allergies at all. After they stopped laughing, most people told me they wanted a copy of the book as soon as it was published. My friends know that if there is an easy, low-maintenance, nontoxic way to accomplish a task, I will find it.

I have been an organic landscaper, gardener, and worm farmer for most of my adult life. One of my great pleasures is to design and set up a miniature ecosystem, tend and tweak it, and watch it balance itself out. During the years I have repeated this process in dozens of gardens, ranging in size from the tiny to the massive, and with hundreds of worm-composting systems for food waste, ranging in size from under-the-sink to large industrial. My goal with each of these projects has been to design a low-maintenance ecosystem that is as self-sufficient as possible.

Both a low-maintenance organic garden and a worm composting system depend upon beneficial bacteria, fungi, and other microorganisms to break down organic waste materials, synthesize vital nutrients, and fend off harmful microorganisms. In this way they resemble all other living systems on our planet, whether that system is a prairie, a blue whale, or a human being. Without bacteria, the surface of much of our planet would rapidly be buried under piles of unrotted wood, leaves, and dead animals. But we would not be here to suffer the consequences because, without our intestinal microbes, we would long since have starved to death.

Unfortunately, many modern cleaning products contain antimicrobial agents. Like all other pesticides, antimicrobials have a tendency to kill off beneficial organisms while allowing harmful ones to proliferate. As they say: "Only the good die young." Our homes are our habitats, and our health depends upon a large population of helper microbes in and on our bodies as well as in our houses.

My housekeeping philosophy and my gardening philosophy are essentially the same: Evaluate the situation; work with what you have; don't make extra work for yourself; and as much as possible, avoid the use of toxic chemicals. In general, I've found that my attitude mirrors that of people who are the most knowledgeable about the effects of chemicals; all of the chemists, hazardous materials workers, emergency workers, and biological researchers whom I've interviewed avoid using synthetic chemicals in their own homes.

If we are to thrive physically, our air, water, and food must be clean. If we are to thrive emotionally, our shelter should be a home filled with love. With the exception of clothing, our basic needs are exactly the same as those of other mammals.

Many of us who live in the developed world have gone well beyond satisfying our basic physical and emotional needs. In fact, we have gone so far that some of those basic needs are no longer being met. We seem to have forgotten what our ancestors knew quite well: The only real reason to do any cleaning at all is in order to maintain our health. If that cleaning happens to make our homes and our clothing look prettier, so much the better. But if we clean just for appearances, rather than for health, we may end up rubbing our burning eyes, scratching our rough, reddened skin, and suffering asthma attacks while wearing soft, fragrant, toxic clothing in gleaming homes that make us dizzy with the aerosolized essence of mountain meadows. Then we can look out the windows and watch the robins fainting on our perfect lawns.

One spring Emily Dickinson wrote this down: "House is being cleaned. I prefer pestilence."

Before the twentieth century, housework was a grueling, full-time job that only the wealthiest householders were able to avoid. Carrying water, tending fires, making clothing, and cooking left very little time for other activities. Wood and coal fires and oil lamps produced soot that built up on walls, furniture, and carpeting each winter, making exhaustive spring cleaning a necessity.

Twentieth-century "labor saving" devices promised to change women's lives beyond recognition. A shirt that used to take months to sew by hand could be machine sewn in a matter of hours; central heating and gas and electric stoves rendered wood piles obsolete; and automatic washing machines and dryers liberated housekeepers from days of heavy labor every week.

Our predecessors knew that the reasons for doing household chores were to keep their families healthily fed, clothed, and sheltered and to protect the house and its contents from damage caused by pests and the elements. They would be shocked at the extra work we are making for ourselves. If a woman living in 1904 was transported one hundred years into the future and was given a washing machine and dryer, a vacuum cleaner, a sewing machine, a dishwasher, running water, indoor plumbing, electric lights, and a gas or electric stove, would she spend all that saved time fretting over bacteria in her drain or garbage pail, or worrying about whether dust mites inhabited her pillow?

In 1900, a newborn American's life expectancy was 47 years, but by 2000, it had increased to 74.8 years. This increase is due to the construction of municipal water and sanitation systems and to the development of vaccines. We are no longer dying in droves from diseases caused by poor sanitation; now we are suffering from chronic conditions such as heart disease and diabetes, caused by our affluent and indolent lifestyle, and allergic diseases such as asthma and eczema, which many researchers believe are induced by too much cleanliness. Many of us seem to be suffering from alienation and depression as well.

Our great-grandmothers' homes were obviously clean enough, or we wouldn't exist. The extra sanitation promised by in-the-tank toilet cleaners, antimicrobial dish liquids, disinfecting sprays, and air fresheners is not making us happier or healthier. There is not a synthetic cleaning product on the market that can improve our health, though there are plenty that can ruin it.

One thing that our foremothers knew only too well is that housework is tedious, repetitious, and boring. Suggesting that housework is fulfilling or satisfying or that you can get exercise by doing deep knee bends while cleaning is disingenuous. The only rational response is to do housework efficiently and as little as possible, then go out and do something you enjoy.

In 2002, researchers at the University of Glasgow officially discovered that doing domestic chores lowers people's spirits; all other known forms of exercise elevate them. Professor Nanette Mutrie, who is on the Scottish Executive's national physical task force, said, "With vigorous exercise, the effect is clear; the more you do, the better it is for wellbeing. . . . With housework it is the opposite—the more you do, the more depression you report."

We cannot afford to assume that industry has our health and best interests at heart. Dr. Benjamin Rush, a signatory to the Declaration of Independence and America's first surgeon general, wrote, "There is a place in Scotland where madness is sometimes induced by the fumes of lead. Patients who are affected with it bite their hands, and tear the flesh upon other parts of their bodies . . ." Yet lead was added to gasoline to improve engine performance until 1976, when it was banned by the federal government. Lead was also a common ingredient in house paints until the government banned it in 1977. Inner-city children are still suffering from the effects of exposure to lead-based paints and lead contaminated soils.

If industry can ignore lead's well-known toxicity, how much more easily can it ignore the as-yet-unknown dangers of newly invented synthetics? More than seventy-five thousand different synthetic chemicals have been formulated in the United States and have been released on to the market and into the environment. An additional two thousand to three thousand new chemicals are introduced each year. Not even the most brilliant and dedicated chemist could possibly keep track of all of them. How can a lay person hope to be well informed enough to make intelligent choices about which products to buy and which to avoid?

I was underwhelmed when I read a December 21, 2000, news release from the U.S. Environmental Protection Agency (EPA), which began as follows: "As part of EPA's commitment to increase chemical information, two notices have been issued directed at voluntary expansion of health and safety testing of chemicals." The release announced the establishment of the Voluntary Children's Chemical Evaluation Program. It continued, "The program identifies 23 chemicals on which manufacturers will be asked to voluntarily generate key testing information. These 23 chemicals were selected because monitoring studies found them present in human tissue samples."

The news release included the announcement of the High Production Volume Challenge program, ". . . which called on the U.S. chemical industry to voluntarily commit to providing the public with basic health and safety data on the 2,800 chemicals produced in highest volume."

Those twenty-three questionable chemicals are already lodged in my body, but I don't remember volunteering to be a chemical guinea pig. One can only wonder why our government is politely asking the manufacturers to volunteer to test their own products for safety.

The 1998 Chemical Hazard Data Availability Study, which is posted on the Environmental Protection Agency's website, stated, "Most Americans would assume that basic toxicity testing is available and that all chemicals in commerce today are safe. A recent EPA study has found that this is not a prudent assumption." This is an interesting statement, especially coming as it does from a governmental agency whose official mission is ". . . to protect human health and the environment."

The EPA looked at a set of 491 chemicals found in commonly used consumer products and found that only 25 percent of them had been tested for toxicity. According to this report, it would cost $427 million to test the toxicity of all of the most commonly used chemicals, a figure equal to "0.2% of the total annual sales of the top 100 U.S. chemical companies." Why hasn't the U.S. government required that this testing be done? Perhaps our ignorance is the chemical companies' bli$$.

In the United States, chemicals—like criminal defendants—are assumed innocent until proven guilty. Only chemicals that have been proven dangerous beyond a reasonable doubt are removed from the market.

The Stockholm Treaty on dangerous persistent organic pollutants (POPs), which was signed by 151 nations including the United States, became legally binding on May 17, 2004. The treaty bans the so-called Dirty Dozen of the most dangerous synthetic chemicals. They are aldrin, chlordane, DDT, dieldrin, endrin, heptachlor, mirex, toxaphene, polychlorinated biphenyls (PCBs), hexachlorobenzene, dioxins, and furans.

Klaus Toepfer, executive director of the United Nations Environment Programme (UNEP), said, "For decades these highly toxic chemicals have killed and injured people and wildlife by inducing cancer and damaging the nervous, reproductive and immune systems. They have also caused uncounted birth defects."

If it took decades to remove these horrifyingly dangerous chemicals from the market, how long might it take to ban a chemical that was merely dangerous? The surest way to protect yourself and your family from the dangers of toxic synthetic chemicals is to choose products made of safe, natural, and preferably food-grade ingredients.

Modern dwellings may contain many synthetic products that can be hazardous to the health. These products can be divided into two categories: those that are built into the house and its furnishings, which can be expensive and time consuming to replace, and consumer products that are used up and replaced on a regular basis, such as toiletries, cleaning supplies, clothing, and bedding. It is relatively easy and inexpensive to switch to nontoxic versions of these consumable products, and the health benefits can be enormous.

Most of this book deals with these easily replaceable, nondurable goods. But it is important to understand the more permanent toxins that lurk in our homes so that we can make informed decisions when we need to replace our more durable belongings.

A quick overview of the average American home may reveal the following toxins:

Living room: Volatile organic compounds (VOCs), which can outgas for five years from new furniture, carpets, carpet pads, upholstery, curtains and paneling; fabric and carpet waterproofing and stain proofing treatments (fluoropolymers); furniture polish; and antique mercury barometer.

Kitchen: Formaldehyde outgassing from particleboard in new cabinets and countertops, toxic gases produced by overheated nonstick cookware, mold and mildew growing under the sink, carbon monoxide emitted from a stove that isn't functioning properly, polycarbonate milk and juice bottles in the refrigerator, plastic-lined tin cans, vinyl flooring, chlorine-bleach scouring powder, antimicrobial dish liquid, chlorine-based dishwasher detergent, spray disinfectant, one-serving microwaveable plastic foam bowls, plastic food wrap, all-purpose cleaner, bleach, drain cleaner, floor wax, oven cleaner, metal polish, lead-glazed dishes, lead crystal decanters, and pewter drinking mugs.

Utility closet: Carpet cleaner, room deodorizer, and mothballs.

Bathroom: Chlorine-based cleansers, toilet bowl cleaners and disinfectants, drain cleaner, room deodorants, antimicrobial soap, body and hair care products, antiperspirants, lotions, cosmetics and perfumes that contain endocrine-disrupting chemicals, mold and mildew, PVC plumbing pipes, and mercury thermometer.

Bedroom: Freshly dry-cleaned clothing emitting perchloroethylene fumes in the closet, mattress outgassing formaldehyde, stain repellent, flame retardant, dust-mite insecticide, wrinkle-resistant sheets, and curtains and clothing emitting formaldehyde fumes.

Basement, garage, workshop: Gasoline, solvents, paints, paint thinner, lubricants, antifreeze, caulk, glue, lacquer, pesticides, herbicides, degreasers, spray paint, water sealant, rubber cement, turpentine, mineral spirits, lighter fluid, and mold.

Laundry room: Spot removers, chlorine bleach, perfumed fabric softeners and detergents, spray starch.

Older homes: Lead-based paint.

Obviously, it's easy to end up with an impressive collection of toxins unless you're selective and creative in your approach to housekeeping. Though the advertisers would like us to believe otherwise, most cleaning products are completely unnecessary and easily replaced with common ingredients that may already be in your pantry or cupboard. Throughout this book, you'll find information on recommended equipment and supplies as well as many nontoxic, timesaving cleaning techniques. In addition, at the end there's a complete bibliography and list of sources and websites that contain information on topics ranging from fire safety and hazardous materials to insulating paint and self-cleaning windows.

They say that if you haven't got your health, you haven't got anything, but I would like to add that once you have your health, having a little space, time, and money is nice as well. Environmentally sound housekeeping minimizes the household's negative impact on the environment. This approach generally leads to fewer things in a house, and thus more open space; having fewer possessions means you're spending less time taking care of them; and buying fewer things saves money. What could be better than being healthy and having more time, money, and space to enjoy?

A home can be developed into a balanced ecosystem, just as a garden can. The biggest difference between interior and exterior ecosystems is that the outdoor ones are largely self-cleaning, while interior ecosystems are not. Because many natural processes are excluded from the indoor habitat, humans have had to perfect activities such as taking out the garbage to do the work of decomposers, and washing the dishes and dusting to replace the cleaning properties of the excluded wind, rain, and snow.

In the pages ahead you'll find all of the information you need to create your own healthy, balanced ecosystem with a minimum of fuss. Knowledge is power. Read on.

First Things First

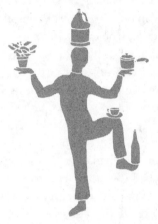

Moderation in All Things

Keeping everything perfect in your home is generally impossible unless you live alone. Being extremely organized may be a simple form of authoritarianism. It was said of Mussolini that "He made the trains run on time."

If you are tyrannizing your loved ones in order to keep your house "just-so," try to relax! Try really hard! Most people will find you much more attractive if you smell like freshly baked cookies rather than Lysol.

Before my friend Sarah-the-Neatnik mellowed, she would say to her son: "Just give Mommy two hours with a clean house! No, you can't use the bathroom."

Because she loves her family, Sarah has learned to ask herself weighty existential questions such as, "Is it important that I put away the laundry right now, or should I read to Maggie?" By the time you get around to asking the question, you already know the answer.

Organizing

You cannot clean a surface that you can't reach. Tidying and cleaning go together like horse and cart: The horse must precede the cart and the tidying must precede the cleaning. Most people are more than capable of applying a suitable cleaner and a reasonable amount of force to a dirty object, thus transforming it into a clean one. Even very young children can do this quite effectively. (So can our dogs, who quite efficiently clean spilled food off our kitchen floor.) Unfortunately, tidying up can stymie even the most well-intentioned cleaner. The key is organization.

A friend who worked in hotel housekeeping for a few years told me about the cleaning routine: Each suite contained a bed (and sometimes a hide-a-bed and a roll-away cot), bedside tables, a dresser, a closet, a bathroom, a kitchenette with a table, a dinette, and a living room with a couch. Every single surface in the suite had to be cleaned every day. By the time the maid left, she had scrubbed the entire bathroom and replaced the towels; sprayed, wiped, and dried the shower curtains; washed the bathroom fixtures, and dried them to prevent water spots. She had changed all the bed linens; emptied and cleaned out the refrigerator and microwave; vacuumed the floors and dusted all the surfaces, including the lampshades. She accomplished all of this in about thirty minutes per suite.

Cleaning at this breakneck speed is only possible because uninhabited hotel rooms are completely devoid of clutter. I find a touch of clutter comforting and homey, but one needs to find a happy medium between a light dollop of the happy clutter that makes a house a home, and the deep sedimentary layers that settle heavily on the soul.

A Place for Everything

"A place for everything and everything in its place" can seem hopelessly out of reach when one is in the throes of disorganization. Mopping a completely bare floor can be accomplished in about five minutes, but if you have to shift dozens of homeless objects back and forth as you mop, the job may take hours.

Anything that is stored on the floor, on countertops, or on tables and dressers will slow down your housecleaning. Unless you are one of the two or three people in the world who actually loves to clean and wants to prolong the process as much as possible, you really don't want to be indoors cleaning at all.

So get those knickknacks locked away in a glass fronted cabinet where you can enjoy them without having to dust them every week (or month, or year). Dusting the top of a cabinet will take a fraction of the time it would take to dust each piece of your extensive collection of snow globes, beer bottles, or porcelain frogs, ducks, penguins, or pigs.

Put the books back on the shelves.

Send those extra toasters to Goodwill. (And speaking of appliances, an appliance garage—a sliding door that closes off the space under an open kitchen counter—is a beautiful thing, especially when compared to a herd of dusty and grease-spattered small appliances on top of the counter. Appliance garages are fairly easy and inexpensive to install.)

This is not a rehearsal. This is your real life. Make it as pleasant as possible.

(If you are naturally tidy, your home is already neat, and your family is helpful, you may want to skip this chapter.)

If You Can't Find It, You Might as Well Not Own It

This is the tale of the marvelous household index file.

The American Demographics Society tells us that Americans waste a collective 9 million hours per day looking for misplaced items. Cleaning professionals estimate that getting rid of clutter would eliminate 40 percent of the housework in the average American home. Perhaps not coincidentally, a report from *The Wall Street Journal* stated that white collar workers waste an average of up to 40 percent of their workday due to disorganization and clutter. (And how much more complex is the average home than the average office?)

It is certainly preferable to retrieve an item from its accustomed place than to go buy a replacement; replacing usable items wastes time, money, resources, and storage space.

The greatest discovery of my housekeeping voyage has been the Household Index File. One day, after spending several unamusing hours trying to find a seasonal kitchen item, I decided that since *my* memory was unlikely to improve, I needed to create an *external* memory. I spent about three hours emptying and cleaning our kitchen storage, jettisoned items we weren't using, and thought hard about which items to put in the most convenient places. Then, as I put each item away, I filled out a Rolodex card for it.

I was quite proud of my new memory aid, and when my family returned home, I happily showed off my system. They laughed. I attempted to explain. This made them laugh harder. Within a week I was lording it over them: When they asked, "Mom, where's the ___?" I would open my Rolodex file with a flourish, look up the item—"tape measure, kitchen" for instance—and find that it was stored in drawer 10/B. Eventually even the biggest skeptics had to admit that the system worked.

I spared myself at least three hours of searching during the first week. Gradually, I've been expanding the scope of my household index beyond the kitchen. Being able to find things quickly and easily gives me a great feeling of power. But the true beauty of the system is that it spreads knowledge and increases everyone's ability to put things away.

When we go on vacation, I leave the file on top of the kitchen counter for the benefit of the house sitter. My ambition is to have a household index system so complete that a house sitter could find everything necessary to run the house by looking it up in the index. *There is no such thing as absolutely obvious!* There are people in my family who can barely find their underwear while they are wearing it. Obvious is in the mind of the beholder.

I consider my Household Index File, and the extra month of time it saves me per year, to be the ultimate in functional beauty. My initial investment of three hours paid off in a savings of more than one hundred hours in the first year, and at least one hundred hours every year since.

Setting Up a Household Indexing System

1. Acquire a small index box or a Rolodex with alphabetized dividers and a lot of blank cards.
2. Decide on a labeling system. My original labeling system was a bit cumbersome; having learned the hard way, I suggest an alphanumeric system such as 1/A, 1/B, 1/C; 2/A, 2/B, 2/C.

3. Label your storage areas. My labels are on the fronts of my drawers and cupboard doors, but you may want to be more discreet and
   write the numbers on the insides of the cabinets.
4. Remove everything from a single storage area. Dust and clean the
   storage area, then carefully inspect each displaced item. Now is
   the time to relocate items to the most efficient storage spaces.
   - Store items by category: If you have two hundred sal-
     vaged buttons together in a cigar box, it's a collection;
     the same buttons in twenty different locations would be
     trash. (Keep matching buttons together by stringing
     them on a length of button thread or on a large safety
     pin.) Resources are resources only if you can find them
     and use them.
   - Heavy or bulky items should be stored close to the ground
     in order to minimize accidents.
   - Frequently used items should be stored in the most con-
     venient locations.
   - Seldom-used items should be stored in the least conven-
     ient locations.
   - Items that no one ever uses should be stored in someone
     else's location. Good, usable items should be sold or given
     away. Useless items should be recycled or discarded.
5. Fill out a Rolodex card for each item that you put in the newly
   cleaned storage area. Write the name of the item across the top of
   the card and its location on a top corner of the card, like so: *top
   left corner:* 11/B top shelf; *middle of card:* Seed Sprouter. There is
   plenty of room on the card for additional information such as
   where to find spare parts. (I am sure that computer-savvy householders can set up a Domestic Index System with a simple database program. Don't ask me how.)

   Put the displaced items near their eventual storage spaces.
   Put the discards, the recyclables, and the Goodwill items in boxes
   and bags.
6. Label, clean, and empty out the next storage space.
7. Continue until all your storage spaces are clean and organized.

8. Index new items immediately. When you finally need those pipe cleaners five years after you acquired them, you will be able to find them.

   Note: Anything not worth writing about isn't worth keeping. If you're having real trouble divesting, try filling out an index card with the name, location, and function of the object. This exercise may make you laugh or blush, enabling you to let go.

9. An empty space in a cupboard means that something was there and needs to be put back. Don't just randomly put stuff in the empty space. If you can't label the object that goes in the space, try writing on the shelf, like so: "Coffee maker goes here."

   Make it obvious where things belong. Don't move them from place to place; keep things consistent. If you have to move things to get to objects you need every day, you need to reorganize.

10. Don't throw things randomly in the garage or basement. The Household Index File system works well for these utilitarian areas, too. Wouldn't you prefer to be able to easily retrieve your own pair of tin snips rather than go to the hardware store because you've misplaced eleven previous pairs?

Home Maintenance Protocols

Many households include one essential person who knows how to shut off the water supply, turn off the gas at the main valve, turn off electrical breakers, relight pilot lights, change water filters, replace faucet washers, and perform other routine maintenance chores. This is knowledge that should be shared before there is an emergency. Ask your expert(s) to write how-to instructions for each of these procedures and start a Household Maintenance binder.

Each how-to page should include the location of the service or appliance, the relevant emergency phone number (electric company, water company, gas company), safety precautions, the location and description of necessary tools, and detailed instructions for completing the job. Either slip each page into a plastic binder-sleeve or have it laminated so that when you take it on the job with you, it will stay clean and dry even if you are getting wet and dirty.

Labeling Tools

We are a multiple-tool family. For instance, we own two pairs of kitchen scissors, a pair of sewing scissors, shop scissors, paper scissors, office scissors, and greenhouse scissors; we also own three tape measures that belong in three different locations, as well as many other duplicate tools. These tools have an irritating tendency to migrate to the wrong floor or even the wrong building, so I have labeled them by location. (Light-colored handles take indelible ink very well, but the label on dark-handled tools may need to be scratched or engraved.)

Labeling tools is very much like putting a tag on a dog: When the dog wanders, the finder can return him.

Junk Drawers and Miscellaneous Storage

Our friend Grace, who has eight decades of housekeeping under her belt, taught me how to divide and conquer junk drawers, cupboards, and closets. Grace's house is so organized that when her brother came to live with her after his wife died, he could easily find everything in the house without assistance. Grace's secret weapon is modified cardboard boxes.

GRACE'S BOX TRICKS

- Use labeled shoe boxes to store things on closet shelves.
- Use cereal, tea, and cracker boxes to divide drawers and cupboards. Gather your pasteboard materials, then divide the drawers and cupboards one at a time. Simplify by putting seldom-used items in a box or bag at the back of the appropriate drawer.
- Put open boxes in underwear and sock drawers.
- Use a utility knife to cut the boxes to fit.

For a short while, customizing pasteboard boxes with a utility knife was my hobby, and "Square Is Beautiful" and "Divide and Conquer" were my favorite mottos. Ready-made drawer organizers just cannot compete with these customized dividers.

Once a space has been divided and its contents categorized, its carrying capacity increases and it tends to resist disorder. When was the last time you saw a disorderly silverware drawer? We don't drop our spoons in with our knives, why should we allow our twist ties to twine around our rubber bands, salvaged string, and spare electrical cords?

- I cut the tops off tea boxes and used them to tame our kitchen junk drawers three years ago. The drawers are just as tidy today as the day I conquered them.
- The bottom of a thin cereal box (from hot cereal, for instance) works well for organizing twist ties and rubber bands.
- Prevent lightweight extension cords from tangling by storing them in the cardboard tubes from paper towels.
- I made cardboard dividers for our overflowing collection of grocery bags; the dividers increased the capacity of the cubby by keeping the folded bags upright. The chaos has never returned.
- Heavy-duty cardboard boxes, such as detergent boxes, can be used to build stacked cubicles for storing lightweight dry goods like dry noodles or lightweight toiletries such as toothbrushes or Band-Aids.
- Square, heavy plastic containers such as liquid detergent bottles can be cut down to make cubby holes and dividers for under-sink and other damp storage. Many of these containers are heavy enough to support some weight. Since I don't use liquid detergent, I scrounged for detergent bottles at our local recycling center.

Absentmindedness

A lot of clutter is the product of absentmindedness. We walk into a room with something in our hand, set it down for a minute while we are doing something else, then forget to put it away. If everyone in the household does this, it isn't long before everyone is running around frantically looking for misplaced items. Acquiring anticlutter habits can make life much easier.

Living in a house is like a giant game of Memory. I don't have enough memory power to waste it on insignificant trivia such as where I left my keys, wallet, hairbrush, or backpack. If I didn't put things back in the same place

≈ A HAPPY MEDIUM

"Happy families are all alike; every unhappy family is unhappy in its own way."
—LEO TOLSTOY, *ANNA KARENINA*

There are myriad paths to messiness, but truly great housekeepers share similar practices:

• They try to find a happy medium where everybody is comfortable.
• They pick things up as they go.
• They generally avoid putting things down temporarily.
• They believe in this saying: "A place for everything and everything in its place."
• They make mental lists of small jobs they can do in a few minutes.

Rather than fuming while on interminable hold—waiting to speak to a computer expert, doctor, or refrigerator repairman, or while waiting for a tardy friend—these experts are busy pouring crumbs out of toasters, polishing kitchen sinks, emptying wastebaskets, cleaning toilets, sweeping kitchen floors, dusting bedrooms, or emptying dishwashers. Being put on hold is a much less frustrating experience if you end up with a clean bathroom!

• They stay busy and don't allow things to get ahead of them.
• They enjoy feeling in control of their homes and their belongings and believe it is important to live in peaceful, uncluttered surroundings. They tend to say things like, "There are so few aspects of life we can actually control that I like to make my home as peaceful and tranquil as possible," or "It's a shame to let your stuff control you and make you unhappy."
• They love, need, and use everything in their homes. This requires regular pruning back of unloved, unneeded, outgrown, and unused items. Even when you don't have much, getting rid of things that you don't like or don't use can give you a real feeling of power, control, and wealth.

In his illuminating and touching book about his life as a homeless person, *Travels with Lisbeth: Three Years on the Road and on the Streets,* Lars Eighner wrote about dumpster-diving: "I find my desire to grab for the gaudy bauble has been largely sated. I think this is an attitude I share with the very wealthy—we both know there is plenty more where what we have came from."

• They buy fewer, but higher quality, things.
• And the cardinal rule of housekeeping: *Do it now, or don't do it*. In many instances, if we don't do it now, we won't do it later, either.

each time, I would have no time left to do anything else each day after I hunted for misplaced items. (Many of my friends assure me that even people with normal memories can get overloaded and stressed and begin forgetting things.)

Here are some useful tips, techniques, and products for the memory-challenged:

- A cordless phone with a locater button on the base so when it is left off the cradle, you can find it again.
- Plug-in rechargeable flashlights that turn on automatically when the power goes out. Our property is impenetrably dark on moonless nights. We have a rechargeable flashlight plugged into a socket in each bedroom, and at least one on each floor of our house. These flashlights are lifesavers!
- A full set of bathroom-cleaning equipment in each bathroom.
- Magnetic clips.(Our elegant steel entrance door sports a couple of these. We clip our outgoing mail, bills, and rented videos to them. (If we clip them right next to the doorknob, we usually remember to take them with us.)
- An erasable white board or chalkboard installed in a prominent location.
- Bags, boxes, pockets, baskets, purses, and backpacks were invented to hold small objects such as keys, wallets, and eyeglasses, which are easily deposited in random locations but difficult to find afterward. The container is one of mankind's greatest inventions: Use one today!
- Label your storage boxes, and make sure the labels are facing out. If you take the time to list every single item in the box, you will save enormous amounts of time and trouble later.

Too Much Stuff

I am married to a packrat. He is not a terrible packrat, but he does save more stuff than we could ever conceivably use. When we were newlyweds about

🌿 RASH CACHES AND STASHES

Some people stash things while tidying for company, and never un-stash them. A friend who grew up in a large and chaotic household told me that when company was coming, her mother would panic and throw things randomly in boxes and bags, then stash them in closets and behind furniture. These bags and boxes were never unpacked, and whatever was in them then needed to be replaced.

When her parents finally retired and were moving out of their home, my friend used up all her vacation days and weekends during a five month period, cleaning and clearing out their house. She typically worked from 6 in the morning until midnight for a total of seventy days. These hours add up to more than half of the average American's work year.

Among the items my friend unearthed during her marathon cleaning sessions was a cubic yard of clean, mismatched, but barely used dress socks in her dad's closet. These abandoned socks had been thrown into the closet in various bags and boxes during panic cleanings. (I couldn't help wondering how much it cost to buy a cubic yard of socks.)

My friend keeps her own house tidy. She says, "Serenity versus chaos. Who would choose chaos?"

Another friend, who is a professional housecleaner, told me that one day a client told her not to touch the oven. The dirty dishes were hidden there because the woman "didn't have time to deal with them." My friend looked in the dishwasher, found it empty, and silently wondered why her client hadn't hidden the dirty dishes there rather than in the oven.

My friend cleaned the house without touching the oven, and went home. When her client's husband came home from work that evening, his wife was out doing errands so he decided to help her by starting dinner. He preheated the oven and cracked all the dishes.

to embark on a romantic cross-country voyage of relocation with our two cats and all our worldly possessions in our work van, I had to dissuade him from bringing along an anvil. I just didn't think it was prudent to carry a 100-pound anvil with us across the Sierras and the Rockies. Walt still misses the anvil, though we have put in a good solid twenty years of not needing it. I am as interested in learning blacksmithing as the next person, but I have faith that if we ever need an anvil, we will be able to find one.

We all have squirrel-like hoarding tendencies, but remember that squirrels often forget where they've hidden those acorns; that's how many oaks get planted. Unfortunately, most man-made objects do not improve with neglect.

There are several different ways of acquiring more things than you can use:

- You need to replace the doohickey in your toilet, but you can't find your doohickey wrench so you go to the store to buy a new one.

  My friend Ann says she has spent $100 buying $5 needlenose pliers because she can never find one when she needs it.

  Solution: Buy duplicate tools, label them, and put them away where they belong.

- You can't resist a bargain.

  There is a big difference between owning a month's supply of toilet paper and owning a twenty years' supply of spackle. We will use up the toilet paper in a month, but the spackle will have dried before we ever get a chance to use it.

  Solution: Take advantage of the bargain, but share the excess with others.

- You can't resist free stuff.

  Solution #1: Learn to say no. Do not accept cast-off items from other people's newly organized homes.

  Solution #2: Don't resist. Figure out who can use the stuff and give it to them.

- You have a hard time discarding things because you get emotionally attached to them.

  Solution: Put neglected items in a bag and put the bag away. If no one misses the items for a year, get rid of them.

- You are inattentively hoarding useless items.

  One day while I was sewing, I noticed that every other pin I picked out of my magnetic pin box was bent. Sewing machine needles break when they run over bent pins. All of a sudden I realized that I had been absentmindedly hoarding cheap, useless items for years, and I threw away half my pins. Later, I asked Grace whether she ever caught herself saving stuff like bent pins. She said no, she tends to get rid of things she isn't using. Then we played cards, and the first two pens she picked up didn't work.

Solution: When you finally realize your pins are bent or your pens are dry, toss them. Everyone occasionally saves worthless items.

- You are purposefully hoarding useless items.

  Don't store things that are broken and cannot be repaired. Why would spare parts that are unavailable now be easier to find in twenty years?

Photos

There is no point in saving photographs of your thumb or unrecognizably overexposed or underexposed photos. As you look at a new batch of photos, throw away the bad ones. (It took me fifteen years to figure this out.)

Photo boxes are a great alternative to photo albums: They are less expensive as well as faster and easier to use and store.

Sorting Papers

Each week a large amount of paper and paperwork enters our homes. If we don't get rid of an equal or larger amount, the sheer volume can rapidly overwhelm us.

When your paper pile is looming large, try this:

1. Gather as many large manila envelopes (at least 9x12) as you can muster. You will be labeling these envelopes by subject, and using them to temporarily file your important paperwork.
2. Sit in a comfortable chair at the cluttered desk or table.
3. Open up a couple of paper grocery bags and set them on the floor to receive recyclable office paper.

4. Pick up each piece of paper and peruse it to determine whether it is recyclable or should be saved.
   - If it is recyclable, put it in the paper sack.
   - If it should be saved, put it in an appropriately labeled envelope.
   - Repeat until the pile is gone.
   - Put the recyclable paper in your recycling container, and transfer the important papers to your filing cabinet.

Weeding Out Junk Mail

Find a convenient spot to store and process your newly harvested mail. (Near a recycling bin is helpful.)

Dealing with incoming mail is similar to weeding a garden: It is very important to identify before culling. Never discard or recycle an envelope without opening it first; it is quite easy to mistake an official envelope with a check in it for a piece of junk mail. If you don't understand part of your mail, make inquiries before getting rid of it.

Bills

- An unopened bill is an incubator for trouble. Open your bills and categorize them right away.
- Designate a place for mail that needs attention, whether it is bills or deadlines, and make sure that nothing else is ever stashed there.
- Do not lapse into using the horizontal, sedimentary-layer filing system for bills. Force them into a regimented filing system.

Office supply stores carry an astonishing array of In and Out Boxes, household files, file boxes, expanding files, and literature sorters; there is a different type of system to suit every human temperament. The most important thing is to find a system that works for you and stick with it.

Note: As society switches from paper-based banking, bill-paying, and checking to online banking, debit cards, and online bill paying, canceled checks and piles of bills are gradually becoming obsolete. These online services are great paper, time, and space savers, but one must still keep careful records in order to avoid trouble at tax time.

Taxes

You should keep all the following paperwork related to your home: purchase price, settlement or closing costs, mortgage records, damage losses, insurance reimbursements for damage, and home improvement bills. You will need all of these for tax purposes when you sell your home. (*Note:* Utility bills are not in this category. Even after you sell your house, the amount of money you paid the electric company twelve years ago is of no interest to the IRS.)

Old bills and receipts can take up a lot of space if you save every bit of paperwork that crosses your desk. Once they have been paid and the relevant ones have been saved long enough to satisfy the IRS, you may safely destroy them.

According to the IRS website (www.irs.gov), "You must keep your records as long as they may be needed for the administration of any provision of the Internal Revenue Code." The length of time you must hold on to your tax records varies with individual circumstances, though the longest anyone needs to keep their records for IRS purposes seems to be seven years.

Though you should consult a tax expert or accountant about your own taxes and what records you need to keep, here is the basic list from the IRS:

KEEP AS BASIC RECORDS

Income
• Form(s) W-2
• Form(s) 1099
• Bank statements
• Brokerage statements
• Form(s) K-1

Expenses
• Sales slips
• Invoices
• Receipts
• Canceled checks or other proof of payment

Home
- Closing statements
- Purchase and sales invoices
- Proof of payment
- Insurance records
- Form 2119 (if you sold a home before 1998)

Investments
- Brokerage statements
- Mutual fund statements
- Form(s) 1099
- Form(s) 2439

For more specific tax information or to print out tax forms, visit the IRS website at www.irs.gov.

For years I saved my business receipts in a shoebox, which is a legal but inefficient practice. By tax time I would have built up an intimidating stack of random receipts. Then one year I encountered a see-through expanding thirteen-pocket file folder with tab markers. It was love at first sight. Tax time hasn't been the same since.

TRANSPARENT TAX RECORDS

1. Buy an expanding file with at least thirteen pockets.
2. Label the file Taxes, and date it.
3. Label the pockets based on your latest tax return: Office Supplies, Shipping, Vehicle Mileage, Medical, Education, etc.
4. Put all your invoices, receipts, and canceled checks in the appropriate pockets. By tax time, all your documentation will be categorized and ready.
5. After your taxes are done, put a copy of your tax return in a file pocket, snap the elastic closer around the file folder, and store it in a safe place.
6. Repeat each year until the other sure thing overtakes you.

If You Ask Them, They Will Come

When large amounts of work needed to be done, people used to hold barn-raisings, quilting bees, and corn-husking parties because a large project made a wonderful excuse for a party. As they say, "Many hands make light work."

Some of us are so busy that control of our houses has slipped away from us. Clearing out a house is just as worthy an endeavor as making a quilt or shucking corn. Why not hold a house clearing party? If your friends truly love you and you humble yourself enough to ask for their help, they will help you. Tell your friends you are trying to regain control of your house, and invite them over for a work party. Ask them to bring along their favorite cleaning tools, rubber gloves, and extra buckets. You can provide the earth-friendly cleaning solutions and rags.

It is certainly true that asking for help in recovering control of your home can be mortifying. It is also true that many people who cannot bring themselves to ask for help have their homes condemned by the health department. Jim Mlodozyniec, the lead housing inspector for the city of Duluth, Minnesota, told me that an average of 5 percent of the homes in every neighborhood in the city are either so cluttered that they are largely impassible, or are so filthy that the Health Department is forced to condemn them for human habitation. This problem crosses all economic, age, and ethnic categories. When given the choice between getting rid of hoarded stuff and losing the house, many people are still unable to clean up. This is tragic. Ask for help if you need it. If you notice that a friend is suffering under these conditions, offer to help.

Banishing Chaos

If you can walk on all your floor space, sit on all your chairs, lie down on all your beds, and most of your belongings can be put away when they are not in use, your cleaning party is likely to be a sociable event rather than a clutter exorcism. Warm up your casserole and get ready to party!

But if, on the other hand, much of your floor is littered with dirty laundry; your tables, chairs, and beds are covered with reading materials; you have old newspapers and magazines stacked up against the walls or you have maintained paths between the stacks so you can get from room to room, you and your friends have a lot of work ahead of you, and you will need to strategize. When most of the horizontal surfaces of a home are being used for storage, it is usually safe to assume that the home is overfilled. You will need to jettison large quantities of material objects before you will be able to gain control of your home:

1. If your house resembles a junk storage facility rather than a home, invite all your biggest, strongest friends. Plan to have your party during a mild season, and have an outdoor barbeque. Schedule a rain date.
2. Call your recycling facility and ask whether they can send a recycling truck to your home to pick up a large quantity of recyclables. If that is not possible, you may need to rent a recycling Dumpster or haul a few truckloads of recyclables to the recycling facility yourself.

   If your excess paper material includes usable books, donate them to your local library, homeless shelter, or nursing home, or try calling a book dealer to see if he is interested in making you an offer. If the dealer tells you your books are worthless, do not bring them to Goodwill; recycle their paper.
3. If you have large quantities of broken, soiled, or otherwise unusable and unrecyclable junk such as old carpeting, broken furniture, or ruined lumber, rent a Dumpster. In cases of extreme clutter, successive Dumpsters may be required.
4. Stock up on garbage bags and paper bags for recycling newspapers. Ask all your friends to bring extra grocery bags.
5. On the day of the party, clean the cat's litterbox, pick up the dogs' droppings in the yard, wash the dishes, and pick up the dirty underwear off the floor and put it in the hamper. Your friends will be a lot more useful if they aren't nauseated.
6. A modified bucket brigade is helpful for removing large amounts of material from a house. Set up a line of volunteers from the door

to the curb, truck, or Dumpster. Start removing materials nearest the door first. As you work, it will become easier and easier to navigate through the house.

7. When you're tired, stop. Rome wasn't built in a day, and you didn't acquire all this extraneous stuff in one day, either.

8. After your house is cleared out and cleaned up, invite your friends over for a celebratory party. I am a strong believer in "party motivation": If you know people are coming over, you will clean and tidy up the house. The trick is to have parties often enough to prevent your house from sliding into chaos again. The friends who helped cast out your household chaos will take great pride in your communal accomplishment and will be your best weapon against recurring chaos.

(Routine preparty cleaning: Do the dusting a couple of days before the party, clean the bathrooms the day before the party, and vacuum up the dog hair at the last minute.)

Hiring Help

If you would rather not impose upon your friends, you might consider hiring a hauling service to remove your piles of junk. Haulers usually work by the job, rather than by the hour, and they will haul away a wide variety of stuff. Check to be sure that the company is reliable and bonded and licensed, and that they will not dump your junk illegally.

Cleaning Outbuildings and Extremely Chaotic Houses

Even the neatest and tidiest of us may find ourselves dealing with chaos occasionally. Cleaning up the aftermath of natural disasters or fires, acquiring a neglected property, or the simple impulse to help someone who is feeling overwhelmed can land us in the midst of a mess that we may feel ill equipped to handle. Here are some tips for coping with extreme disorder:

1. Work with a friend. Coping with chaos can be depressing: Don't attempt it alone.
2. Before you begin cleaning or moving things, do a quick survey and move hazards out of the way. Broken glass should be swept up immediately.
3. If the room or building is extremely dusty, is very moldy, or contains large quantities of rodent droppings, wear a dust mask or respirator while you work. Use a shop-vac to remove dust from each tiny area as it is cleared of clutter.
4. Many people who lived through the Great Depression make a

☙ AN AVALANCHE OF PRINTED MATERIALS

MAGAZINES

Most of us subscribe to magazines because we are vitally interested in their subject matter, which is exactly why getting rid of old periodicals can be so difficult. Force yourself. If you don't recycle constantly, you may be crushed by a slippery avalanche of magazines.

• Keep only the magazines you need for reference, then process them as quickly as possible: Take notes, copy information into your computer, or rip out useful articles and file them away. After you have saved the information you need, donate the magazines to schools, artists, or other people who will use them; recycle the leftovers.
• *Do not* read materials you are attempting to recycle. Yes, you probably didn't read every single word in every single magazine, but life is short and recycling piles up. If you missed an article, you can read it at the public library.
• Don't store dated material. Your computer magazine is nearly obsolete as soon as it rolls off the presses. It is unlikely to be more timely when you take it out of storage.
• Many magazines offer online subscriptions. *Consumer Reports,* for instance, has a searchable online archive of all their articles, reports, and ratings, and you can subscribe to the online service without receiving the actual magazine. With an online subscription, you can easily find any article and need never fear losing information.
• Everyone has a complete collection of *National Geographics*! Yes, they are gorgeous, but they have no resale value. Unless you are going to use them in an art project within a year, give them to a school or an artist who will. Our public library not only possesses a complete collection of the magazine—dating back to its first issues in

practice of saving materials that might be useful some day. It is much easier to let go when one knows that these potentially useful things will be sent to someone who needs them.

These objects have usually been saved with a specific use in mind: glass jars to be used for canning, scraps of fabric for quilts or hooked rugs, lumber for carpentry projects. If the materials are still intact and usable, try putting an ad in the paper: "Free quilting scraps" or "Free canning jars."

5. Mixed piles are trash; sorted piles are resources. Build segregated piles: garbage, Goodwill, recycling, cider jugs, glass, lampshades . . .

---

the late nineteenth century—they also have a complete index. This means that I can go to the library, look up any subject I'm interested in, fill out a request form, and have the issue I need in a few minutes. Finding the same issue in a home collection is unlikely to be as quick and easy.

NEWSPAPERS

• Share your newspaper with a close neighbor; you'll cut your costs and your recycling chores in half.

• Home collections are not usually indexed, catalogued, or systematically shelved, and an organized collection of newspapers in a private home is the least likely scenario of all.

• If you are working on a research project and need clippings, mark the page and the article while you're reading the paper (brightly colored Post-it notes, which can be stuck to the edge of the paper, work well and can be reused several times). After everyone in the household has finished reading the paper, you can clip the article, file it, and recycle the rest of the paper.

• Don't keep piles of papers so you can read them later. You won't. Piles of newspapers will choke the life out of your home. I can guarantee that once you have saved a stack of newspapers to read later you will not be able to find the information you are looking for.

• Many articles are available on the Internet, and many libraries maintain extensive collections of newspapers on microfiche. Your librarians are trained professionals who can help you find any issue you need.

• Piles of newspapers are like flammable underbrush in a forest; they need to be cleared out or they endanger the rest of the ecosystem.

(I delivered almost one hundred beautiful glass cider jugs to an amateur cider maker after one cleaning session at a farm.)

6. Disuse encourages rodents, insects, rust, mold, mildew, and fungus. There will be large quantities of ruined materials in a disorderly building. The following are not salvageable:
   - Fabric, carpeting, upholstery, bedding, insulation, books, papers, and other porous materials that have been contaminated with rodent droppings and urine
   - Objects that have begun growing fungus or mildew
   - Compacted or wet insulation
   - Rotten wood
   - Rusty cans or jar lids
   - Dried out or age-thickened paint
   - Expired medicines and desiccated cosmetics
   - Obsolete appliances and electronics

7. Don't start fixing things while you are still clearing out the building. That old aquarium has been languishing for ten years; you don't need to fix it now.

8. Don't get rid of things you use all the time. They are part of your life, and you will miss them immediately. The aim of decluttering and clearing out is to give you more room to live your life, not to deprive you of the things you need.

9. Keep a running list of things to do, such as "Clean out bedroom closet," "Clean out medicine cabinet," "Take old cans of paint to the Household Hazardous Waste Facility." Cross tasks off as you accomplish them.

10. Keep a running list of things to save and their ultimate destination. For instance, "Box up old eyeglasses. Deliver to Lions Club."

Post-Clutterectomy Care

Space—living space—is much more valuable than the clutter it contains. Do your best to maintain and preserve your domestic open space.

If something is bothering you, do something about it! If you trip over it,

> 🐝 Perhaps for the savers out there, finding good homes for the items they have lovingly stored for so many years is as imperative as finding good homes for a litter of puppies. Finding a cider maker who can use glass jugs, artists who can use various saved materials, or schools that can use plastic containers with working lids may make the difference between cleaning out a garage and not cleaning it out.
>
> Waste is never a good thing, but wasting space is no better than wasting glass jugs or usable fabric. Building a new structure to house a collection of potentially usable junk is far more wasteful than recycling the materials.

move it out of the way for the hundredth time, notice it's nonfunctional and impossible to repair, have grown out of it, or realize that it stinks—move it, put it away, sell it, jettison it, recycle it, or send it to Goodwill. If you do this every day, your house will be in better shape than ever before.

A bit of clutter will inevitably creep back into most households. If you frequently and consistently put things back where they belong, you can fend off chaos. To sort misplaced objects, set out garbage bags, grocery bags, or cardboard boxes, and label them Discard, Recycle, Donate, Sort Pile (this container is for items that are in the wrong location). As you pick up objects, throw them in the appropriate container for later dispensation.

> 🐝 ·A very effective way to convince children to pick up the tiny pieces of their toys is to announce that you are going to vacuum, and anything small enough to be vacuumed up, will be.

Your house did not get trashed all in one day. If you do a little more cleaning every day than you do messing, eventually your house will gather itself together.

If you cannot decide which of your belongings are truly important to you, try this trick: Empty your home out one drawer, cupboard, closet, or room at a time and carry the items as far from where they started as possible. Pile them at the other end of the house or even in the garage. Vacuum and wipe down the cupboard, closet, or drawer and paint that empty room, then get rid of the items that you don't want to bother to carry back. Put the usable items in boxes

and cart them off to Goodwill that very day. Recycle the recyclables. Throw
the rest in the trash.

Storage Protocol

- Unless you are running a junkyard, avoid saving large objects in
  order to salvage small parts. If you want to save the tiny screws from
  your broken eyeglasses, remove the screws immediately, then throw
  away the eyeglasses. (Eyeglasses with usable frames can be donated
  to the Lions Club.)
- Don't store things so you can throw them out later. While assisting
  at a clutterectomy, I discovered two cut-down, carefully taped milk
  cartons, both labeled in beautiful copperplate handwriting. One

---

STORAGE HAZARDS

SHARP EDGES

A split length of rubber garden hose makes a fine protective sheath for a saw blade:

1. Cut a piece of hose the same length as your saw blade.
2. Draw a straight line down the hose—this will be your cutting line.
3. Use a razor knife or other very sharp blade to cut through the hose. Be careful to
   cut through only one wall of the hose. You now have a length of hose that has been
   sliced from end to end. The natural curl of the hose wall will maintain the cylindrical shape of the split hose.
4. Slide the split side of the hose over the jagged edge of the saw blade. Be careful
   not to slide your hand or fingers against the saw's teeth.
5. This blade guard will work for most carpenter's and gardener's handsaws.

CONFUSION

- If you start a random pile, people think it's a random pile and throw random things
  on it randomly. Soon it will be a rubbish pile. Set up obvious and convenient storage
  areas for specific items.
- Install shelving, cabinets, and tool hangers in shop, garage, laundry, and utility areas.
  The classic method of drawing the outlines of tools on a pegboard is a wonderful
  technique for banishing chaos.

---

carton said Broken Glass Candlestick. Very Sharp. The label included information on the origin of the candlestick and the date (more than thirty years previously) on which it had been shattered. The other milk carton was similarly labeled. I immediately threw the milk cartons in the trash. I had no doubt that the pieces were still sharp, and the candlesticks were still not repairable.

- If you dismantle something for parts, keep the parts together (Ziploc bags and baby food jars work well) and label them very carefully as to what they are and what they're from. The label might look something like this: Kenmore Vacuum Cleaner, 2001. Spare Parts.

    If you don't label parts before you store them, you might as well throw them out immediately because unless you have a perfect

DETERIORATION

There is no point in carefully saving items if you are going to allow them to mildew in the basement.

- When the weather is humid, set out shallow pans of garden lime to absorb dampness and musty odors. Replace every few weeks. The used lime can then be put in the garden.
- Storage does not improve the smell of mildewy books.
- Leather does not store well; it needs to be cleaned and oiled regularly or it will either stiffen and crack or turn to dust. Use it or lose it. It is better to give leather items away than put them in storage.
- Concrete floors ooze dampness. Things stored on the ground will tend to rot or rust, even under a dry roof. Anything that can be damaged by water should be stored on a pallet, on a shelf, or hung on the wall.
- Banishment does not agree with furniture. No matter how carefully you wrap it or how dry the outbuilding, furniture suffers when it is evicted from a house.
- While clearing an outbuilding, I helped move a couch that had become a home, nursery, and cemetery for a family of mice, as well as a favored hunting ground for a cat that had also used it as a litter box. The couch's owner said, "I guess we should have given it away while it was still good. It was nice when we put it in here." My husband and I once wrecked a perfectly nice headboard by trying to hang on to it when we moved and had no room to store it in the house. *Moral:* Give it away while the giving is good.

memory, it will be very difficult to recognize exactly what they are if you ever need them.

- Our friend Tim uses an old steel filing cabinet to store spare parts and small tools such as screw drivers, wire, packages of washers, and salvaged electronics components. He puts the small parts in a Ziploc bag then files it in a flat-bottomed hanging file folder.
- People who live on boats or in very small houses quickly learn to maintain an equilibrium of stuff. Most of the rest of us could also benefit by practicing similar restraint.
- If you don't have anywhere to put something, don't bring it home.

  My husband and I once bought a tiny little end table with a drawer at a garage sale. We had to move every stick of furniture we owned just to find a place to put it.
- Make a practice of getting rid of something old every time you bring home something new. Holidays are an excellent time for this: Put on the new fuzzy slippers and throw out the old ones that Fido chewed.

Habits

Habits are the things we do so automatically, so unconsciously, that we may not be aware we are doing them. Sometimes we need to be jolted out of our accustomed rut in order to even recognize these habits. If you are extremely unhappy with the amount of clutter or disorder in your house, you may need a fresh eye to help you see things as they really are rather than as they were, as they should be, or as they could be.

If you have a friend whose housekeeping style you admire, you might think about asking that friend for help. Bear in mind that the state of our housekeeping can be a very sore spot or source of embarrassment. If the thought of having a friend help makes you uncomfortable, you might want to hire a professional housecleaner or home organizer. You may need to rein yourself in, hold your tongue and your temper. Take notes. Put them away and look at them again in a week. Remind yourself that this person is trying to help, not insult you. Truly constructive criticism is one of the most valuable commodities in the world.

You are What You Do;
You are What You Think

Not long ago, scientists were absolutely positive that adult brains were incapable of growing new cells. Though the structure of immature brains evolved and changed in response to the environment and experiences, the structure of adult brains could only change for the worse. It was further believed that brain damage in adults was irreparable. In the past few years, as new brain-imaging techniques have shown that adult brains can grow, change, evolve, and heal in response to stimuli, that pessimistic view of the brittleness of adult brains has changed.

Research done by Dr. Edward Taub showed that stroke victims who had been unable to use one arm for years were able to regain the use of the arm when their "good" arm was tied down and immobilized, and they were forced to use their afflicted arm in intensive physical therapy sessions. After only two weeks of this treatment, patients were able to use their afflicted arm in a relatively normal fashion. Brain scans taken before and after the therapy showed significant changes in these patients: The therapy had induced their brains to rewire themselves.

If stroke patients are able to rewire their brains and regain the use of their crippled limbs, certainly those of us who are struggling with counterproductive habits should be able to change them. Interestingly, though it takes only two weeks to regain the use of a crippled arm, experts agree that it takes a minimum of three weeks to make or break a habit.

There are two different types of habits that adversely affect housekeeping: slovenly habits and excessively neat habits. Though it is unlikely that the Health Department or Child Protection Services will be called because a house is overly neat, both housekeeping modes can cause much familial suffering. I have friends who have overcome both extremes: The neatniks decided to calm down and relax their housekeeping standards because they realized they were terrorizing their families in order to satisfy their own cravings for order; the slobs decided to tighten up their housekeeping because extreme disorder was affecting their family's ability to function.

The only good reason for housekeeping is to make all the inhabitants of a home as comfortable, healthy, and happy as possible. If your housekeeping style is making you and/or your family or housemates miserable, it's time for a change.

How to Change

Ask yourself this question: "Why should I change my housekeeping style?" My friend Sarah changed her neatnik ways after her five-year-old son said to her, "You never play with me because you're always cleaning that house!"

Now ask yourself this question: "Who will benefit if I change my house-keeping style?"

Beware: Answering these questions may make you sad because uncomfortable housekeeping styles are not usually the product of rational thought. I try to do this type of self-interrogation while hiking alone and carrying a big hankie. It can be quite painful to admit that one is not in control of one's own behavior.

Talk to your family or housemates and explain that you intend to change your ways, and why. It is always harder to abandon a project that has been announced.

Remember that you are responsible for your own behavior. Other adults are responsible for their own behavior. Adults are responsible for training children.

Once you have organized the troublesome spots in your home, you need to learn how to maintain your hard-won order. You will need to form orderly habits. Here are a few tips contributed by my friend Sarah, whose orderly habits are so ingrained that she practically cleans house in her sleep.

Setting Orderly Habits

Being organized is a way of paying attention to what you're doing. It also enables you to see what you're doing.

1. Remember that it takes twenty-one days to "set" a habit. Decide which one you want to instill, and consciously work to keep up the activity for at least a month. After that, the habit should have acquired some momentum of its own.

2. Don't use the horizontal filing system! Horizontal is the position of death! Use files, bulletin boards, inboxes, etc.
    • If you don't already have a household filing cabinet, get one.
    • File! File! File! If you don't already have a file for a bit of paperwork you need to save, immediately set up a new file for your filing cabinet and use it. The time you will spend creating a new folder and filing your bit of paper is insignificant compared to the time you will waste if you allow that piece of paper to go into the horizontal file on your countertop or table. Clean out material in files when you notice that it's obsolete.
    • Set up file folders for each child's school work. File your child's report cards, school projects, administrative paperwork, art work, and other important information in these active files. At the end of the school year, you can transfer the report cards, the outstanding reports, and the choicest artwork to a file box for long-term storage—one file box per child. Later in life, when your child's biographer is hard at work, you will be able to grant him access to a wonderfully well-preserved record of your progeny's formative years.
3. Keep a pocket-size notebook handy to jot down ideas and to keep track of chores that need to be done. If your life is not filled with heavy, wet, and messy chores, you can substitute a PalmPilot for a pocket notebook.
4. Get a calendar with lots of writing room. I favor the kind with separate columns for each family member (including the dogs); these calendars are not pretty, but boy are they handy!
    • Immediately after making appointments or receiving invitations, transfer all the essential information—phone numbers, names, and addresses of contact people—to your calendars, then recycle the paperwork.
    • Write in to-do's, (dog's heartworm pills, call dentist, pay insurance, etc.)

- Notate children's first words, first steps, and funny incidents on the calendar, and save your old calendars as family diaries. (I find it impossible to keep a journal or a diary, but I can keep a calendar.)

5. Housework can be lonely. Make a habit of doing chores while you're talking on a cordless phone.

6. Objects often end up on the wrong floor of multilevel dwellings. Put displaced items on the stairs or in a basket near the stairs, and carry them with you when you go up or down.

7. Put dirty dishes in the dishwasher rather than on the counter. This takes a whole thirty seconds. If everyone did this, there'd be no washing up to do.

8. Slow and steady wins the race. Once your house is under control, you can pick up a few things at a time and clean a few surfaces every day. If you do a little bit of housework every day rather than a lot at once, cleaning is a lot less onerous.

   Don't think about the entire, huge task: Pick a drawer, pick a room, and clean it up. Bag stuff up and get it out of the house. You don't have to do all your cleaning in one session, as long as you tidy up faster than you clutter.

9. Act! Don't just move things around—put them away. If grime is bothering you, clean it. Unlike other projects, which always take way more time than I think they will, cleaning, once I really get down to it, always takes far less time per job than I'm anticipating. I think it's the reverse of the time-flies-when-you're-having-fun phenomenon.

10. Keep drawers and storage area doors closed to keep the contents clean. It is much easier to wipe grease off a cupboard door than off every utensil inside the cupboard. (When we moved into our country home, every single kitchen drawer contained a disgusting collection of crumbs.)

11. Enjoy your home. Overly clean and tidy is intimidating; overly dirty and cluttered is depressing. Find your happy medium and try to stay there. When you become uncomfortable, take action.

Health, happiness, and security are our goals. Organization is only a tool that we can use to help us reach these goals.

May all the objects in your home be either useful, necessary, or well loved; if they are not, read on.

Living Lightly and Happily

Chaos is a silent and sneaky enemy. In order to maintain order, it is of the utmost importance that, once you have identified the materials and items you no longer want, you work quickly to remove them from your property.

The U.S. Environmental Protection Agency (EPA) recommends that solid waste be dealt with in the following order: (1) waste prevention, (2) recycling, and as a last resort, (3) disposal.

If you aren't using it and you aren't enjoying it, get rid of it in the most ecological way possible. This means sell it or give it to someone who can use it; retool it into something else so you can use it; or repair it. Next down the line is recycling, so the raw materials can be reused (this includes composting). Worst of all is throwing something away.

Waste Prevention

- Eschew processed food in individual serving-size packages. This is the most expensive way to buy food, and many individual packages create far more waste than a single, larger package.
- Buy items in recyclable packaging or, better yet, without packaging.
- Buy products in bulk whenever possible, then store your bulk products in reusable containers. Recycling is an onerous chore, especially when the containers pile up really high. You will save money as well as recycling time by reusing your containers and buying in bulk.

Our co-op buys shampoo, cream rinse, hand lotion, dish liquid, etc., in large containers, and we bring our own containers and fill them up. This costs less per pound and we drastically reduce the amount of recycling we must do.

Reusing bags, bottles, jars, and other food containers is not allowed in many stores. Check with the store before making assumptions. Food safety laws mandate that containers must be thoroughly washed and rinsed before they can be refilled, and some laws require container "matching" (for example, maple syrup can only be poured into maple syrup bottles; shampoo refills must be in shampoo bottles). Even if you don't have a nearby store that sells in bulk, you can still bring your own bags to the store. I am rather partial to strong but lightweight string or nylon grocery bags.

A huge box is not necessarily an indication that the product inside is being sold in bulk. Many buying clubs such as Sam's Club and Costco sell large boxes that contain many smaller packages that contain individual servings. Read the label before buying. (A rule of thumb from my friend Jean, the co-op queen: "If buying in bulk doesn't require some small but extra effort on your part—repackaging, bringing your own packaging, etc.—then it may not be reducing or reusing.")

- Leave all hazardous or poisonous materials in their original packaging and containers with the labels intact. The labels contain vital emergency information in case of accidental poisoning.

    Never store poisonous liquids in beverage containers. Many young children are poisoned each year when they drink household chemicals out of soft drink bottles and other beverage containers.
- Buy only as much as you can use in a reasonable amount of time. The enormous, institutional-size box of cereal may seem like a good deal, but if you don't finish the cereal before it goes stale, you will end up discarding it. The beauty of buying in bulk is that you purchase the item for a reasonable amount per pound, yet you don't end up with more than you can use.
- Buy durable, high-quality goods. Buying a more expensive item once may be less expensive than buying a cheaper version several times. Since you will be buying fewer items, your house will be less cluttered. Whenever possible, buy consumer products that are repairable and have easily available replacement parts.
- Buy rechargeable alkaline batteries; they last far longer than disposable batteries and are less hazardous. Avoid buying disposable items

such as cameras and flashlights whose more durable counterparts can last a lifetime.

- Owning more than you can take care of is not only uneconomical, it is unenvironmental. If you have more lumber than you can store successfully, you might as well give it to someone who can use it. If you think you are saving money by keeping it, you are mistaken. After plywood, for instance, has warped due to weather exposure, you will have to pay to dispose of it. If you had given it away while it was still usable, the recipient would probably have been happy to pick it up.
- Take care of your possessions. Keep them clean and in good repair so that when you are done with them, other people may be able to use them. If there is no room in your home, garage, or storage shed for that lumber and those antique chairs and tables, maybe it is time to sell them. If you leave them outdoors long enough, they will turn to trash.

Conserving Paper

The average American uses more than 300 kilograms (660 pounds) of paper per year. Americans are responsible (or is it irresponsible?) for consuming one-third of the world's annual paper production.

Here are some easy ways to cut down on your paper consumption:

- Choose lightweight paper to minimize the amount of material per page.
- Do your editing on the computer screen, not on paper.
- Make double-sided copies.
- Use the blank sides of copies for draft copies and note paper.
- Store your reams of paper up off the ground in a dry location. Leave the paper lying flat in its wrapper until you need it. Properly stored paper is less likely to jam your printer.

Reuse

Living sustainably requires more than simply loading empty containers into a recycling bin and waiting for someone to take them away. Processing raw materials into usable form requires a lot of energy; reusing materials conserves all the original processing energy. Before the Industrial Revolution, people were painfully aware of how much effort went into the objects that made up their material world. When more of the work was done by hand, people tried to reuse everything: Scraps of cloth and old clothes were turned into patchwork quilts or cut into strips for rag rugs; hand-me-down clothes were remade into smaller items for children; sweaters and coats with worn-out elbows were turned into vests; pants were turned into skirts or shorts; lumber, bricks, and building stones were used and reused. Many people made their living by collecting and selling discards that ranged from old rags to cooking grease.

Nowadays, material goods are relatively cheap and easy to come by and we are discarding ever-increasing volumes of stuff, but it is becoming increasingly obvious that we live in a finite world with finite resources.

As our foremothers used to say: "Use it up, wear it out, make it do, or do without."

Disposable Food Packaging and Tableware

Disposable food packaging and tableware constitutes a large percentage of this country's solid waste. A few simple changes can make a big difference at home.

- Use cloth napkins. Inexpensive dishcloths, bought by the dozen, make perfectly serviceable everyday napkins.
- Use unbleached waxed paper rather than plastic wrap. Waxed paper can be composted, plastic wrap cannot.
- Pack lunches in sturdy, reusable, insulated lunch bags rather than in disposable paper bags.
- Avoid buying individual servings of packaged foods; repack snack foods in small reusable containers.

Party Waste Reduction

When we have large parties at our house, we use inexpensive, durable, and dishwasher safe colored plastic plates, cups, and goblets of the type that are sold for summer patio use. We bought our party plates for very little at an after-summer sale.

We have been using the same partyware for well over a decade, and no one has ever had clothing ruined by food spilling from a collapsed plate. (The savings in garbage costs, disposable plates and cups, and dry cleaning have been enormous.) We also invested in sturdy, inexpensive party cutlery, though most garden-variety plastic cutlery is strong enough to be washed and reused several times.

Biodegradeable Cutlery Sources

Even the most lovingly preserved plastic cutlery will eventually give up the ghost. Biodegradable, compostable cutlery is an environmentally preferable alternative to unrecyclable plastic cutlery.

Nat-Ur, Inc. (formerly Biocorp North America) produces corn- and potato-based biodegradable, compostable garbage bags, leaf and yard bags, cups, bowls, plates, drinking straws, cup lids, boxes, food containers, and cutlery. I have used all of these products and they work quite well. The bioplastic cutlery is far stronger than most plastic cutlery; we washed and reused the same bioplastic spoon in bag lunches for almost a year until my husband finally snapped and broke the spoon just to see how strong it was. I composted the broken pieces in my worm bin. Website: www.nat-ur.com.

Companies in other parts of the world are working on plant-based bioplastics made from plants such as seaweed, tobacco, soybeans, potatoes, and wheat, and on bioplastics produced by bacteria. Many of these packaging materials will be edible as well as biodegradable, so one day we may be able to eat our cake and its wrapper, too.

Gift Waste Reduction

Wrapping paper, which is often used only once, is wasteful and expensive. Pretty gift bags can be sent back and forth between friends and family for years. Cloth gift bags made of velvet, satin, or other beautiful fabrics make presents look elegant.

If you are giving a gift to someone who is low on cash, why not make the wrapping part of the present?

- New pillowcases in a pretty pattern make wonderful gift bags. New bedsheets can be used as extra large gift wrap.

- A new silk scarf makes an attractive gift wrapping.
- Many quilters would welcome a present wrapped in a small square of nice cotton fabric.
- Package the gift in a container that you know the recipient can use, such as a new canvas tote bag, a colander, an attractive wastebasket, a diaper pail, or a fancy planting pot. Use your imagination; the recipient will be impressed.

Recycling: Reducing Things to Their Basic Elements

Unless human beings get in the way and impede natural processes, recycling is the way of the world. Mother Nature not only abhors a vacuum, she also abhors waste: Elements are used and reused to form new organisms and new minerals. Bedsprings rust, flake, and stain the ground orange; paper rots and molders back into the earth from whence it came unless it is kept under a solid roof. Perishables perish unless they are preserved or kept refrigerated or frozen, and in the end, it's "ashes to ashes and dust to dust" for us, unless a mortician gets to us first.

If we don't protect our "durable goods" by keeping them clean and dry, we soon discover that some aren't so durable after all. And therein lies the problem: Our dry, comfortable homes are designed to thwart this process of biodegradation, so we must take out the trash or smother under its weight.

It is certainly easy to throw unwanted items into the trash. Unfortunately, our landfills are filling up and nobody seems to want new landfills near their homes, nor do they want to live near garbage incinerators. Many brilliant people are working very hard to figure out how to create a zero discharge society in which nothing is thrown away permanently—everything is either reused, recycled, or composted. We humans have traveled very far toward making everything disposable; we have a long way to go before we return to our starting place, older, wiser, and less likely to toss our trash by the side of the road.

> Though only 5 percent of the world's population lives in the United States, we use 25 percent of its natural resources.

The Law of Supply and Demand

If we as consumers insist on buying products made of recycled materials, manufacturers will continue to develop and produce them. If we do not buy recycled products, the market for them will disappear, and the recyclables that we have so carefully rinsed, packed, stacked, saved, and recycled may end up in the landfill after all; this would be a shame because the amount of energy saved by reusing these valuable materials is considerable.

Glass

Molding new glass containers from recycled glass requires only half as much water as making glass from *raw materials*, and produces 20 percent less air pollution. Recycling a single glass bottle, rather than manufacturing a new one from sand, saves enough energy to light a 100-watt light bulb for four hours.

Glass bottles and jars are typically recycled back into glass bottles and jars, but can also be used to make fiberglass insulation, glass beads for reflective paint for road signs, and construction material.

To recycle, rinse out glass containers and remove metal or plastic rings, lids, and caps. Clean, unbroken containers are recyclable; broken glass, tempered glass, and window glass are not.

Aluminum

Making new aluminum cans from old cans uses 95 percent less energy than making aluminum cans from raw bauxite ore. This is why aluminum cans are a valuable commodity.

- Recycling a single aluminum can saves enough energy to run a television or a desktop computer for three hours or a notebook computer for an entire day.
- Throwing away a single aluminum can rather than recycling it wastes the energy-equivalent of half the can's volume in gasoline. Throwing away the average aluminum can, which weighs 12 ounces, wastes the equivalent of 6 ounces of gasoline.

All aluminum, whether foil or cans, should be clean and free of food residues before it is recycled.

Paper

Making paper from recycled paper uses 60 to 70 percent less energy and 55 percent less water than converting virgin pulp to paper.

- A four-foot stack of recycled newspaper can save the life of one pulp tree.
- One tree equals seven hundred paper grocery bags.

Recycling paper, then buying recycled paper products, does not necessarily save the life of a single, specific, farmed tree on a pulpwood plantation. Conserving paper may, however, reduce the acreage of natural forest that is cut down and planted with pulp trees. Natural forests help improve air, soil, and water quality and provide a rich, diverse habitat for wildlife; pulpwood plantations (which are treated with agricultural chemicals) do not.

Dark colored and fluorescent papers are difficult to recycle, and the dyes are toxic. Try to use only white or light-colored papers.

Recyclable materials should be recycled regularly. If you wait long enough to recycle your newspaper, it will oxidize and become brown, brittle, and fit only for the compost heap, the woodstove, or the trash.

Cardboard

Cereal boxes, wrapping paper, and egg cartons are considered mixed paper. They can all be recycled. Corrugated cardboard is a separate category. Cardboard must be clean to be recyclable.

Choosing Copy Paper and Office Paper

The U.S. General Services Administration (GSA) requires that federal agencies use postconsumer recycled-content copier paper. The U.S. Government Printing Office (GPO) has tested recycled content paper and maintains a list of paper brands that meet its recycled-content and performance specifications. Approved copy paper must contain a minimum of 30 percent postconsumer recycled fiber, must have caused fewer than one paper jam per five thousand continuous copies, and must be lint- and fuzz-free.

Green Seal, a nonprofit organization that promotes the use of environmentally friendly products, encourages the use of paper products that are produced without chlorine because paper mills that use chlorine release large amounts of dangerous dioxins into the environment. Here is a list of paper products that satisfy the GSA, the GPO, and Green Seal as ranked by Green Seal:

Environmentally Friendly Copy Paper Brands

THE BEST BRANDS

Badger Envirographic 100 (100 percent recycled postconsumer content, processed chlorine free) (Badger Paper Mills)

Encore 100 (100 percent recycled postconsumer content, processed chlorine free) (New Leaf Paper)

Eureka! (100 percent recycled postconsumer content, processed chlorine free) (Georgia-Pacific, Fort James)

NEXT BEST

New Life DP 100 (60 percent recycled postconsumer content, processed chlorine free) (Rolland)

ACCEPTABLE

Geocycle (30 percent recycled postconsumer content, processed chlorine free) (Georgia-Pacific)

Windsor Copy Recycled (30 percent recycled postconsumer content, processed chlorine free) (Domtar Papers)

Great White Xerographic (30 percent recycled postconsumer content, processed chlorine free) (International Paper)

Exact Multipurpose (colored paper, 30 percent recycled postconsumer content, processed chlorine free) (Wausau Papers)

Recycled Husky Xerocopy (30 percent recycled postconsumer content, processed chlorine free) (Weyerhaeuser)

Willcopy (30 percent recycled postconsumer content, processed chlorine free) (Willamette)

Plastics

Because there are so many different types, not all of which are recyclable, plastic is the most difficult material to recycle. The only way to accurately tell the types of plastic apart is to look at the symbol on the bottom of the object. If you do not want to be stuck with large amounts of plastic containers that you cannot recycle, avoid buying products that are packaged in plastic that is not recyclable in your area. Ask for information about which materials are recyclable at your local recycling facility. Though the manufacturers may claim that their product or packaging is recyclable, if no facilities will accept it, it is not recyclable.

Here are the recycling codes for plastic containers:

1-PETE (Polyethylene Terephthalate) is used to make clear soft drink bottles, as well as bottles for dish detergent, ketchup, and mouthwash.

Recycled PETE plastic is used to make luggage, synthetic fabric, shoes and boots, carpeting, and fiberfill for clothing, bedding, and sleeping bags.

Note: Plastic beverage bottles are one of the fastest-growing components of the waste stream. (Almost 3 million water bottles are being thrown in the trash every day in California!) The water contained in these bottles is generally no better than the water that emerges from most household taps—and is frequently worse—and PETE bottles may leach small amounts of chemicals into the water. Reduce your volume of recyclables and drink cleaner water by filling your own reusable water bottle at home. HDPE is the safest material for unbreakable, reusable plastic water bottles.

2-HDPE (High-Density Polyethylene) is used to make milk jugs, juice bottles, water jugs, and detergent containers.

Recycled HDPE plastic is made into such products as carpeting, clothing, nursery plant pots, detergent bottles, coat hangers, video cases, drainpipes, floor tiles, fencing, plastic lumber, and road barriers.

3-PVC (Vinyl/Polyvinyl Chloride) is a ubiquitous material that is made into plumbing pipes, vinyl siding and windows, electrical wire insulation, and vinyl flooring among other things.

Recycled PVC is used to make packaging, decking, paneling, mud flaps, flooring, speed bumps, and floor mats.

4-LDPE (Low-Density Polyethylene) is turned into flexible lids and bottles.

Recycled LDPE is used to make shipping envelopes, garbage can liners, floor tiles, furniture, compost bins, paneling, trash cans, plastic landscape timbers, and plastic lumber.

5-PP (Polypropylene) is used for flexible and rigid packaging, synthetic fabrics, and large molded parts for cars and consumer products.

Recycled PP is turned into auto battery cases, battery cables, brooms and brushes, ice scrapers, oil funnels, rakes, and pallets.

6-PS (Polystyrene) is formed into either thin and rigid or puffy Styrofoam. PS is used to make protective packaging, containers, lids, cups, bottles, and trays.

Recycled PS is used to make light switch plates, thermal insulation, egg cartons, foam packing, carryout containers, and spray foam insulation.

7-"Other" is the catch-all recycling category that is used to collect plastic made of resins other than the previous six, or plastic that is made of more than one resin.

Once recycled, this material is used to make custom products and plastic lumber.

Plastic Bags

Plastic grocery bags and produce bags are the bane of my existence. Washing out the plastic bags for reuse is one of my least favorite jobs. (We store our clean produce bags in a narrow cloth bag with an elastic opening in the bottom and a drawstring at the top.)

Some retail stores accept clean, dry plastic bags for recycling.

The easiest way to reduce the drudgery of too many plastic sacks is to bring your own bag to the store. Sturdy canvas, string mesh, or rip-stop nylon bags can be reused practically forever. Try keeping a few of the supermarket variety in the car to bring into the store with you when you shop.

Foam Packing Peanuts

Opening a package that spews packing peanuts all over the room is almost annoying enough to dull the delight that accompanies opening a present. Not only are the peanuts numerous, light, and easily blown around, they are also full of static electricity, so they don't necessarily stay on the floor where they are easily swept up.

If you have been afflicted with synthetic peanuts, you may either want to retaliate by returning them to the sender in your next package, or take advantage of the recycling program sponsored by the Plastic Loose Fill Council to collect small loose-fill polystyrene packing material (aka packing peanuts). Consumers can drop off their packing peanuts at Mail Boxes Etc. and other retail locations. To find the nearest packing peanut collection location, visit www.loosefillpackaging.com.

If you don't want to afflict your distant loved ones with packing peanuts, use egg cartons or plain air-popped popcorn to cushion delicate items in their shipping packages.

Tin Cans

Tin cans are actually steel cans coated with tin to keep the steel from rusting.

Recycling steel uses 74 percent less energy than refining steel from iron ore.

To recycle these, remove the top and the bottom, then squash the cylindrical body flat by stepping on it.

Steel or iron in other forms, such as metal roofing and scrap iron, can be recycled at a scrap yard, as can other metals such as copper, brass, aluminum, and tin. Look up Scrap Metal in your phone book to locate the nearest scrap yard. (Copper and brass are valuable, and you will actually make some money on the transaction.)

Computers, Phones, and Other Electronics

The best way to deal with old computers is to sell or donate them while they are still new enough to be useful. The longer you let a computer sit, the less useful it is and the more likely it is to need to be recycled rather than reused.

If you have waited around long enough for your computer to become obsolete, you will be faced with a disposal problem. Old computers and electronics not only take up a lot of room, they may also contain heavy metals such as lead, mercury, cadmium, and toxic flame retardants. When electronics are put in landfills, these toxins can leach into the groundwater. Some states have banned old computer monitors from landfills, and more will surely follow suit, but no matter where you live, the responsible thing to do is to recycle your old electronics.

The best source for local information on computer recycling is your community's Solid Waste Management facility. If there is no local computer recycling program, try some of the following sources for information that will help you recycle your old electronics and computer equipment:

International Association of Electronics Recyclers (IAER)
(www.iaer.org/search)
Offers a comprehensive list of electronics recyclers.

National Recycling Coalition (www.nrc-recycle.org/programs/
electronics)
Hosts a database of electronics recyclers, reuse organizations, and
municipal programs that accept old electronic equipment.

Carnegie Mellon University's Green Design Initiative
(www.ce.cmu.edu/GreenDesign/index.html)
Provides a comprehensive international resource list for information
about end-of-life options for electronic products. The website
includes links for computer, software, component, and diskette
recycling; federal, state, and local recycling/donation programs;
electronics manufacturers' programs; dealers of used and refurnished
equipment; and school and charity donation coordinators and
academic and research institutions.

Recycler's World (www.recycle.net/computer)
Lists computer and telecommunications equipment recyclers
and refurbishers and hosts a worldwide electronics materials
exchange.

Manufacturers' Asset Recovery and Recycling Programs

Frankly, none of the manufacturers' recycling programs are as easy or as
cheap as they should be. European countries require that all manufacturers
accept their products for recycling at their retail outlets. The United States
should follow their example, but until then, these computer manufacturers
will accept their outmoded computers for a fee (typically about $30), but
you will need to pack up and ship the computer back to its maker at your
own expense.

Go online to a search site and type in the brand name of your computer
and "recycle." Or try these websites:

COMPAQ Computer Asset Recovery Services (www.hp.com/hpinfo/
globalcitizenship/environment/recycle/hardwarerecycle.html)

IBM Product End-of-Life Management (PELM) Service
(www.ibm.com/ibm/responsibility/world/environmental/
products.shtml)

Apple Computer, Apple Recycles Program (http://www.apple.com/
environment/recycling/nationalservices/us.html)

Dell Computer, Dell Recycling (http://www1.us.dell.com/
content/topics/segtopic.aspx/dell_recycling)
Dell Computer offers free recycling of your old computer when you
buy a new Dell computer, and they also offer a slight discount on a
new Dell computer when you recycle your old Dell computer
through them.

Hewlett-Packard, Hardware Recycling (www.hp.com/hpinfo/
globalcitizenship/environment/recycle/hardwarerecycle.html)

Ink Jet and Toner Cartridges

An estimated 400,000,000 printer cartridges are dumped in landfills annually. It takes approximately 2.5 ounces of oil to manufacture each ink jet cartridge and about 3.5 quarts of oil to produce each laser cartridge. These cartridges cost more to destroy than to remanufacture. Quite a few companies pay for used cartridges, which they remanufacture and sell back to consumers:

www.empties4cash.com
"Empties 4 Cash" sends collection boxes with prepaid shipping labels. The company pays an average of $2 to $3 per ink jet cartridge, and up to $4 on some cartridges, but the cartridge must retain its print head (the copper metal on the end of the cartridge) in order to be recyclable. Any organization, business, or individual can fund-raise by participating in this program.

http://www.fundingfactory.com/
Funding Factory accepts empty ink jet and laser ink cartridges, as well as old cell phones, and they pay in gift certificates or cash. Nonprofit organizations, schools, and businesses can participate for fund-raising purposes.

www.inkjetcartridges.com
Inkjetcartridges.com is a company that pays for old ink jet cartridges, then remanufactures them.

http://www.c-rep.net/
C-REP (Cartridge Recycling for Environmental Protection) is a company that pays for empty ink jet and laser cartridges and old cell phones. Organizations can fund-raise by collecting these items and sending them to the company.

Construction, Demolition, and Redecorating Debris

Many construction materials are reusable, such as paneling, framing wood, roofing materials, hardware, doors, windows, cabinets, countertops, bathroom fixtures, light fixtures, molding, tile, building stones, and brick. If you don't want to reuse them yourself, place an ad in the newspaper advertising "free building materials," and you are likely to find willing takers.

Concrete, asphalt, steel, and sheet rock can all be sent to recycling facilities, where they will be crushed and processed for reuse.

Caveat: Lead paint was outlawed in the United States in 1978. Construction debris that contains anything painted before 1978 should be treated as hazardous waste. Don't pawn off your lead-contaminated materials; it isn't neighborly to give hazardous materials to the unsuspecting.

Treated Wood

Most wood is rather appetizing to insects and susceptible to rot. In order to adapt plentiful, rot-prone, inexpensive woods such as fir and pine for use as decking material and posts, manufacturers have learned to pressure treat them with chemicals that are toxic to insects and fungi. Unfortunately, chemicals that are toxic to pest organisms often turn out to be toxic to other organisms—such as humans, for instance. Such has been the noxious fate of wood treated with pentachlorophenol (Penta), creosote, and chromated copper arsenate. Newer, less toxic pressure-treated wood is now on the market; it is treated with the preservatives Alkaline Copper Quat or Copper Azole, which are water based and just as effective at preserving wood as the older, more dangerous preservatives.

Wood that has been treated with these water-based compounds can be disposed of at the landfill, but if you have scraps of the older, more toxic pressure-treated wood laying around, gather them up in your rubber-glove clad hands, put the scraps in garbage bags, throw the bags into your vehicle, and make a visit to your local hazardous waste facility.

Never burn treated or painted wood! Even the newer, safer preservatives will create toxic smoke and ashes.

Asphalt

Asphalt is a petroleum product, and therefore nonrenewable. The 4 million miles of paved roads in the United States hold 270 billion gallons of petroleum.

It is no longer economically or morally feasible to bury large amounts of petroleum in landfills. Many companies have developed techniques and machinery that can recycle old asphalt paving and old asphalt shingles into new hot-mix asphalt for road construction. If you are tearing out old asphalt, contact a local asphalt company and ask whether they can recycle your asphalt for you, or do a web search for "asphalt recycling."

Rugs, Carpets, and Wall-To-Wall Carpeting
Though high-quality antique hand-knotted rugs are quite valuable and newer high-quality throw rugs are saleable items, used synthetic wall-to-wall carpeting is worth less than nothing. About 3.5 billion pounds of unwanted, mostly synthetic carpeting is sent to American landfills every year. Can we really afford to discard 3.5 billion pounds of oil per year?

Try to buy carpeting that is either made of natural fibers or of recycled nylon.

Natural fiber carpeting that is beyond saving can either be composted or used as a weed-suppressing mulch that can be hidden under a layer of bark or landscaping gravel.

Recycling synthetic carpeting is often not as easy as it should be. Try contacting local carpet outlets and ask whether they participate in a carpet-recycling program. Or, search the web using your state's name and "carpet recycling." You can also try the following websites:

http://www.earthsquare.com
Milliken & Company refurbishes carpeting. The renewed carpet
even comes with a renewed warranty.

http://www.lafiber.com/sys-tmpl/recycleprogram
The Los Angeles Fiber Company recycles waste carpeting into
synthetic carpet cushion. The company will accept carpeting from
all eleven western states. The company doesn't charge a disposal fee,
but the customer pays the freight.

http://www.antron.net
Antron Carpet Company uses recycled nylon fibers to manufacture

its carpeting, and it has been recycling old carpeting through its
Invista carpet reclamation program since 1991.

http://www.infinitynylon.com or call 1-877-N6-CYCLE
The Infinity nylon renewal program will accept any carpet made
with nylon 6 fiber. The carpet must be tested and identified as nylon
6 by your local carpet collection service.

Recycled Infinity nylon is used to make carpets, athletic turf,
car and truck components, fibers for airbags and tires, and plastics
for tools, electronics, and appliances.

Appliances

Have appliance deliverers, mattress deliverers, and carpet installers haul
away the old material. They are far more likely to have systems in place for
recycling/reusing your discards than you do.

The Future

A combination of recycling, buying in bulk, and composting reduces the
amount of trash my family sends to the landfill. We often don't bother to put
our nearly empty garbage can out on collection day. Most of the trash that
ends up in our garbage can is unrecyclable plastic food packaging and plastic wrap. This distresses me. I am delighted with the rapid progress that is
being made in developing biodegradable, plant-based, nontoxic bioplastic
food packaging, and I look forward to the day when I am able to recycle or
compost all of our trash.

For information on composting, please refer to the chapter on gardening on page 358.

Keep Moving

Life is movement; cessation of movement is death. It is vitally important to
keep materials flowing into and out of the house at a nearly equal rate; a

stagnant house, like a stagnant pond, is an unpleasant phenomenon. Recycling our unwanted materials allows us to keep our homes as well as the environment in working order.

The kitchen is the heart of the home—a clog in the works of either can wreak havoc. Reading chapter two will help you create a smoothly flowing kitchen.

CHAPTER 2

The Kitchen:
You Are What You Eat

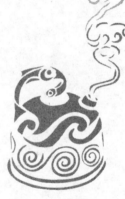

It is of the utmost importance that kitchen surfaces, cookware, and utensils are clean and free of chemical contamination. There is no point in buying organic food, bringing it home, and then preparing it in a chemically contaminated kitchen. But looking clean and being clean are not necessarily the same thing . . .

It is entirely possible to have a kitchen that looks less than clean and pristine, yet is a completely safe and healthy place to prepare food. One kitchen may contain wooden cutting boards that are rough and stained, a fifty-year-old oven with impregnable baked-on stains, and a copper kettle that rarely gleams, but the surfaces are clean and free of chemical and microbial contaminants. Another kitchen may sparkle and gleam from its stainless-steel sink and refrigerator to its convection oven and granite countertops, yet its plastic cutting boards harbor dangerous bacteria and its counters are coated with a thin film consisting of pesticides, disinfectants, and antimicrobials.

Kitchens R Us

Our dogs are very efficient predators and scavengers. They think nothing of snapping up an errant mouse or chewing off a piece of dead deer. On the other hand, I would certainly starve to death if I had to process my food with just my teeth.

The art of cooking helps us humans compensate for our small teeth, weak jaws, and delicate digestive systems, allowing us to digest what would otherwise be inedible. If we learn to regard our kitchens as extensions of our own bodies, we may be less willing to contaminate them with dangerous chemicals.

Organic Cleaning

The main goal of organic kitchen cleaning is to preserve human and environmental health by avoiding the use of synthetic chemical cleaning products and pesticides, which are very harsh (see chapter eight, "Hazardous Materials," page 301). Using them is the cleaning equivalent of calling in the special forces because things have gotten completely out of hand. It is always better to use intelligence and timing to deal with problems before they get too big and recalcitrant. In almost every instance, the cleaning technique that uses the least amount of energy and resources—whether human, electrical, or petrochemical—is the most effective. Extra chemical ingredients such as fragrances and dyes, which contribute nothing to a product's cleaning ability, are generally to be avoided.

Though there are many household chores that can be neglected for long periods of time without causing much difficulty, most kitchen chores are not in that category. The combination of heat, grease, food, and moisture makes the kitchen one of the main domestic battlegrounds in the fight against pests and grime. Our most effective weapons in this battle are grime prevention and frequent cleaning.

⚘ DESIGN GRIME OUT!

Some kitchen surfaces are much easier to keep clean than others. In an ideal world, we would all have kitchens that were designed to minimize grime collection. If you do have the chance to design a new kitchen or rehab an old one, here are some time-and-energy-saving suggestions:

• Choose smooth rather than textured surfaces. A refrigerator with a smooth white surface can be wiped clean easily, but a dirty textured surface must be scrubbed clean with a brush. A smooth floor is easy to mop clean, but getting the grease out of the creases of a textured floor may require some really hard scrubbing.

• Unless you really enjoy polishing things, choose white or light-colored appliances. Appliances with dark shiny surfaces are very reflective and show streaks and smears as if they were mirrors; streaks are invisible on white appliances.

   The only exceptions to this rule are stove tops and drip pans. Though built-up grease is a fire hazard, stains are just stains. If you would rather not spend time scouring stains off your stove, choose a black stove top and/or black drip pans, which don't show stains at all. Black enameled replacement drip pans are available at appliance stores.

• Fiberglass sinks scratch and mar easily and are much more difficult to keep clean than sinks made of harder surfaces such as stainless-steel, enamel, or porcelain.

• If you don't want to spend a lot of time polishing your faucets, choose dull "gun-metal" surfaces that will hide hard water spots, which are very obvious on shiny stainless-steel or chrome.

• Open shelving may be chic, but a closed cabinet door is one of the best grime-prevention devices yet invented. I would much rather wipe down a cabinet door than clean the interior of a cabinet along with its contents.

• The open space between the tops of kitchen cabinets and the ceiling is a haven for grease and dust, and most cabinet tops are unfinished and can't be scrubbed or washed. Boxing off this area will greatly reduce the amount of grime in your kitchen. A cheaper solution is to cut corrugated cardboard to fit inside the recessed top of the cabinets. The cardboard will be invisible to anyone who is under seven and a half feet tall. When the cardboard gets really dirty, replace it.

• Cabinets and cupboards should be installed at the right height for the adults who will be using them. It is very common for tall architects and builders to design kitchens that fit themselves and not the people who will actually be using them.

What Is Clean?

There is no such thing as cleaner than clean. A clean surface is just the surface, with nothing else on it; a lingering fragrance, no matter how sweet and pleasant, signals that a chemical has been left behind.

Organic cleaners are made of natural, often food grade, materials. Most synthetic cleaners and detergents are petroleum products. Soaps are manufactured from natural animal or vegetable fats. Plain soap is usually made from rendered animal fats and lye; castile soap is the term for soap made from vegetable oil. Regular soap reacts with the minerals in hard water to form a very stubborn soap scum that doesn't dissolve in water. Castile soap is gentler, dissolves more completely, and doesn't form a hard scum. Petroleum-based detergents also don't form soap scum—in fact, that's why they were invented—but petroleum products are toxic.

The dish liquid I use is made from water, edible oils, and salt. All the ingredients are listed on the label. I find the labels of synthetic dish liquids to be rather indecipherable and uninformative.

Drinking soap is never a good idea, but if your two-year-old is going to get into the dish liquid, it would be far better if he drank a natural castile soap made from vegetable oil rather than a petroleum-based detergent. And I like the fact that even if I do a sloppy job of rinsing my dishes, the residues left behind by my organic dish liquid are nontoxic.

If everything could be cleaned using only the universal solvent—water—the environment would be far healthier than it is!

The Products

Chlorinated and antibacterial products can wreak havoc on septic systems by killing the bacteria that make the systems work. If you are having trouble finding natural or organic cleaning products in your area, choose products that are labeled Safe for Septic Systems.

When you are buying cleaning products, especially ones that will be used in the kitchen, choose products that are labeled 100 percent biodegradable; do not contain chlorine, antimicrobials, phosphate, dyes, or artificial fragrances, and are safe for septic and greywater systems. Many of these products, such as Murphy's Oil Soap and Bon Ami cleanser, have been on the market for generations. Newer companies such as Seventh Generation, Ecover, and Restore specialize in environmentally friendly products; these companies produce dish liquid and dishwasher detergent that are efficient and nonpolluting.

Commercial kitchen degreasers can contain volatile chemicals such as perchloroethylene and toluene, which are neurotoxins and are considered human carcinogens. These products emit dangerous fumes and their residues may contaminate work surfaces.

Dish liquids are designed to cut grease, and they are very good at their job. A solution of any good organic dish liquid can be used to remove cooking grease from just about any washable surface including your kitchen appliances and kitchen floor. (*Caveat:* Never use any type of dish liquid inside a dishwasher. It makes too many suds and will wreak havoc on the machine.)

If you find the writing on product labels too small or too confusing, you might consider buying your cleaning products at your local health food or natural food store. Many of these stores have carefully vetted their merchandise because they cater to clientele who suffer from chemical sensitivities. There are also many online sites that carry environmentally friendly cleaning products. Remember that unscented products are generally easier on sensitive skin since even natural fragrances can cause allergic reactions.

> Distilled white vinegar is the solvent of choice for many nontoxic cleaning jobs. A few years ago I was astonished to learn that in some countries white vinegar is made from petroleum. The best way to make sure that white vinegar is not made from petroleum—especially if you are outside the United States—is to look for Made from Grain on the label.

Many common foods can double as cleaning products. Vinegar, salt, baking soda, lemons, cabbage leaves, potatoes, mayonnaise, olive oil, apple peels, ketchup, and vodka can all be used for cleaning. If it's safe to eat, it's certainly safe to clean with!

Cleaning Tools

I prefer simple, reusable, multipurpose cleaning tools. The following standard cleaning tools are easily purchased: a soft bristle broom and dust pan, a bucket, a vacuum cleaner, and spray bottles for homemade cleaning solutions.

I also use a couple of less common but extremely useful cleaning tools:

The Dutch Rubber Broom is a long-handled rubber floor squeegee with a short-fingered rubber rake on the other side. I bought mine at a home show a couple of years ago, and I have used it at least once a day ever since. The Dutch Rubber Broom can be ordered online through Euroshine USA, Inc. (www.euroshine.net)

Another extremely useful piece of equipment is a small portable steam cleaner with a shoulder strap and various attachments; I bought mine at a department store. Steam cleaning is a very effective nontoxic cleaning method that removes grease and grime from most surfaces.

Recycled cleaning tools are key components of the organic housekeeper's toolkit:

- An old toothbrush is the perfect tool for scrubbing small spaces, seams, and cracks. Never throw an old toothbrush away before you have used it to clean up something really greasy, grimy, and filthy.
- Voltaire wrote: "If God did not exist, it would be necessary to invent Him." Likewise, if cotton rags did not exist, it would be necessary to invent them. Luckily for me, my family is very hard on clothing, so we are always well supplied with useful rags.
- Clean absorbent cotton rags are the foundation of environmentally sound housecleaning. There are two types of rags: valuable ones such as cloth diapers, kitchen dishcloths, old cotton T-shirts, and old terrycloth towels; and lesser rags such as holey underwear and old socks. The valuable rags are used and washed again and again until they wear out and become disposable rags. The disposable rags can be used for really filthy jobs like oven cleaning and are then thrown away or composted. Keep a stack of each type of rag in or near the kitchen and in each bathroom.

Wham, Bam, Thank You Ma'am

When I am cleaning my kitchen, my objective is to leave the kitchen clean and as soon as possible. Here are a few very effective techniques that help me reduce my cleaning time:

- Prevention is the first rule of environmental housekeeping, and preventing pest infestations is a very basic goal. Household pest prevention starts with keeping the kitchen clean and dry, in order to render it less attractive to vermin such as cockroaches and rodents. These varmints are very similar to teenagers: They follow the food.

  It is extremely important to wash the dishes and clean up food scraps every day.

  If you already have a pest problem, you will need to make all your food inaccessible to pests: Store your dry goods in glass, ceramic, or metal containers with glass, ceramic, or metal lids. Store your bread in an airtight container, and keep all your fresh produce in the refrigerator. Keep crumbs and grease cleaned up, don't leave pet food out all day, and fix all plumbing leaks.

- It's much easier to clean up fresh spills and spatters than to clean up crusty old ones. If you really want to reduce your cleaning time, don't allow spatters and spills to dry and harden. Jam does not get easier to clean up after it has been drying on the kitchen floor for a week.

- Use your rags progressively, starting with the least soiled areas and progressing to the dirtiest. For example, you can use a clean damp rag to wipe the baby's face, then her highchair, then—if the rag isn't totally saturated with strained squash—use a clean corner to clean the floor under the baby's chair.

  If you are worried that somehow your rags won't get clean enough in your washing machine if you use them on the kitchen floor, you might need to consider getting a new washing machine. There is no reason why a hot, heavy-duty wash cycle shouldn't be able to wash out normal household grime.

- Avoid spreading grease around. If your floor is extremely greasy in a specific spot—for instance, where the roast turkey slid after it fell off the platter—wash the greasy spot with a wet rag and a bit of dish liquid, then rinse the rag before washing the rest of the floor.

- One of the best ways to reduce your kitchen cleaning time is to keep drawers and cupboard doors closed. It is easier to clean grease splatters off a cupboard door than out of the interior of the cupboard, and it is far easier to wipe counters and sweep the floor than to clean cereal or milk out of a junk drawer.
- The kitchen is the one room in the house where postponing the dusting actually makes a difference. Kitchen dust will eventually combine with airborne grease to form a fibrous, puttylike goo. Keep the top of the refrigerator and the range hood dusted off. You will never regret it.
- It is not necessary to buy specialized kitchen cleaners to clean kitchen surfaces. Dish liquid is designed to cut grease. Wipe down greasy cabinets and appliances with a solution of 1 tablespoon dish liquid per gallon of water. Particularly greasy spots can be scrubbed down with a folded plastic-mesh produce bag.
- Whoever invented kitchen carpeting was a sadist: The surface that jars of jam, full milk cartons, and peanut butter sandwiches land on should be smooth and easily cleaned. If you have kitchen carpeting, try to replace it. No one wants to shampoo carpeting every other day.
- One of the main roles of a canine in a human dwelling is floor cleaner. If you'd rather not bend over to clean up kitchen spills, consider hiring a dog.

Mopping Up

The Dutch Rubber Broom is my instrument of choice for cleaning large surfaces. I use it to squeegee water into the floor drain in the basement and to push glass shards and juice or milk into a dust pan after kitchen accidents.

Most of all, I use my rubber broom instead of a mop. I was overjoyed when I first realized that I could keep my floor perfectly clean without lugging around a heavy bucket of filthy water. The beauty of this method is that you never have to wring out a mop head or touch dirty water:

- If your dog tracks mud all over your floor or you spill something, wet a clean rag under the hot water tap, wring it out a tiny bit, and drop it on the floor. If the floor is really filthy, wet the clean rag in plain white vinegar and spread it out on the floor. Put the head of the rubber broom on it. Scrub the dirty spot with the wet rag. When the rag gets dirty, throw it in the kitchen laundry basket. Repeat.
- If you want to mop the whole floor, fill a household bucket with hot water, a cup of white vinegar, and one drop of dish liquid or Murphy's Oil Soap. If you are having ant problems, add a pinch of borax to the vinegary wash water; when the floor dries, the slight residue of borax will act as an insect repellent. This cleaning solution does not need to be rinsed off.

  Drop a clean kitchen rag into the water, pull it out, and wring it out a little. Drop the rag and swab the floor with it. When you need more wash water, throw the used rag in the kitchen laundry basket and drop a clean rag in the bucket. Because only clean rags are put in the wash water, the wash water stays clean and the floor gets cleaner.

  There are wet mops with removable terrycloth heads that work the same way, but I like multipurpose tools because my storage space and budget are extremely limited.
- If you want to dust the walls or the ceiling, put a thick rubberband around the handle of the rubber broom, near the head. (The rubberbands that hold broccoli heads or celery stalks together are the perfect size for this.) Stretch a dry dust cloth or dust rag over the broom head and hold it on with the rubberband.

  You can attach a clean damp rag over the broom head in the same way to wash the walls or the ceiling.

Get Steamed

A small steam cleaning machine is a phenomenal tool for cleaning dirty kitchen surfaces. It loosens dirt, grease, and grime so they can be wiped off with a clean cloth, and it uses pure water, so it leaves no residue. Because the steam is hot enough to burn skin and some parts of the appliance get very hot, it is very important to read and follow all the directions and safety instructions before using the appliance.

Steaming Floors and Counters

- To steam clean a wood, vinyl, or tile kitchen floor, attach a clean terrycloth towel to the floor brush, then put the floor brush on the end of the steamer's extension tube. Use a mopping motion to steam the floor clean, moving quickly to prevent heat damage. When the towel gets dirty, turn it over or replace it with a clean towel.
- Clean tile grout by using the steamer's detail brush, then use a towel-covered floor brush to remove excess moisture and residue. If the tile is very dirty, use the floor brush without a towel, then wipe the steamed area with a clean towel. You can use this technique for tiled counters as well as tiled floors.
- Strip off old wax by using the floor brush to steam a small section of floor at a time. Wipe off the dissolved wax before moving to the next section. When the job is done, clean the brushes with hot water before the wax has a chance to harden. Wipe down the floor with a clean dry towel before applying new wax. (See page 248 for information on environmentally preferable floor waxes.)

Environmentally Friendly Dishwashing

Dishwashing Supplies

Scrubbers

Don't use sponges for dishwashing. They are bacterial incubators. Instead, use a clean, dry dishcloth each time you wash dishes. If you need convincing, read on.

Carlos Enriquez and Charles Gerba, microbiologists at the University of Arizona at Tucson, collected and tested sponges and dish rags from one thousand kitchens in five American cities. They found dangerous bacteria, including *E. coli*, salmonella, pseudomonas, and staphylococcus, which can cause food poisoning, living on at least two-thirds of the sponges tested. One spectacularly contaminated dish rag was harboring enough bacteria to sicken almost anyone unwise enough to touch it.

Maybe Dogs are Smarter than We Thought . . .

> *"You'd be better off eating a carrot stick that fell in your toilet than one that fell in your sink. Your dog is right."*
>
> —CHARLES GERBA

The scientists were more likely to find dangerous bacteria in kitchen sinks than they were to find bacteria in and on flushed toilets. Carlos Enriquez said, "Consistently, kitchens come up dirtier. We have swabbed the toilet rim, for instance, and seldom do we find fecal coliform bacteria there . . ."

"We found that the most germ-laden object in your home is actually your kitchen sponge or your dish rag," said Gerba. One milliliter of liquid squeezed from a particularly lively sponge contained 10 million live bacteria!

At first, Enriquez and Gerba were surprised by their findings, but later realized that moist cellulose sponges provide a perfect culture medium for bacteria. Bacteria have very simple needs: a porous surface to cling to, a stable food supply, and moisture. A damp sponge can nurture a healthy bacterial population for two weeks. Bacteria can't survive more than a few hours on a dry surface.

Further study revealed that the cleanest-looking kitchens often contained the most bacteria. Tidy people wipe up so often that they tend to spread bacteria all over the place. "You think you are cleaning, but you're actually spreading the bacteria," said Gerba. The research showed that the healthiest, most sanitary kitchens were kept by bachelors who never cleaned at all. Sloth emerges victorious.

Dirtying Up the Kitchen

The average kitchen sponge contains millions of bacteria because it stays damp from the moment it is put into service until it is retired.

Elizabeth Scott, a microbiologist who specializes in food-borne pathogens, found that washing kitchen sponges with detergent and hot

---

🐜 IS THE SKY FALLING? OR IS THAT JUST A STAIN ON THE CEILING?

Are we all doomed? Should we prepare our food in the bathroom? Must we emulate slovenly bachelors in order to stay healthy? Probably not. If our great-grandparents hadn't managed to stay alive despite their total lack of modern disinfectants, we wouldn't be here. A recently retired friend of mine was a micro-biology professor and researcher for more than thirty years. She has a Ph.D. in microbiology and prefers to remain anonymous, so I will refer to her as Dr. Micro. I asked her what she thought people should know about keeping kitchens sanitary. Her answer: "Don't worry about it I don't."

This is actually a carefully formulated opinion based on her years of meticulous laboratory observation. Dr. Micro told me, "I always observed that the people who were the most fanatical about sterile techniques always had the biggest infections in their experiments."

She went on to explain that microbiologists who are total slobs tend to end up with a lot of uninvited bacteria in their experiments; the researchers who are moderately careful generally have uncontaminated experiments; but people who try to run absolutely pristine experiments consistently have worse luck than the total slobs.

Dr. Micro also told me that the world is a lot cleaner than people think it is. She said that it's usually impossible to culture anything off a floor. Perhaps the saying, "That kitchen is so clean that you can eat off the floor" should be taken literally, since scientists have proven that neat and tidy kitchens often have really filthy countertops!

---

water does not kill the bacteria, it merely breaks the colonies up into smaller, more efficient missionary units that are ready, at the swipe of a sponge, to colonize every surface they encounter.

These tiny colonists can live for a couple of hours after a plastic or laminate counter dries. If you have improved the habitat by using your plastic counter as a cutting block, live bacteria may lurk for many hours in the small chips and nicks of a damaged countertop.

A Bacterial Playground

Some people regularly throw their kitchen sponges in the dishwasher. The sponges look cleaner afterward, but most dishwashers do not get hot enough to kill bacteria, and the dish drying cycle is certainly not enough to dry out a sponge. Washing a bacteria-infested sponge in the dishwasher will successfully redistribute bacteria all over the dishes, where they will remain alive as long as they stay moist. (Never put wet or damp dishes back into your dish cupboard.)

Many people try to sterilize cellulose kitchen sponges by heating them on high power in the microwave. The entire sponge must reach boiling temperature; recommended lengths of time range from 30 to 90 seconds based on the size of the sponge and the oven's power. If you can figure out the appropriate amount of time that works for your microwave, this method will probably kill the bacteria.

I must admit that I am quite biased against microwaving sponges: I don't like the idea of microwaving anything as filthy as a kitchen sponge. I think microwaving sponges is a waste of energy. And last, but not least, if the sponge or dishcloth dries out, it can ignite in the microwave.

Some experts recommend sterilizing kitchen sponges by boiling them for three minutes. I don't even want to think about the comments this activity would generate in our household! I would rather just take a nice clean dishcloth out of the cupboard and put the used one in the wash.

If you miss the wonderful combination of absorbency and a tough scrubbing surface that a scrubbing sponge can provide, here's a cheap, easy, and clean substitute: Cut the label end off of one of the plastic mesh bags that oranges or onions come in, thus transforming the bag into a tube. Fold a standard one-foot-square dishcloth twice and slip it into the plastic mesh tube, then fold the whole thing until it is the size of a dish sponge. This homemade dish scrubber works beautifully and never scratches or mars shiny pans or glasses. When the dishes are done, remove the cloth, wring it out, and throw it in the laundry. Rinse off the mesh bag and hang it up so it will be clean and dry the next time you need it. If you don't feel like rinsing off the mesh bag, throw it out; it's easily replaced. Using these bags for scrubbing duty postpones their trip to the landfill or incinerator while reducing the volume of dish scrubbers that must be manufactured and eventually discarded.

Dish Liquids

The American Medical Association (AMA) released a report in 2000 which stated that bacteria are developing resistance to the antimicrobials which are increasingly being added to consumer products such as dish soaps, bath soaps, hand soaps, toothpaste, and hand lotions, and that the use of these products may lead to antibiotic resistance. The report stated: "Ultimately, antibiotic resistance is a major public health concern that has to be controlled . . ." "The use of common antimicrobials . . . in consumer products should be discontinued . . ."

All the bacteria that survive antibacterials become the foundations of new, improved, bacterial Superraces. Ironically, research has shown that regular hand soap and liquid dish soap are just as effective at killing bacteria as antibacterial soaps are. One of the most effective disease prevention techniques ever devised is frequent hand washing with plain soap and hot water. Buy plain regular soap and use it often.

It is not just their salutary effect on dangerous bacteria that makes antibacterials hazardous: In 2002, the U.S. Geological Survey published a study of chemicals detected in our nation's surface waters. Triclosan, the most commonly used antibacterial, was found in 58 percent of the water bodies tested. Inspired by this information, professors Kristopher McNeill and William Arnold at the University of Minnesota decided to examine what happened to triclosan once it entered the natural environment. They exposed triclosan-laced river water to ultraviolet light and discovered that the triclosan degraded into a form of dioxin.

Never assume that "biodegradable" means harmless. Many synthetic compounds biodegrade into more dangerous compounds.

Avoid dish liquids that contain antibacterials. There are many fine brands of biodegradable dish liquids that are easy on the environment and don't jeopardize our medical use of antibiotics. If you can't find a natural dish liquid, use a pure liquid castile soap such as Dr. Bronner's. (For more information about castile soap, see page 63.)

Automatic Dishwasher Detergents

Many dishwasher detergents contain chlorine, phosphorus, and antimicrobials, which are potentially dangerous, completely unnecessary, and very hard on the environment. Whether you are concerned about the health of our waterways or are merely trying to keep your septic system working properly, it is a good idea to choose a dishwasher detergent that does not contain any of these ingredients.

Look in the health food store for environmentally friendly dishwasher detergents that utilize enzymes, washing soda (sodium carbonate), and borax. Or you can make a batch of homemade dish detergent by mixing equal parts of laundry borax and washing soda. Follow your dishwasher's instruction manual and use the same amount of the homemade detergent as you would of a commercial detergent. Do not wash aluminum or teflon pans with this homemade detergent.

Using too much dishwasher detergent, whether it is commercial or homemade, will make your dishes dull and dingy. My very efficient dishwasher requires only one tablespoon of detergent. If your dishwasher has a detergent dispenser and a rinse dispenser, fill the rinse dispenser with vinegar to help prevent mineral buildup on your dishes and glassware.

Dishwasher Technique

While working on this book, I interviewed an appliance repairman who told me that most dishwasher detergents contain enzymes that react with and break down organic material (food waste). These enzymes make the detergent very hard and porous. If dishes are nearly clean when they are put into the dishwasher, the enzymes have nothing to stick to and are flung about the

---

～ THE SCOOP ON DISHWASHERS

The best dishwashers are so energy efficient and require so little water that using them is actually better for the environment than washing dishes by hand.

Some dishwashers have built-in water heaters; using the temperature boost setting will allow you to set your household water heater at about 120° Fahrenheit (50° Celsius), which will save energy, money, and prevent accidental scaldings. Many dishwashers also have settings that allow you to choose heated drying or air drying; choose the air dry setting to save more energy. When the wash cycle is over open the dishwasher door and let the dishes sit and dry in the dishwasher. Run the dishwasher only when it is full; doing partial loads wastes water.

Most dishwashers do not get hot enough to kill microbes. Bacteria can survive in water in the dishwasher, so be sure to dump out the water that sits in the bottom of cups and goblets, then dry off the bottoms before putting the dishes away.

inside of the dishwasher, effectively sandblasting the dishes and glassware. This sandblasting effect can permanently cloud glassware and wear the decorative paint and glazes off of dishes.

Here is the recommended way to load a dishwasher:

1. Use a rubber spatula to scrape large chunks of food off the dishes and flatware. (I scrape my food scraps into my compost bucket, from whence they are tipped into my vermicomposting bin. For more information on vermicomposting, please refer to page 359.)
2. The dishwasher may not remove hardened bits of food. Anything that is crusty or hardened should be removed.
3. Brush off all bits of cheese before loading dishes or utensils into the dishwasher. The heat of the dishwasher will bake cheese right onto a fork or plate, where it will cling like a limpet until it is forcibly removed.
4. Don't prerinse your dishes before you load them into the dishwasher. Leave that light glazing of turkey juice, spaghetti sauce, and gravy on the plates. Your dishes and glassware will last longer if they are not sandblasted by underemployed dishwasher enzymes.
5. Read the directions on your dishwasher detergent, then use the least possible amount. A scum of excess detergent is just as dirty as a scum of milk or grease, and may be harder to rinse off.
6. If your dishwasher begins to stink, clean the filter according to the manufacturer's instructions. Then pour 2 cups of white vinegar into a bowl and set the bowl face up on the bottom rack of the dishwasher. Run the machine through a wash cycle to clean the inside of the appliance. The vinegar will deodorize the dishwasher as well as dissolve hard water deposits.
7. To remove hard water spots from dishes and glassware, use the normal amount of detergent and run the dishes through the wash cycle. Remove all the cutlery and other metal items from the dishwasher, then pour 2 cups white vinegar into a bowl and set the bowl face up on the bottom rack of the dishwasher. Run the dishes through the wash cycle again, with just vinegar as a cleaning agent. Allow the dishes to dry completely before putting them away.

Keep These Out of the Dishwasher

Never put your good kitchen knives in the machine—the dishwasher will dull the edges. I usually try to wash my kitchen knives as soon as I finish using them so they don't get buried in the sink and I don't cut myself.

The dishwasher will eventually crack and ruin any wood that is put into it. Wooden cutting boards, wooden handled knives, and wooden salad bowls should all be lovingly washed by hand then towel dried. If the wood begins to look dry, rub it down with a little olive oil.

Antique tableware, fine china, hand decorated china, delicate glassware, glass with metallic decoration, real silverware, pewter, and cutlery with bone, ivory, bakelite, or wooden handles are all too delicate for the dishwasher.

Glass measuring cups will quickly lose their painted markings if they are washed in the dishwasher.

Cast iron and tin will rust in the dishwasher. (You can remove rust from tinware by rubbing it with a peeled potato dipped in baking soda or salt.)

Aluminum will darken in the dishwasher. (Boiling apple peels in aluminum pots will remove the discoloration from the metal.)

Heat and abrasion can cause plastic to break down and release chemicals. All plastic tableware and containers, whether they are labeled "Dishwasher Safe" or not, should be washed by hand.

Dishwashers are designed to wash hard, durable, impermeable materials. Soft items, such as paint brushes, air filters, dishcloths, or sponges, may damage the dishwasher.

Washing Dishes by Hand, Saving Water

Water is an infinitely precious yet finite resource. Just ask anyone whose water comes from a private well or who has lived through a drought. There was a severe drought while I was growing up in California. We all learned to wash using a minimum of water and consequently less soap. "Drought washing" is much easier on the environment than the water-wasteful kind, and I think it is far less disgusting than washing dishes in a sinkful of greasy, scummy water.

The Hand Washing Technique

The perfect sink for hand dishwashing has a big, deep, single bowl and built-in drain boards on both sides. Most double sinks are annoyingly small and cannot accommodate large roasting pans or long-handled skillets.

The perfect hands for manual dishwashing are clad in rubber gloves.

1. Keep greasy pots and pans away from dishes. Greasy dishes are much harder to wash than nongreasy ones, and why make more work for yourself? You can put hot water and dish soap in the greasy pots and pans and let them soak on the stove until you're ready to tackle them.

   Filling a sink with soapy water to wash dishes is wasteful as well as inefficient. Not all the dishes used at a meal will be equally dirty, but if they soak in a sink together, the dirty dishes get a little cleaner, while the nearly clean dishes get a lot dirtier.

   If your water is really hard, letting the dishes soak in the sink can get truly disgusting. A sinkful of mineral-laden water, dishes, and dish soap can congeal overnight into a sinkful of greasy, gelatinous scum.

2. To remove a hardened, burned-on crust from a pot or pan, fill it with a solution of 2 tablespoons baking soda per quart of water and bring to a boil. Turn off the heat and let the pan cool. The carbonized crust will lift right off.

   To clean burned crust out of a large roasting pan or glass baking dish that cannot be heated on top of the stove, pour in the baking soda solution and heat the pan in a 350 degree oven. When the water begins to steam, turn the oven off and let the pan cool.

3. If you have somewhere to stack your dirty dishes other than in the sink, do so.

4. Scrub your sink with a clean, soapy dishrag.

5. Put all your dirty cutlery in the sink, run hot water on the dishcloth, then squirt some dish soap (preferably organic) on the dishcloth.

6. Scrub the cutlery pieces and stack them in a corner of the sink or in a rinse basket. When all the cutlery is scrubbed, rinse it with hot tap water and put it in the dish drying rack. (Researchers who have studied these things have concluded that air-dried dishes are far more sanitary than dishes that have been dried with a towel. Air-drying dishes is also, perhaps not coincidentally, less work.)

7. Next, start washing dishes, taking them off the counter, or wherever they are stacked; wash them with a soapy dishcloth, and stack them in the sink.

8. When your sudsy stack reaches the top of the sink or you've washed all the dishes (whichever comes first), rinse the dishes with hot water and put them in the dish drainer.

9. After the dishes are clean, wash the glasses and stack them in the sink. Rinse them off and put them in the dish drainer.

10. After you have washed all the dishes, you can start washing the pots and pans. They have been soaking awhile by this time, and should be a little easier to tackle.

Kitchen Odors

It is a rare kitchen that always smells sweet. Some foods are just plain smelly, others reek only after they have been burned. And most of us conduct the occasional refrigerator "experiment." Here are some ways to exorcise those unpleasant odors without poisoning yourself with synthetic "air fresheners."

Track down the source of the smell. If it is not a member of the family, get rid of it.

Eliminate Odors

Clean Out Your Refrigerator

Throw slimy vegetables and rotting fruit in your compost bucket. Wash the slime out of the fruit and vegetable drawer. Put rotting meat in your freezer until garbage day. Wash sour milk off the refrigerator shelves.

Put an open container of baking soda in the refrigerator. The baking soda will absorb odors. Replace it after about six months. Use the old baking soda for cleaning jobs or to unclog a drain.

Empty the Garbage

If the inside of the can is wet, wash it out and let it dry. Sprinkle some baking soda in the bottom of the garbage pail to absorb odors.

Burned the Dinner?

If something has burned but is no longer producing actual flames, turn on the range hood to suck the smoke out of the house. If the weather is above freezing, open some windows.

You can try to placate your smoke alarm by whirling a vinegar-dampened towel over your head. Some of the smoke will catch in the towel, and the vinegar will help neutralize the smell.

Damp and Dank

Molds and mildews are often rather malodorous. If they are growing in your undersink cabinet, you need to fix the leak and dry out the cabinet. Wash out the cabinet with vinegar and borax to kill the mold and mildew. A portable fan can be used to speed up the drying process.

Garlic and Onion Odors

Hot water sets in these odors. Cold water removes them. Wash your odoriferous cutting boards and hands in cold water. Rinse well.

Add Better Smells

Warm a little vinegar on the stove while you are cooking fish, cabbage, or other strong smelling food.

Burn an unscented candle to help dispel odors. Be careful to keep the candle out of the reach of children, pets, and mischievous breezes. (For information on nontoxic candles, please read page 282.)

Pour equal amounts of vinegar and water into a spray bottle. Spray a little vinegar water into the air to dispel strong cooking odors.

Pour a little vanilla extract on a cotton ball in a saucer and set it out on a countertop.

Heat cinnamon sticks and cloves or cut-up lemons in a saucepan of water on the stove. If the smell is too tantalizing, make mulled cider instead: Heat apple cider with a cinnamon stick and a few whole cloves in a saucepan over a burner turned on low. Do not allow the cider to boil. Let the cider smell permeate the house until you can't resist it any longer. Pour the cider into a mug. Drink.

Growing Clean Air

Green plants are the only true air fresheners. They produce oxygen and also remove toxins and particulate matter from the air.

Houseplants with scented leaves can make indoor air smell wonderful. Stroke the leaves of fragrant houseplants such as scented geraniums, lavender, thyme, rosemary, and mint to release their fragrance into the room. Or pick a couple of scented leaves and simmer them in a saucepan of water.

(For more information, see chapter eight, "Domestic Odor Control," page 279.)

Sink Cleaning

Stainless-Steel Care

1. Do not use abrasive cleansers or metal scrubbing pads on stainless steel; they scratch its polished surface and make it harder to keep clean. Do not use your stainless-steel sink as a cutting board; the knife will scar the surface.
2. Stainless steel is damaged by contact with chlorine and other strong chemicals. Organic cleansers, soaps, detergents, and bleaches do not contain chlorine, but plain old table salt (sodium chloride) can damage stainless-steel. Don't allow food or beverage residues, especially salty ones, to sit and dry on your stainless-steel sink. Rinse your sink clean after each use. When you scrub your

sink, use a plastic netting scrubber and a gentle, non-chlorinated dish liquid, or a nonabrasive cleanser such as Bon Ami or baking soda, and rub in the direction of the finish lines.

3. When water dries, it can leave mineral deposits behind. Hard water leaves a white film and water with a high iron content leaves a rusty brown stain. If you wipe the sink with a clean dry cloth after use, you remove these minerals and prevent stains. It is much easier to prevent stains than to scrub them off.

Porcelain Enamel Sinks

Enameled surfaces are composed of glass melted onto a metal base. This surface, like other glass, is easily damaged by acids and harsh abrasives, and will chip or crack if it is hit with a hard object.

1. Don't allow food or beverage residues or metal cans to remain on the porcelain surface.
2. Clean your enameled sink with hot water and mild dish liquid or baking soda, then rinse well with plain water.
3. If you need to scrub the sink, use a plastic netting scrubber that won't scratch it.
4. If your sink gets stained, pour a little consumer strength (3 percent) hydrogen peroxide on a clean, wet cloth, rub it on the stain, and rinse it off immediately. Don't allow it to sit on the surface for more than a couple of seconds.

Artificial Stone, Corian, or Acrylic Sinks

These man-made materials are easily damaged by strong chemicals such as oven cleaners, drain cleaners, and paint removers that shouldn't be poured down the drain anyway.

1. Do not allow food or beverage residues or metal cans to sit on the man-made surface.
2. Do not cut on the man-made surface.

3. Do not set hot pans in the sink; you will melt the surface. Run cold water while pouring boiling water into the sink.
4. Clean the sink with hot water and mild dish liquid or baking soda, then rinse well with plain water.

Faucets

Clean faucets by wiping them with a vinegar-soaked rag, then wiping them dry.

Dissolve mineral deposits by wrapping a vinegar-soaked rag around the faucet and letting it sit for a couple of hours. If the rag won't stay put, hold it in place with a rubber band. Rub the deposits off with a clean wet cloth, then dry with a clean cloth.

If you wipe your faucets with a cloth dipped in water and a wee bit of Murphy's Oil Soap, they stay shiny longer.

Wipe faucets and other shiny metal fixtures clean with 100-proof vodka. (100-proof vodka has a 50 percent alcohol content, and is a safe alternative to rubbing alcohol or denatured alcohol.)

Down the Drain

Researchers have investigated kitchen drains and found live bacteria (no surprise).

Water usually runs down my drain, not up, so bacteria living in the drain don't tend to contaminate my sink. Here is how to keep the bacteria down where they belong:

1. Grease build-up is the biggest cause of sewer overflows. Hardened fats can also clog pipes, so refrain from pouring grease down the drain. Scrape meat drippings and used cooking oil into a can. If you store your drippings can and meat scraps in the

freezer until garbage day, animals will not be attracted to your garbage.

2. Unless you have a garbage disposal, do not put food down your drain.

Garbage disposals are of dubious value. Though disposals are convenient for householders, the excess organic material they wash down the drain can strain the capacity of sewage treatment systems, deplete the oxygen in waterways, prematurely clog septic systems, and last but not least, feed sewer rats that thrive on the prechewed, piped-in diet delivered to them via garbage disposals.

Composting your kitchen waste is a much more environmentally friendly way to deal with food waste. Some progressive metropolitan areas are developing municipal food composting programs because composting food waste is really the most environmentally sound way to process food wastes. Other areas are encouraging residents to compost their own food wastes in vermicomposting (worm composting) bins.

As long as we regard materials as waste rather than as raw materials awaiting future use, we will continue to be wasteful. Please refer to page 358 for more complete information on composting.

If you do use a garbage disposal, you can clean, deodorize, and sharpen its blades at the same time by grinding up ice with lemon or orange peels.

3. Use a drain strainer to prevent bits of food from washing down the drain.

4. Chemical drain cleaners are extremely dangerous. Avoid them. See page 146 for emergency information on spilled drain cleaner.

5. If your kitchen drain begins to stink or slow down, pour a half cup baking soda down the drain and chase it with a cup of white vinegar. An impressive amount of fizzing will ensue as the vinegar and baking soda react. When the fizzing stops, pour a kettleful of boiling water down the drain. Your drain will be left clean, fast, and sweet smelling. If it is not, it is time to warm up the drain snake.

Drain Snake

A drain snake, or auger, is a flexible metal shaft that is attached to a hand crank that makes it spin.

A hand-cranked snake is more than adequate for dislodging minor clogs beyond the J trap under the sink.

Here's how to use a snake:

1. Remove the sink stopper.
2. Push the end of the snake into the drain opening and keep pushing until it meets an obstruction.
3. Turn the crank clockwise, while pushing and pulling the snake until it moves easily in the drainpipe.
4. Run water down the drain. If it runs freely, you have vanquished the clogged. If not, you may need to remove the J trap and run the snake into the drainpipe just past the trap. If you're not comfortable doing this, it's time to call a plumber.

Choosing a Refrigerator

In most homes, the refrigerator is second only to the furnace in energy consumption. Though refrigerators are energy hogs, they were much worse before federal efficiency standards went into effect in 1993; even stricter energy standards were mandated in 2001. A typical refrigerator sold in 1973 used more than three times as much energy per year than the average 2001 model.

Refrigerators that are at least 10 percent more efficient than the federal standard qualify for the Energy Star label. The most energy efficient refrigerators and freezers use 80 percent less electricity than their average competitors.

If your refrigerator is more than ten years old, it's like running a 300-watt lightbulb night and day. A new refrigerator is like running a 75-watt lightbulb. If you want to save money and energy, get a new refrigerator!

🌿 **SELECTION, CARE, AND FEEDING OF LARGE KITCHEN APPLIANCES**

The energy costs of running any appliance tend to dwarf its initial purchase price. Though it may cost more to purchase, using an efficient appliance is an ongoing bargain.

The American Council for an Energy Efficient Economy has a website that contains energy efficiency ratings for appliances: www.aceee.org. They also sell a booklet called *The Most Energy-Efficient Appliances*.

The Consumers Union, which produces the magazine *Consumer Reports*, has a free website called "Consumer Reports Greener Choices: Products for a Better Planet," which contains information on choosing environmentally friendly products and appliances: www.eco-labels.org/greenconsumers/home.cfm.

Fridge Maintenance

The working parts of refrigerators should be cleaned every year. *If you need to be reminded that an appliance needs to be unplugged before you attempt to clean it, you should let a technician do the work.*

Refrigerators work by removing heat from inside the refrigerator, then the condenser coils release the heat into the room. The sleepy golden retriever absorbing the heat blowing from under the refrigerator is making the machine work harder and get dirtier faster. Try to discourage your pet from lying there. Pet hair should be vacuumed out from under and behind your refrigerator two or three times a year.

Older refrigerators need to be pulled away from the wall so the condenser coils at the back can be carefully and gently vacuumed. If dust is allowed to build up on the coils the compressor can give out, which is the refrigerator equivalent of blowing the engine. Older refrigerators have been known to catch fire, so it's a good idea to have your aging appliance checked annually by a technician.

The coils of newer refrigerators are usually sealed, but you should pull your newer refrigerator away from the wall and vacuum under it at least once a year anyway. Or, if you can't move the fridge, slide a small washable cotton throw rug under the refrigerator and move it from side to side to capture and remove dust bunnies.

Inside the Fridge

Refrigerators should stay between 35 and 40° Fahrenheit. Use a thermometer to check the temperature, then adjust the controls as necessary.

A good refrigerator door seal keeps cold air in and hot air out. If you allow your door seals to get sticky, they will eventually rip and need to be replaced, so wipe smears and spills off the seals immediately. Harsh chemicals can cause refrigerator seals to dry out and crack. Use water and a little dish liquid on a toothbrush to gently clean between the folds, then wipe off the residue with a clean, damp cloth. If mildew tends to grow on your refrigerator seals, wipe them down with a cloth dampened with vinegar and water. A quick spray from a steam cleaner is another good way to clean refrigerator seals without damaging them.

Clean as You Go

Emptying and cleaning the refrigerator is not my idea of fun. Here are some very effective ways to make this chore easier:

- Put raw meats on plates before you put them in the refrigerator. Meat should be stored on the bottom shelf of the refrigerator where its juices can't drip down on other foods.

  If your refrigerator has wire shelves, you might also want to consider putting your milk cartons on small plates or coasters to prevent drips from running all the way to the bottom of the refrigerator.
- Wipe up spills, crumbs, and smears immediately with a clean damp cloth, then dry the area with a clean cloth. A puddle of milk can be wiped up in a few seconds, but a dry crust of milk must be scrubbed off.
- Clean off bottles and jars before you put them back in the refrigerator. It is much quicker to rinse off a ketchup bottle than to wipe ketchup out of a narrow door shelf.
- A semiempty refrigerator presents a wonderful opportunity to wipe down the shelves with a wet soapy dishrag or water and vinegar.

- If a piece of fruit melts down in your produce drawer, pull the whole drawer out and empty it. Wash the drawer in the sink, dry it, then slide it back into place.
- Wipe spills and crumbs out of the freezer immediately. If you are lucky, you will catch the spills before they freeze.

Refrigerator Wash Day

If your refrigerator gets past the point of no return, you will need to remove the food, pull out the shelves and drawers, and unplug the refrigerator. If its freezer section needs to be cleaned, take out all the frozen food and put it in an insulated cooler. To speed up the defrosting, put a pot of hot water in the freezer and close the door. As always, when in doubt, read the instruction manual.

1. Wash the shelves and drawers in the sink with warm water and dish liquid. Rinse and dry them.
2. The interior surfaces of refrigerators are easily damaged. Do not use cleaning products that contain abrasives, harsh or concentrated detergents, bleach, or petroleum products. Do not scrub the surfaces with paper towels or metal or plastic scouring pads; they are also abrasive. Do not scrape the surface with metal tools.

     Here are some recipes for refrigerator cleaning solutions. Apply one of them with a clean rag:
     a. A dash of dish liquid in 1 quart warm water.
     b. 2 tablespoons baking soda in 1 quart warm water.
     c. 1 tablespoon borax in 1 quart warm water.
     d. 1 tablespoon salt and 1 tablespoon baking soda in 1 quart warm water.
3. Really hardened food deposits can be softened up with warm water, then gently scrubbed off with a plastic-mesh onion bag folded to scrubber size. The plastic mesh is quite gentle and will not mar the refrigerator's surfaces.
4. After it is washed, wipe the interior clean with a damp cloth, then dry it with a clean cloth before plugging the refrigerator back in

and repatriating the washed and dried shelves and drawers. Now you can move on to the job of cleaning the freezer.

5. Cleaning the freezer section of a modern self-defrosting refrigerator is a fairly straightforward operation:

    a. If the freezer shelf is removable, take it out and wash it in the sink.

    b. Wash out the inside of the freezer with warm water and a tiny bit of mild dish liquid on a clean rag.

    c. Wipe the interior down with a clean wet cloth, then dry it with a clean cloth before reinstalling the shelves and the food.

6. Freezers that are not self-defrosting will eventually build up enough frost to prevent them from functioning properly. When this happens, even the most reluctant householder will be forced to tackle the job. If you live in a cold climate, winter may be a good time to defrost the freezer: You can store your frozen venison in a box outside or on an unheated porch.

    1. Transfer the food to another freezer or to a well-insulated cooler.

    2. Disconnect the power to the freezer.

    3. Gently remove the drain plugs at the bottom of the freezer. Put a pan under the drain(s).

    4. Put some pans of hot water in the freezer to speed up the melting.

    5. Once the freezer is defrosted, clean it as described in point number five, above.

    6. Replace the drain plugs.

    7. Reconnect the power and put your food back in the freezer.

Clean, Clean the Range

Cleaning the oven is not one of life's supreme joys. Neither is cleaning the stovetop. Many people avoid these jobs until food residues have heat-cured into durable, varnish-like substances that can be difficult to remove. Overzealous cleaning can also cause trouble by ruining smooth enamel, porcelain, and shiny metal surfaces, leaving them rough and even more difficult to clean.

There are a couple of exceptionally good reasons to avoid using commercial oven cleaners. Most of these cleaners contain sodium hydroxide, which is extremely corrosive and can react violently if mixed with other chemicals. Oven cleaners can dissolve almost any organic material they contact, including your skin and eyes. The mist from aerosol oven cleaners can cause lung damage. (See page 148 for emergency information on spilled oven cleaner.)

You can make your life much easier by doing frequent preventive cleaning.

Oven Grime Prevention

- Put a baking pan underneath pies, sweet potatoes, casseroles, and other foods that might spill or bubble over.
- Put a sheet of aluminum foil on your oven floor. Do not let it touch heating elements or cover the vents. When the foil gets dirty, take it out and replace it. (This foil will probably be too irremediably greasy to be recycled.)
- If something bubbles over in the oven, sprinkle salt on the spill to make it easier to clean up. As soon as the oven is cool enough, wipe up the spills and spatters. Don't leave them there to bake on the next time you use the oven.
- Wipe grease off the oven interior with a cloth dampened in vinegar and water. If you wipe the grease off before you use the oven again, it won't have a chance to bake onto the oven surfaces.

Safer Oven Cleaning

If you have a self-cleaning oven, count your blessings and use the cleaning cycle whenever the oven starts looking dirty. Don't wait until the grease bakes on and becomes a hard, black, carbonized coating.

Many people are afraid of the high heat of the self-cleaning cycle and are hesitant to use it. If the intervals between cleanings are too long, large amounts of grease and food residue can build up, which will produce a lot of smoke and may even catch fire during the cleaning cycle. This can be alarming (in more than one sense of the word) and thus the cycle of "avoiding-the-self-cleaning-cycle" is perpetuated.

Here is how to take full advantage of the self-cleaning cycle:

1. Minimize smoke production by wiping up new spills, splatters, and crumbs as soon as the oven cools.
2. It is time to use the cleaning cycle when the oven interior acquires a thin film of grime.
3. The self-cleaning cycle will not clean outside the oven door. Use a clean rag dipped in hot water and a dash of dish liquid to clean the frame around the oven door and the edge of the door outside the gasket.
4. Remove the oven racks. If you don't, the high heat of the cleaning cycle will ruin their finish, leaving them rough and dull. Use a gentle dish liquid to wash the racks in the sink.
5. Remove the broiler pan and wash it in the sink. A grease-laden broiler pan may catch fire during the cleaning cycle.
6. Remove built-up food residues from the oven surfaces to prevent them from baking on during the cleaning cycle. Dip a folded plastic-netting produce bag into a solution of warm water and dish liquid, and use it to scrub off spots of built-up food residues. The plastic netting will not scratch the enameled finish.
7. Read your oven's instruction manual and follow the instructions exactly.
8. When the oven has cooled off after the cleaning cycle, wipe down the oven interior with a damp cloth to remove the fine ash left behind by the incinerated food residues.
9. Never use commercial oven cleaners, abrasive cleaners, or scrubbers in a self-cleaning oven. They will ruin the enameled finish and make the oven impossible to keep clean.

Cleaning the Oven by Hand

Cleaning the oven by hand is a filthy job. Put on your lowliest work clothes and wear rubber gloves. If you have inherited an oven with a large build-up of baked-on grime, you may need to accept the fact that you can remove the new layers of grease, but the old ones have become part of the oven's structure.

1. Remove the oven racks. Take them outside and put them in a garbage bag with a cup or two of cleaning ammonia. Close the bag tightly and let the racks sit overnight. The ammonia fumes inside the tightly closed bag will loosen the grease. Open the bag, remove the racks, then hose them off and scrub them. This technique also works for pots and pans with really tough baked-on grease.
2. Use one of the following recipes:
   a. Mix 2 tablespoons dish liquid, 2 teaspoons borax, and 1 quart warm water. Sponge the mixture on the inside of the oven. Let it sit for 20 minutes, then scrub with a plastic scrubbing pad and Bon Ami cleanser.
   b. Pour 2 tablespoons liquid castile Dr. Bronner's Soap or Murphy's Oil Soap and 2 tablespoons borax into a pint spray bottle. Fill the bottle with hot water and shake it well. Spray the mixture on the oven surfaces and let it sit for 20 minutes before scrubbing it with a plastic scrubbing pad.
3. A metal spatula can be used to scrape off hardened deposits. Old rags or newspaper are perfect for removing loosened grime from the oven. Rinse the surfaces with a wet soapy rag, then finish the job by wiping with a wet rag dipped in vinegar. The vinegar helps slow the build-up of grease.
4. If the weather is warm and your oven is impossibly filthy, open all your windows, fill a small glass bowl with half a cup of full strength sudsing ammonia, and put the cup in the oven.

   Close the oven door and let the ammonia work overnight. In

the morning, put on your rubber gloves and wipe out the loosened grime with newspapers or old rags. Rub the tough stains with a plastic scrubbing pad, then wash the oven with warm soapy water and rinse.

Steam Cleaning the Oven

This is the quickest, easiest way to clean an oven I have ever seen. If you steam clean your oven often enough to prevent grease build-up, you will never have to scrub it at all.

1. Follow your steam cleaner's operating instructions.
2. Remove the racks and the broiler pan. You can steam them clean in the sink.
3. Use the spray nozzle of a portable steam cleaner to spray down the oven's interior. Start at the top and work down.
4. Spray a small area at a time, then wipe it with a cloth before moving to the next area.
5. After you've cleaned the oven, check the broiler and steam clean it as necessary.
6. After you steam clean the oven, you may need to relight the pilot light.

The Stovetop

Frying and sautéing can scatter grease far and wide; your kitchen will stay a lot cleaner if you cover that skillet of hot oil with a mesh splatter guard. If you don't already have one, you can make a simple homemade version by punching holes in a pie tin with a small nail or skewer.

Running the over-the-range exhaust fan while you cook helps remove smoke, grease particles, and moisture and keeps your kitchen cleaner. Exhausting cooking fumes may also improve your health: Lance A. Wallace of the Environmental Protection Agency in Gaithersburg, Maryland, measured pollution levels and particle sizes in his own kitchen when he cooked without running the exhaust fan. He found that cooking produces ultrafine particles which remain airborne for between two and four hours. Inhaling these particles has been associated with breathing and heart problems. (See chapter eight, "Indoor Air Pollutants," page 280, for more information on ultrafine particles.)

Cleaning the Stovetop

Read the appliance manual and follow the cleaning instructions.

Smooth Glass Electric Stovetop

This is very easy to keep clean, but it must be wiped after each use. If food residue builds up, it can ruin the surface. Sugary foods must be wiped off the stovetop immediately because they can stain and pit the glass. Wait until the stovetop cools, then wipe it clean with a warm sudsy rag. Vanquish tough deposits by smothering them under a wet rag for fifteen minutes. Rinse the stovetop with a clean wet rag and wipe it dry.

If you have a choice, choose a gas or electric stovetop with sealed burners—that way you will have only one level of the stove to clean. Bits of food fall through the openings of unsealed burners; an unsealed stovetop must be lifted up periodically so the greasy, crumby goo can be cleaned off the stove floor underneath the burners. (A metal spatula is a handy tool for scraping out crumbs and goop in the stove's "basement.")

Sealed Stovetop

Never clean the stove while the burners are on. Wipe it down after you are finished cooking. Wait until the stove cools, then take out the grates and wipe the top and the drip pans with a clean rag dipped in sudsy water. Rinse with a clean wet rag, then wipe it dry. Put the grates back in place. If you never allow food or grease to build up, the daily wiping is all you'll ever need to do to keep your stovetop clean.

Unsealed Electric Stovetop

Unplug the stove, pull it away from the wall, and read the instruction manual. Follow the instructions for removing the electric elements and tilting or removing the top. Do not immerse the electric elements in water.

Unsealed Gas Stovetop

Take out the grates, then read the instruction manual and follow the instructions for removing and cleaning the burners, tilting or removing the top, and moving the stove away from the wall without damaging or disconnecting the gas line.

Always check to make sure that all the pilot lights are still lit after you have washed the stove or oven.

Clean greasy stove rings and drip pans by putting them in a large stock pot and submerging them in a solution of half a cup baking soda per gallon of water. Put the lid on the pot, bring the water to a rolling boil, then turn off the heat. Let the rings and drip pans soak until the water cools, then wash them in hot soapy water. Whatever deposits haven't already floated off can be easily detached with a slight bit of persuasion from a plastic scrubber. Rinse and dry the rings and drip pans before putting them back in place.

Soften the goop on a stovetop by covering it with a hot soapy dishrag. Wait for five or ten minutes before you begin to scrub with a plastic mesh scrubber.

Molded Gas Cooktops

This type of cooktop lacks removable drip pans and can be especially difficult to clean. If left long enough, built-up cooking oil and fat in the built-in drip bowls can form a durable varnishlike coating that is nearly impossible to scrub off. To remove this hardened grease, cover the area with baking soda, then fill the drip bowls with boiling water, pouring very slowly and carefully so the bowls don't overflow and extinguish the pilot lights. Let the water sit for a few hours, then sop up the water with an old sponge or rag before carefully and gently pushing the loosened goop off with a metal spatula.

The Range Hood

You need to clean the range hood regularly to prevent grease build-up, which can pose a fire hazard. Turn off the fan and the light before washing the hood inside and out with a rag dipped in warm, soapy water. Rinse it with clean water, then wipe it dry.

Exhaust fan filters need regular cleaning to remove grease and grime. Read the instruction booklet and follow the directions for cleaning the exhaust hood, filters, and fan. Here are some general instructions on how to clean metal filters.

1. Remove metal exhaust filters.
2. Let them soak in hot sudsy water. Scrub them with a nylon dish brush and swish them through the water to remove dirt and grease. Never use scouring powders or abrasive pads on a metal filter.
3. Rinse well and shake dry.
4. Put the filters back in place.
5. If you have a steam cleaner heated up anyway, you can steam clean your filters in the kitchen sink.

Charcoal fan filters must be replaced about once a year. They cannot be cleaned.

The Microwave

Minimize your cleaning liability by following cooking instructions and keeping food covered while it is in the microwave. Consult the instruction manual for cleaning directions.

General Cleaning

Wipe up spills and spatters with a wet sudsy rag each time you remove food from the microwave. Rinse with a clean, damp rag, then dry the interior of the microwave before closing the door. Do not allow food and grease to build up where it can prevent the door from closing properly.

Steam will soften hardened food spills or splatters. Put some lemon juice or vinegar in a cup of water and boil it in the microwave. Let the boiling water sit for a few minutes before you take it out of the oven. Wipe the interior of the microwave with a sudsy rag, rinse with a clean wet rag, then wipe dry.

Toaster

Shock Prevention

Unplug the toaster before attempting to extract wedged pieces of toast.

Fire Prevention

Don't allow crumbs to build up in the toaster. Unplug it and turn it upside down over the sink to pour the crumbs out. (More complete information on kitchen fire safety can be found in chapter eight, beginning on page 311.)

Polishing

Unplug the toaster and wipe it down with a clean sudsy dishrag. Rinse with a wet cloth, then wipe it dry. Polish with a vinegary cloth.

Coffee Makers, Teapots, and Kettles

Clean coffee pots and percolators by filling them with water, adding 4 tablespoons salt, then bringing the salt water to a boil. Let the hot water sit and cool, then pour it out and rinse well.

Clean a coffee maker by pouring 1 pint white vinegar in the reservoir and topping it off with water. Turn on the coffee maker and let it brew a cup of the vinegar and water. Turn it off and let it stand for half an hour, then turn it back on. Let it finish brewing the pot of vinegar and water, then empty the pot, rinse it out, and fill the reservoir with water. Brew the pot of water. Empty, rinse, then brew another pot of water.

Boil white vinegar in tea kettles and coffee pots to clean out the mineral deposits. Let the vinegar cool before pouring it down the drain. Rinse with clean water.

You can kill two birds with one stone by pouring baking soda down the drain before pouring out the vinegar.

Remove coffee stains from cups or counters by scrubbing with a paste made of baking soda and water.

Now that the kitchen is clean and free of chemical contamination, we can go out and buy some nice healthy food . . .

Why Buy Organic Food?

Cynthia Curl and her colleagues at the University of Washington tested the levels of organophosphate pesticide contamination in preschool children in Seattle. The study showed that children who ate conventionally grown food had pesticide concentrations that were six times higher than those found in the children who ate organic food. The researchers concluded, "Consumption of organic produce appears to provide a relatively simple way for parents to reduce their children's exposure to OP pesticides."

Organic food can be relatively expensive. (Though as my friend Jean points out, it is only more expensive if you don't factor in the health and environmental damage done by chemicals.) Very few of the families studied ate organic food exclusively, so the researchers defined an organic diet as one that consisted of 75 percent organic foods. It is not necessary to attain organic perfection in order to improve your family's health!

Save Your Health and Your Money

These recommendations are based on more than one hundred thousand tests conducted by the U.S. Department of Agriculture and The Food and Drug Administration. The tests measured the pesticide levels on washed and peeled nonorganic fruits and vegetables.

High Level Contamination

You can significantly reduce the amount of pesticides your family ingests by buying the organic versions of these heavily contaminated fruits and vegetables:

Contaminated fruits: Peaches, strawberries, apples, nectarines, pears, cherries, red raspberries, and grapes.

Contaminated vegetables: Spinach, celery, potatoes, green beans, winter squash, and sweet bell peppers.

For more detailed information, read *Diet for a Poisoned Planet,* by David Steinman, which lists pesticide residues by food category.

Clean and Healthy

These fruits and vegetables are relatively free of pesticide residues. You can stretch your organic food budget further by buying the following produce at the conventional food market.

Clean fruits: Pineapples, mangos, bananas, kiwis, and papayas. (Pineapples, mangos, kiwis, and papayas are well equipped to fend for themselves: They all contain protein-dissolving enzymes that digest hapless pests.)

Clean vegetables: Sweet corn, avocado, cauliflower, asparagus, onions, peas, and broccoli.

❧ CORN AND BEANS

Tortilla chips and soybean protein made from Monsanto's genetically modified (GMO) Roundup Ready corn and soybeans have been on the market for quite a few years now. The jury is still out on whether these products cause allergic reactions in sensitive people. The only way to be sure that one is not eating genetically engineered foods is to buy products that are labeled as such: "Made with NO Genetically Engineered Ingredients."

These genetically modified organisms were not invented for the consumer's benefit. The Roundup Ready plants were designed to be resistant to the effects of Monsanto's herbicide, Roundup. This means that the chemical giant can sell seeds and herbicide to the farmers, and the farmers can spray larger amounts of herbicide directly on their fields without killing the growing crops.

If you want to decrease your exposure to toxins, buy organic corn and soybean products.

Preventing Food Poisoning

"If you haven't got your health, you haven't got anything." The kitchen is where health and happiness are born, and often where they perish. There's nothing quite like a juicy case of food poisoning to make you wish you'd never been born.

And many Americans are stricken: The Centers for Disease Control (CDC) estimates that each year approximately 76 million Americans are sickened by food poisoning; of these, 325,000 require hospitalization and 5,000 die. Most food poisoning originates in home kitchens and is easily preventable.

The only weapons that are effective against food poisoning microbes are proper food handling, cooking, and storage techniques, and careful, thoughtfully executed kitchen sanitation.

Real Cleaning for Real Kitchens

Many of the bacteria, viruses, and parasites that cause food poisoning are already on raw food before it enters the kitchen. Other bacteria grow in cooked food. In many cases, it takes large numbers of bacteria to cause illness. If the bacteria can be prevented from multiplying, the disease can be prevented.

Bacteria propagate very rapidly. For example, *Staphylococcus aureus* bacteria split in half every thirty minutes, forming two daughter cells. Given comfortably warm, moist conditions and a food source, a lone staphylococcus bacterium becomes a clan of more than 8 million in just twelve hours. *E. coli* bacteria are even more prolific: One can produce more than 68 billion daughters in twelve hours. Only intelligent and conscientious food storage, handling, cooking, and clean up can protect us from the gut wrenching-and-emptying effects of food poisoning. Food preservatives were invented to stop or slow bacterial growth in food. This means that fresh organic food is more likely to support bacterial growth than is food that contains preservatives. Proper food handling is essential in the natural foods kitchen.

Wash These Germs Right Off Your Hands

Shigella bacteria are found only in the human gastrointestinal tract. Prevention involves washing hands after using the bathroom or changing babies' diapers. If you pass this infection along, shame on you!

Norwalk virus and *hepatitis* A virus can contaminate food when infected food handlers do not wash their hands after using the bathroom.

Blinded By the Refrigerator Light

Staphylococcus aureus is a very common bacteria that is found on humans, animals, and food and in sewage, air, water, dust, and milk. In other words, it is everywhere. Staphylococci produce endotoxins that can cause food poisoning, which usually is not fatal to healthy adults, but can kill infants and elderly people.

Staphylococcus thrives at room temperature; cooking kills the bacteria but doesn't destroy the toxins it has already produced. Temperatures below 40° Fahrenheit stop its growth.

Prevention: Staphylococcus is a microbe that really loves picnics! Its favorite foods are meat, poultry, milk, dairy, and egg products, cream-filled pastries and pies, potato salad, tuna salad, and sandwich fillings. Avoid postpicnic suffering by cooling these creamy foods quickly and keeping them cold.

Bacillus cereus is a bacteria whose spores are common in soil, dust, and spices. Its spores are heat-resistant and survive cooking temperatures; they begin to grow as soon as a suitable food source reaches room temperature. Cooked foods such as rice, macaroni, and potatoes are this microbe's favorite host foods.

Prevention: The best way to prevent this type of food poisoning is to serve starchy cooked foods hot, or cool them quickly and keep them cold. Starchy food that has been allowed to sit at room temperature should be discarded.

Clostridium perfringens is a bacteria commonly found in dust, soil, and inside the intestinal tracts of humans and animals. Its favorite foods are meat, poultry, sauces, and gravies. Though the bacteria is killed by cooking temperatures, its spores are not. It cannot grow at temperatures below 40° Fahrenheit.

Prevention: Halt the growth of *Clostridium perfringens* by keeping hot foods hot until they are served, dividing leftovers into small portions before refrigerating them, and reheating leftovers to at least 165° Fahrenheit before serving.

The Really Scary Bacteria

Clostridium botulinum is a common bacteria found in soils all over the world. It produces botulism toxin, the most poisonous natural substance known to man.

Clostridium botulinum is an organism with very simple needs: Give it an airless environment, moderate temperatures, and voilà! The live bacteria and the toxin it produces are destroyed by heat, but botulism spores are very tough and heat-resistant and can survive temperatures up to 240° Fahrenheit. To top it off, the spores can live for up to one hundred years.

Botulism spores are ubiquitous on most root vegetables and are also found on other produce. The spores remain dormant in the presence of oxygen, but when canning temperatures are not high enough, the spores awaken inside comfortably airless canning jars. They then colonize the canned food and transform it into deadly poison.

Canned botulism is most commonly found in home-canned meats, fish, and poultry, as well as in low-acid vegetables such as corn, green beans, lima beans, mushrooms, sauces, and soups.

Here are the steps you can take to preserve yourself from toxic canned goods:

1. Commercial canned goods are generally just fine unless the can is damaged or the jar's seal has failed. Canned goods should suck air when they are first opened; if they do not, their vacuum seal has failed and the contents are not safe to eat. Never eat out of cans that are bulging, dented, rusty, or otherwise damaged. Any foods that are bubbling or smell bad should be discarded.

2. Unfortunately, food that is contaminated with botulism does not always stink, spew, bubble, or bulge. This is why food safety experts recommend boiling all home-canned corn, spinach, and meats for twenty minutes, and all other home-canned foods for ten minutes before eating it. Never taste canned food before it has been boiled; do not even lick the spoon!

3. Low-acid foods such as corn, beans, carrots, and meat must be processed in a pressure canner that can be heated to 250° Fahrenheit. No other canning method is safe enough. Follow your canning recipes religiously. If you have doubts about any canned food, throw it out. Don't rely on an old hand-me-down pressure cooker or canner. Older models can be quite dangerous. See page 315 in the fire safety section for further details.

4. High levels of sugar, salt, and acidity all prevent or slow bacterial growth. This is why pickles, jams, and jellies can be safely processed in a water bath canner, though the recipes and directions must be followed exactly to ensure a safe product. Contact your County Extension Office or Community Garden Program for detailed information on canning.

Other Botulism Sources

Though many of us never preserve any food at all, we are still more than capable of producing a crop of homegrown botulism.

In April 1994, thirty diners in El Paso, Texas, who had had a nice Greek dinner landed in the hospital suffering from botulism poisoning. Four of the victims had to be put on ventilators. Sleuths from the Centers for Disease Control determined that the offending food was *skordalia*, a mashed potato and garlic dip.

The potatoes used in the dip had been wrapped in foil and baked. These foil-wrapped potatoes were then left at room temperature for several days before their innards were scooped out to make the dip.

Aluminum foil reflects heat very nicely; a foil-wrapped potato never gets hot enough to kill botulism spores on the skin. From a botulism bacteria's point of view, a room temperature, airtight, foil-wrapped baked potato is an ideal stomping ground.

🌾 THE DANGEROUS GREEN POTATO

Potatoes are in the Deadly Nightshade family, the Solanaceae. When potatoes are exposed to light, they turn green and produce an alkaloid poison called solanine. Potato eyes and shoots also contain solanine.

Always peel the green skin off your potatoes before cooking them.

If the greening is shallow enough, it can be peeled off along with the skin, but if the flesh has begun to turn green, the whole potato should be discarded.

While eating small amounts of green-fleshed potatoes *may* not harm you, green flesh can be very dangerous or even fatal to people with sensitivities to solanine. It can also be dangerous to pregnant women and children, and to virtually anyone if consumed in large amounts. For that reason, I never eat potatoes that have turned green.

Preventing Potato Botulism

1. Scrub raw potatoes thoroughly under running water before cooking. Don't use soap.
2. Bake your potatoes in their own skins, not wrapped in foil. Eat them before they have a chance to cool. Refrigerate the leftover potatoes.
3. Don't let cooked potatoes sit at room temperature for more than an hour; either refrigerate them or discard them.
4. If you are camping and want to roast foil-wrapped potatoes in the fire, unwrap them and eat them while they are still hot. Any potatoes that are not eaten right away should be discarded.

Oily Poison

Oil makes a very efficient oxygen barrier. Any food that is covered with oil and left at room temperature can incubate botulism. Steeping herbs, tomatoes, or garlic in olive oil can be a recipe for disaster. Fried onions soaked in oil, butter, or margarine have also been implicated in botulism poisoning.

Homemade flavored oils should be thrown out even if they were given to you by your best friend. Commercially prepared oil-immersed foods can be kept as long as they are stored in the refrigerator at all times, and the oil level is kept high enough to completely cover the food.

Remember to refrigerate all cooked foods promptly and throw out all leftovers that have been in the refrigerator for more than a week.

Sweet Baby Poison

Infant botulism can strike babies younger than a year if they ingest honey that is contaminated with botulism spores. It is the most common type of botulism poisoning.

Though honey is a perfectly safe and wholesome food for adults and older children, whose more mature intestinal tracts contain enzymes that destroy the bacteria, botulism thrives in infants' immature intestinal tracts. The botulism toxin is produced in the baby's intestine, then is absorbed into the bloodstream. A very tiny amount of honey can endanger an infant's life in just a few hours by paralyzing him and preventing him from breathing. European infants have been poisoned by sucking on honey-sweetened pacifiers.

Though infant botulism is most likely to occur in children less than six months of age, no child under the age of twelve months should be given even the tiniest amount of honey under any circumstances.

Note: Hummingbirds are also susceptible to honey-induced botulism poisoning. Never put honeyed water into a hummingbird feeder. The recipe for hummingbird nectar is the following: ¼ cup white sugar per 1 cup water. Replace the nectar every three days to avert hummingbird poisoning. Don't add food coloring! Synthetic colorants are not healthy for hummingbirds.

Carnivore's Food Safety

Safe Meat Handling

Bacteria grows rapidly at room temperature. All meats—whether beef, lamb, pork, poultry or fish—must be stored in the refrigerator or freezer. Refrigerator temperatures should be kept between 35 and 40° Fahrenheit. The freezer should be kept at 0° Fahrenheit.

Frozen meats should either be thawed in the refrigerator or cooked immediately after being thawed in the microwave.

Meat should be refrigerated while it is marinating. Don't save used marinade; it contains raw meat juice and may harbor dangerous bacteria. Never put cooked meat on the plate it sat on while raw.

Keep cooked or ready-to-eat foods separated from raw meat, poultry, and fish. When you buy fresh meats, bag them separately from all other foods, and pack them in the car where they can't drip or leak on the other groceries. Don't buy precooked lunch meats, cooked shellfish, or smoked fish that are displayed in the same case as raw fish or meat. The cooked food may have become contaminated by the raw meat.

Understanding the Enemy

Disable these bacteria by cooking all meat until well done. Consult your cookbook for appropriate cooking times and temperatures, and use a meat thermometer to determine the internal temperature of the meat.

Campylobacter jejuni bacteria is frequently found in birds' intestines, and it can contaminate their meat. Campylobacter infection sometimes leads to meningitis, arthritis, or Guillain-Barré syndrome, an autoimmune disease that causes temporary paralysis.

Escherichia coli bacteria (*E. coli* for short) is an essential component of the normal intestinal tract and is not usually a health hazard. Unfortunately, it has evil siblings, among them *E. coli* 0157:H7, which can cause dangerous, and sometimes fatal, food poisoning. The evil siblings are also found in the intestinal tracts of animals and can contaminate the meat when animals are slaughtered.

Salmonella bacteria is commonly found in the intestinal tracts of mammals, birds, and fish. Salmonella usually causes classically unpleasant food poisoning symptoms. Meat and eggs can be contaminated by salmonella.

Fashionable Diseases

Vibrio parahaemolyticus bacteria is found on raw seafood. People who eat sushi and sashimi are often exposed to the gastrointestinal turbulence caused by these seafaring microbes. If you want to avoid being sickened by this bacteria, you will have to forgo the sushi.

Listeria bacteria have been found in raw milk, soft cheeses, ice cream, raw vegetables, raw meats, raw poultry, raw and smoked fish, and processed meat. Listeria can cause very severe blood poisoning and brain inflammation, and it is extremely dangerous to pregnant women and very young children. You can prevent listeria poisoning by keeping your kitchen clean, storing food properly, and avoiding raw meat and raw milk products.

Parasites

Diners who eat raw or undercooked meat, fish, shellfish, or poultry can end up with tapeworms, toxoplasmosis, or trichinosis.

- Tapeworms, though disgusting, are the only members of this group that cannot cause permanent disability.

✺ WHERE'S THE CHICKEN JUICE?

Janet Anderson, a professor of nutrition and food sciences at Utah State University, filmed more than one hundred people preparing dinner. Only two of the subjects didn't cross-contaminate their fresh vegetables with juice from raw meat.

It doesn't take many bacteria to cause illness: Swallowing fifteen to twenty salmonella bacteria or about five hundred campylobacter bacteria will do it.

In another experiment, Professor Anderson covered a chicken with a dye called Glo Germ, which is only visible under ultraviolet light. She asked an unsuspecting home cook to prepare the chicken. After the fowl was done, an ultraviolet light was turned on and the cook's sink, counter, and cabinet handles all lit up with a chicken-juicy glow; as did the resident toddler's sippy cup.

- Toxoplasmosis is caused by a protozoa that infests the brain and muscle tissue of infected animals. It can cause neurological damage, vision loss, and birth defects.
- Trichinosis is caused by ingesting raw or undercooked meat that is infested with the larvae of the trichinella worm. Trichinosis causes symptoms ranging in severity from nausea and abdominal discomfort to breathing difficulty, heart trouble, and death.

Parasite Prevention

- Cook red meat, pork, poultry, fish, and shellfish until it is well done. Wash utensils thoroughly after cooking meat. Never taste raw meat or lick raw meat juices.
- Cook wild meat such as deer, bear, elk, possum, squirrel, boar, porcupine, moose, or whatever else you may have killed in the great outdoors until it is well done. Freezing wild game does not kill all parasites.
- Raw pork or bear meat can carry the worms that cause trichinosis. Cook all pork products until they are well done, and buy pork from small producers of grass-fed pigs, preferably those that are certified organic. (Organic growers do not feed meat to their animals. Many nasty diseases can be avoided if you do not eat animals that have eaten other animals.)

Choosing Fish

Fish and shellfish are excellent sources of low-fat, high-quality protein and essential nutrients. However, almost all fish and shellfish contain trace amounts of mercury. These amounts are generally not enough to harm adults who eat fish, but unfortunately even tiny amounts of mercury are enough to damage the developing brains and nervous systems of fetuses, infants, and young children. Eating mercury-contaminated fish is the main source of mercury exposure for humans.

In order to protect our children, scientists have measured the contamination levels of different fish species and have developed fish consumption advisories. These advisories list fish by species, size, and location and include recommendations about how much of each species can be safely eaten, so people can make informed decisions about which fish to eat and which to avoid. The Environmental Protection Agency and the Food and Drug Administration recommend that women of childbearing age, pregnant women, nursing mothers, and young children follow these general recommendations:

- Do not eat shark, swordfish, king mackerel, or tilefish because they contain high levels of mercury.
- Eat up to 12 ounces (two average meals) a week of a variety of fish and shellfish that are lower in mercury, such as shrimp, salmon, pollock, catfish, and canned light tuna. (Albacore, or "white" tuna, has more mercury than canned light tuna.)
- Check local advisories about the safety of fish caught by family and friends in your local lakes, rivers, and coastal areas. If no advice is available, eat up to 6 ounces (one average meal) per week of fish you catch from local waters, but don't consume any other fish during that week.

Most of our mercury pollution comes from the combustion of fossil fuels such as gasoline and coal, and during iron ore processing, concrete manufacture, and chlorine production. The solution is not to quit eating fish, but rather to clean up the environment and conserve energy and resources, thus reducing the amount of mercury that is released into the environment.

Putrescine, Cadaverine, and Histamine— the Rotten Meat Sisters

Animal-based food, such as beef, pork, fish, or cheese, spoils when bacteria breaks the proteins down into toxic amines. The names of these amines — putrescine, cadaverine, and histamine—give some idea of their charm. This trio causes histamine poisoning, which is what your dog gets when it eats a moldy mouse.

Histamine poisoning is violent but mercifully quick; its victims may double over just a few minutes after eating spoiled food, though it may take up to two hours to strike; it is usually over in four to six hours and almost never lasts more than two days.

The symptoms of histamine poisoning include facial flushing and sweating, burning sensations in the mouth and throat, dizziness, nausea, and headache. The reaction can progress to rash, hives, edema, diarrhea and abdominal cramps, blurred vision, swollen tongue, and breathing difficulties.

Once animal products have spoiled, there is no way to make them safe to eat. Cooking does not destroy these toxins, nor does it stop the spoilage process.

Fending Off Spoilage

Aquatic Food

The only defense against these toxins is proper cold storage. Fish and seafood should never be stored at temperatures greater than 40° Fahrenheit for more than four hours.

- Buy only from reputable vendors who keep their products refrigerated or on ice at all times. Never buy fish that feels soft or slimy, smells fishy, or has opaque eyes.
- Fresh fish feels firm and smooth and has clear, bulging eyes, red gills, and very little smell.
- Refrigerate your fish and seafood as soon as possible. If your drive home is long, transporting the fish in a cooler full of ice may be a good idea.
- Those of us who live in the middle of the continent find that frozen saltwater fish and seafood, which is frozen immediately after it is caught, is far fresher than "fresh" seafood. There is no such thing as fresh halibut in Kansas, Minnesota, or Utah.
- If you will be eating your fish within two days, put it in the coldest part of the refrigerator, usually right under the freezer or in the meat keeper. Don't pack it in tightly with other items; leave space for air to circulate around it. Do not store raw fish in the refrigerator for more than two days.

    If you won't be eating the fish within this time frame, remove it from its packaging, wrap it in freezer paper or foil, and put it in the freezer. Frozen fish will keep indefinitely.

Fresh shellfish is extremely perishable and must be cooked alive or it is unsafe to eat. Don't cook shellfish that have cracked or broken shells.

Bivalves such as clams and oysters can be packed on ice and stored in the refrigerator for a couple of days. Live bivalves have tightly closed shells. If you can open the shell with your bare hands, your mollusk has probably bitten the sand and must be discarded.

Crustaceans are extremely perishable and should be cooked the same day they are caught or purchased. Lobsters, crayfish (or crawdads), and crabs must be cooked alive. Keep them in the refrigerator or on ice until you are ready to sacrifice them. Live lobsters, shrimp, and crawdads are greenish in color, as are fresh frozen ones. Crustaceans are much livelier than shellfish, and it should be quite obvious if they are alive before you begin to cook them.

Researchers believe that the most humane way to cook crustaceans is to chill or ice them before dropping them into water that has come to a rolling boil.

Packages of frozen seafood should be intact and free of frost and ice crystals. Ice formation may indicate that the fish has been thawed and refrozen. Refrozen seafood may not be safe to eat.

Warm-Blooded Meat

When selecting fresh meat, look for the following:

- All meat should be firm and springy in texture.
- No raw meat should have a strong smell.
- Fresh beef should be bright cherry red.
- Lamb should be bright brick red.
- Pork should have pink meat and white fat.
- Poultry should be light and even in color.

Store meat in the coldest part of your refrigerator. (This is usually the meat drawer.) If you need to keep meat longer, remove it from its packaging and rewrap it tightly in impermeable freezer wrap, aluminum foil, or freezer paper; or slide the whole retail package into a plastic freezer bag then put it in the freezer.

Depending upon the temperature of the freezer, frozen meat will maintain its quality for up to a year. After a year, the food will still be safe to eat, but its flavor may suffer due to freezer burn. The colder the freezer, the better the meat will keep. Meat will last only a third as long in a freezer that is 10° Fahrenheit (−12° Celsius) as in a freezer that is −22° Fahrenheit (−30° Celsius).

The maximum refrigerator storage time for raw beef is five days; raw ground meat, two days.

Do not store raw poultry in the refrigerator for more than two days.

🐜 CANNIBAL COWS

"Mad cow disease," scientifically known as bovine spongiform encephalopathy or BSE (translation: cows' spongy-brain disease), has infected more than 179,000 cattle in Great Britain since it was first diagnosed in 1986. By January 2004 there were a total of 145 human cases of mad cow disease, and 139 of the victims had already died.

Mad cow disease is particularly frightening because it is believed to be caused by a newly discovered type of infectious agent, a misshapen protein named prion, that misleads other proteins into deforming. Mad cow disease attacks the brain and central nervous system and eventually causes death. Scientists have been unable to discover anything that disables prions.

Cattle become infected with mad cow disease in a spectacularly loathsome manner: These gentle herbivores are infected when they are fed ground-up parts of BSE-infected animals.

To put this into perspective, however, consider the 480 people in England and Wales who died of plain old bacterial, viral, or parasitic food poisoning in the year 2000. Then we can bow our heads and ponder the fate of the 90,000 Americans who died of traditional food poisoning between 1986 and 2004, while mad cow disease raged across Europe, infecting 145 people.

To help protect yourself from mad cow disease, try to buy certified organic or kosher beef (cattle feed that contains meat products is neither kosher nor organic). But remember, you are far more likely to die from a food-borne disease caused by bacteria, viruses, parasites, or fungi than you are to be infected by the prions that cause mad cow disease! The most spectacularly gruesome hazards are pretty unlikely to be the ones that do us in.

Cheese

If you are immuno-compromised or pregnant, buy cheeses made from pasteurized milk, and try to avoid soft cheeses altogether.

Not So Raw, Please

Raw milk poses a significant health hazard. Unpasteurized milk can harbor dangerous bacteria, including listeria, campylobacter, yersinia, salmonella, staphylococcus, *E. coli,* and the tuberculosis bacteria. Do you really know where that dairy cow has been?

Buy certified organic pasteurized milk and milk products, or choose dairy products that are certified free from synthetic bovine growth hormone (rBGH or rBST). Synthetic bovine growth hormone puts a huge stress on cows and makes them more susceptible to infection, so their milk is more likely to contain antibiotics.

Antibiotics, Breakfast of Champions

Since the 1950s, antibiotics have been fed to farm animals in order to fatten them more quickly, reducing the growers' feed costs. Interestingly, this dubious use of antibiotics began a decade after penicillin resistant *E. coli* bacteria was first recognized in 1940.

Some particularly prolific bacteria become grandparents in just a few minutes, while the most sedate bacteria may take a few hours to produce offspring. These accelerated organisms are able to adapt to changing conditions and evolve very rapidly. Bacteria can evolve far more quickly than the drug companies can develop new drugs. Research and development is slow, painstaking, difficult work, while reproduction is, after all, easier than falling off a log.

In spring 2002, *Consumer Reports* conducted tests on 484 fresh, whole broiler chickens bought in stores nationwide. Twenty-nine different brands of chickens were tested. The tests revealed that half the chickens were contaminated with salmonella or campylobacter bacteria, the most common causes of good old American food poisoning. But the news gets worse. To quote from the *Consumer Reports* article: "Ninety percent of the campylobacter bacteria tested from our chicken and 34 percent of the salmonella showed resistance to one or more antibiotics."

Here in the United States we have cheap food, but really expensive health care. Infections caused by antibiotic-resistant bacteria cost an estimated $4 billion per year. Curing these infections is becoming increasingly more difficult and expensive and, in some unfortunate cases, impossible. Prevention is the key.

✎ THESE AREN'T YOUR GRANDMOTHER'S CHICKENS

Once upon a time, when backyard chickens were commonplace, tiny, fuzzy baby chicks wandered around outdoors and acquired normal intestinal bacteria by keeping company with adult chickens. These normal bacteria completely colonized the chicks' intestines, leaving no room for dangerous bacteria.

As time went on, fewer and fewer people raised chickens and the number raised by each grower increased. Eventually, for convenience, most chickens were raised indoors and most chicks never had any contact with adult chickens. These lonely little chicks didn't acquire the friendly bacteria that could protect them from disease-causing bacteria. Many of them grew into plump broilers or roasters that were unwholesome unless they were very thoroughly cooked. So many eggs were contaminated with salmonella that innocent pleasures such as drinking homemade eggnog, eating eggs cooked sunny side up, and licking raw cake batter off a mixing spoon became activities for daredevils.

Finally, in 1998 the USDA announced the release of a new product called "Preempt" that prevented contamination by salmonella, campylobacter, listeria, and the deadly *E. coli* 0157:H7 bacteria in chickens. The product is a blend of twenty-nine different bacteria that normally inhabit the intestines of healthy adult chickens. This chicken yogurt is sprayed over newly hatched chicks, which ingest the bacteria as they preen their fuzz. The good bacteria grow very quickly and out-compete the pathogenic bacteria, greatly improving the health of the chickens, therefore, one assumes, improving the health of the humans that eat poultry products.

Foods that contain beneficial bacteria are called probiotics. Researchers are also working on probiotic treatments for cattle and swine, and are finding that the probiotics that work for cows and pigs are the same as those that work for humans: Lactobacillus and bifidobacteria, which are both yogurt bacteria, are some of the most common. Probiotically treated pigs and cattle are healthier, grow more quickly, and are less likely to need treatment with antibiotics.

Probiotics for People

We are not just part of an ecosystem; each of us is an ecosystem.

A healthy human lives in symbiotic bliss with legions of bacteria. There are at least four hundred friendly species of intestinal bacteria. These beneficial bacteria crowd out and inhibit the growth of dangerous bacteria, prevent food allergies, strengthen the body's defenses against viral diseases, protect against inflammatory bowel disorders, increase the absorption of essential minerals, and improve digestion. Taking antibiotics can decimate beneficial bacteria and leave us vulnerable to colonization by harmful bacteria.

Easily available probiotic foods include yogurt, cheese, buttermilk, kefir, sauerkraut, kim chee, Kosher pickles, and other fermented or cultured foods.

High-fiber foods that help feed beneficial bacteria have been dubbed "prebiotics." These include whole grains, flax, oatmeal, barley, greens, berries and other fruit, dry beans, lentils, and garbanzo beans.

Feed the bacteria and they will feed you.

Food Choices

The type of food we choose to buy has an impact on our own health as well as on the environment. Everybody loves a bargain. Farmers need cheap feed to grow cheap meat. Antibiotics make animals grow faster, and what feed could be cheaper than roadkill and dead dairy cows? So, we chose cheap beef and poultry, and now we have antibiotic-resistant bacteria, and we have created mad cow disease. We like cheap eggs, but they are frequently contaminated with salmonella because factory hens lead such unhealthy lives.

If you want a real bargain, pay a little more for your food and buy organic. Vote with your pocketbook for humane treatment for farm animals, for antibiotics that can still kill dangerous bacteria, and for clean water and healthy soil. If our food costs a little more maybe we'll eat a little less of it, and that wouldn't necessarily be a bad thing.

Clean Cooking

Susan Sumner, a food scientist at Virginia Polytechnic Institute and State University in Blacksburg, developed an environmentally friendly method of decontaminating beef carcasses that turned out to be more effective than the standard method, which utilized chlorine bleach. She then turned her attention to a much more difficult challenge: removing dangerous microbes from fresh produce. Even if raw beef is heavily contaminated with bacteria, careful handling and thorough cooking will make it completely safe to eat. Lettuce, on the other hand, is very delicate and easily damaged, and is usually eaten raw.

The solution to the problem turned out to be the same for meat and vegetables. Sumner contaminated fruits and vegetables with salmonella, shigella, or *E. coli* bacteria, then sprayed the produce with hydrogen peroxide, vinegar, or both. Hydrogen peroxide was one hundred times as effective as vinegar, but vinegar and hydrogen peroxide worked together to kill ten times as many bacteria as were killed by peroxide alone.

This is a very elegant and simple solution to a vexing problem. The bacteria are not just moved around to cause trouble elsewhere; they are—to paraphrase from the movie *The Wizard of Oz*—not just merely dead, they are really, most sincerely, dead.

Implementing a Domestic Spray Program

I have been using this dual spray system for years, and frankly, it couldn't be easier. Vinegar and hydrogen peroxide are natural substances that are produced by living organisms. Our own bodies produce hydrogen peroxide (H_2O_2) as a byproduct of metabolism. Hydrogen peroxide is essentially a water molecule with an extra oxygen atom attached. When hydrogen peroxide is exposed to heat, light, or organic material, it releases its extra oxygen; pure water and oxygen are produced by this reaction. Pure oxygen is extremely toxic to microorganisms, which is why hydrogen peroxide is such an effective antiseptic. It is rather gratifying to watch hydrogen peroxide bubbling and foaming as it kills bacteria; when the bubbling stops and cannot be restarted by the addition of more peroxide, the deed is done.

Vinegar and hydrogen peroxide are utterly harmless to humans, pets, and the environment. The dual sprays don't linger on surfaces, so rinsing is unnecessary, and microbes can't acquire resistance to them.

Setting Up the System

1. Buy two plastic spray bottles in two different colors. One bottle must be completely opaque, and as dark a color as you can find. (My bottle is black.) This dark opaque bottle is for the hydrogen peroxide, which degrades if it is exposed to light or heat.

   Vinegar and hydrogen peroxide cannot be kept in the same bottle because hydrogen peroxide is delicate and readily breaks down into pure water.

2. Buy a big bottle of consumer strength (3 percent) hydrogen peroxide at the drug store or grocery store. Fill your dark spray bottle with hydrogen peroxide and store it in a cool, dark place. (Do not attempt to use laboratory strength—30 percent—hydrogen peroxide. It is a very strong oxidizer that starts fires.)

3. Buy a gallon of distilled white vinegar at the grocery store.

Using the System

1. Disinfecting raw foods:

   PRODUCE

   When you are washing fruits and vegetables, rinse off the dirt and grit, then spray them with vinegar and then with hydrogen peroxide. The peroxide, which has no taste, rinses the vinegar off the produce. No further rinsing is necessary.

   MEAT

   Spray red meat, fish, or poultry with vinegar, then with hydrogen peroxide. No rinsing is necessary.

2. Disinfecting processed foods:

   If you are really worried about germs, you can spray down your food packaging when you bring it home. (Waterproof packaging only, please!) Dry the package with a clean, dry kitchen towel after you spray. This will work for milk cartons and bottles, yogurt containers, cheese, and processed meat packaging. Do not spray any type of cardboard. It is not waterproof and is also very dry, and hence probably sterile.

I do not spray all the food packaging I bring into the house because I believe in giving my immune system a chance to flex its muscles. But if I find that meat juice has leaked onto a yogurt container on the way home, I will certainly wash off the yogurt container and spray it with the dual sprays.

3. After you clean meat, fish, or poultry, wash the sink with a dish cloth and dish liquid, then wring out the cloth before you throw it in the kitchen laundry basket. (I usually hang damp kitchen towels on the side of the kitchen laundry basket to dry.) Next, spray the sink with one bottle, then the other. Use the sprays on any handles and doorknobs you touched while your hands were full of meat juice. If you dislike the lingering smell of vinegar, spray vinegar first, then chase it with hydrogen peroxide.

4. Use the sprays to disinfect the countertops, refrigerator, stovetop, or any other kitchen surface that worries you. There's no need to rinse afterward.

Do not use these sprays on marble countertops. Vinegar dissolves marble, and hydrogen peroxide may damage it. Clean your marble countertops with dish soap and water. (Vinegar dissolves calcium-based stone such as marble, limestone, dolomite, and calcite, and may etch the surface of other natural stone.)

It's Mostly in the Timing

It's easy to avoid contaminating your food if you pay attention to the order in which you do things.

- Use wooden cutting boards. Avoid cross-contamination by using different cutting boards for meat and produce. Wash and prepare fresh produce before you prepare raw meat. Any bacteria on the meat will be killed by the heat of cooking; your mission is to avoid contaminating the produce.

Remember that bacteria need moisture in order to thrive. Use clean, dry wooden cutting boards when you are cutting bread, cheese, or other foods that will not be cooked before they are eaten.

- Before you start preparing meat, set out all the cooking utensils, pots, pans, condiments, and cleaning supplies you will need so you won't have to open the refrigerator, drawers, or cabinets with dirty hands. Clean up immediately after you have prepared the meat so you can remember everything you might have touched while your hands were contaminated with raw meat juice.
- If you've just petted the dog, diapered a baby, changed the cat litter, cleaned a chicken, blown your nose, fixed your hair, answered

---

⚜ IT MAY BE COMMON, BUT IS IT SENSE?

For many years the Food and Drug Administration (FDA) recommended the use of plastic cutting boards, as did the U.S. Department of Agriculture (USDA). Wooden boards were not prohibited, but plastic was obviously more sanitary because germs could be more easily washed off smooth plastic surfaces, while wooden cutting boards, being porous, offered an ideal habitat for bacteria that could cause illness.

In 1992, Philip H. Kass and his colleagues at the University of California, Davis conducted a study which showed that people who used plastic or glass cutting boards were twice as likely to contract salmonella poisoning as were people who used wooden cutting boards.

A year later, at the University of Wisconsin, Madison, food-microbiologists Dean O. Cliver and Nese O. Ak began studying cutting boards in an attempt to develop decontamination techniques that could make wooden cutting boards as safe and sanitary as plastic ones. If they had been aware of Kass's findings, they might not have been so startled by the results of their study.

Cliver and Ak inoculated wooden cutting boards with raw chicken juice fortified with up to 10,000 salmonella, listeria, or *Escherichia coli* (*E. coli*) bacteria. At least 99 percent of the bacteria on the wooden boards were missing and presumed dead within three minutes of inoculation. The bacteria on plastic cutting boards were still hale and hearty. This was a great surprise to Cliver and Ak.

the door, talked on the telephone, potted some daffodils, or used the toilet, you need to wash your hands thoroughly and dry them well on a clean towel before you prepare food. When I cook, I wash my hands every time I touch anything other than the food I'm preparing.

We are all in this together. When you eat at a restaurant, wash your hands before you visit the buffet table!

Clean and Dry

Cleaning is supposed to make you healthier, not sicker. Wet towels are likely to breed molds and bacteria. Don't let your kitchen towels or dish cloths stay wet; hang them up to dry, then throw them in the kitchen laundry basket.

The researchers then left their damp and unwashed experimental subjects overnight at room temperature. The next day, the wooden cutting boards were completely bacteria free, while the plastic ones were hosting a very happy and greatly increased bacterial population.

Cliver and Ak then tested boards made from more than ten species of hardwoods and four different plastics. They found that all the wooden cutting boards killed bacteria, while all the plastic ones encouraged bacterial growth.

Wood fibers absorb and kill bacteria. Plastic behaves differently: "When a knife cuts into the plastic surface, little cracks radiate out from the cut," Professor Cliver said. The bacteria, he said, "seem to get down in those knife cuts and they hang out. They go dormant. Drying will kill, say, 90 percent of them, but the rest could hang around for weeks."

While new, unscarred plastic boards can be successfully cleaned with hot water and detergent, Cliver found that used plastic boards cannot be successfully cleaned. Vigorous scrubbing with hot water and detergent does not remove or kill the bacteria that have lodged in knife scars on plastic boards; running contaminated plastic cutting boards through a dishwasher simply spread bacteria around without harming them; microwaving the plastic boards didn't do anything to the bacteria either, since the boards never got hot no matter how long they were nuked. Even after cleaning, lurking bacteria easily contaminate any food that is prepared on the clean plastic board.

Bacteria on dry cloth are like fish out of water. If you want a clean, sanitary kitchen, throw out your sponges and replace them with a flock of dishcloths. Use a new, clean dishcloth every time you wash a batch of dishes. Wipe, clean, and shine your kitchen counters and sink with a clean dishcloth, then rinse the dishcloth and use it to spot-clean the floor. When you're done, throw the dishcloth in the laundry.

A few dozen cotton dishcloths will last for years. After my dishcloths attain holeyness, I give them a decent burial in my compost pile.

Kitchen Laundry

Kitchen towels and dishcloths tend to be somewhat greasy and should be washed separately from other laundry. When doing the kitchen laundry, turn the water temperature to the hottest setting and choose the longest wash cycle.

I segregate my kitchen laundry from our other laundry by throwing dirty kitchen towels, cloth napkins, dishcloths, placemats, and tablecloths into a small openwork kitchen laundry basket that I keep just outside my kitchen. I wash kitchen laundry about once a week. (Any container that allows air to circulate will work for a kitchen hamper.)

Using cloth towels and napkins rather than their paper counterparts saves money, trees, and landfill space. A single weekly load of kitchen laundry keeps my family happily supplied with all the towels, dishcloths, and napkins we can use. My family uses fancy dishcloths for everyday napkins. They work magnificently, though we must remember not to use them when company comes.

Choosing Cookware

The food containers and cookware we use can have a big effect on the purity of our food.

Pots, pans, bakeware, and storage containers should be strong, sturdy, and react as little as possible with food.

THE CANARY DIED

Fumes from overheated Teflon-coated cookware have been known to kill caged birds. Studies conducted by the Environmental Working Group, a research and advocacy organization, have shown that overheated nonstick pans emit a toxic mixture of chemicals that may cause cancer and birth defects.

Although DuPont, the maker of Teflon, insists that the test conditions were "abusive" and that the product is safe for normal use, it is very hard to predict or control what will happen when synthetic materials are exposed to high heat. In my opinion, items that will be exposed to high temperatures should be made of metal, ceramic, glass, or stone.

In January 2005, the EPA announced that chemicals used to manufacture Teflon pose "a potential risk of developmental and other adverse effects." According to the Environmental Working Group, these "other adverse effects" may include cancer, immune system suppression, and increased risk of heart attack and stroke.

The chemical culprits are fluorine compounds (PFCs), which are slippery compounds used in water- and stain-repellent coatings on carpets, clothing, ironing boards, ovens, and pots and pans.

Flexible Bakeware

Flexible silicone bakeware, baking sheets, and Silpat hotpads are relatively new products. Silicone is nonstick and supposedly nontoxic, though some brands may begin to smoke and emit fumes when subjected to baking temperatures of about 450° Fahrenheit.

Call me an old fuddy duddy, but I am quite nervous about the fumes emitted by hot plastic. Teflon was also once a wonder material. I'll stick with my good, sturdy, inflexible tin bakeware that doesn't collapse as I load it into the oven.

Caring for Stovetop Cookware

Stainless steel is the workhorse of the kitchen. As my friend Jean says, she rides her stainless pans hard. High temperatures don't faze stainless steel. It can be hand scrubbed or thrown in the dishwasher, and unlike coated cookware, it's easy to tell when it's clean. (But don't put wooden handled pans in the dishwasher because the wood will eventually crack.)

Stainless steel is the least reactive metal, so it is the material of choice for general purpose frying pans, sauce pans, and soup pots. Good quality stainless-steel cookware doesn't have to be expensive. Just look for "18/10," (the numbers refer to the percentages of chromium and nickel in the alloy) with an aluminum core for good heat conductivity. Stainless-steel cookware is perfect for cooking acidic foods and liquid foods such as soups and stews.

Woks, cookie sheets, roasting and pizza pans, and other cookware that will be exposed to high heat should never have a nonstick coating. Oil is the original nonstick coating. Eating a little oil is a lot healthier than eating a little Teflon.

Copper cookware is fine as long as it's lined with stainless steel so food never contacts the copper. Though a tiny amount of copper is an essential part of a healthy diet, acidic foods that are stored or cooked in copper vessels can absorb enough copper to become toxic.

Copper items are often given a protective lacquer coating at the factory to prevent tarnish. This lacquer must be removed before copper utensils are used. To remove the lacquer, boil 2 gallons water in a large stock pot and add 1 cup baking soda. Soak the copper item in the hot solution until the lacquer peels off. (Fill your copper teakettle with water first so it won't float.) Rinse well and polish dry.

Polish copper items by dipping them in boiling white vinegar. The tarnish will vanish very quickly. As soon as the copper turns shiny, take it out and rinse it in clean water; wipe dry.

Remove tarnish from copper by rubbing it with a lemon slice dipped in salt or baking soda, then rinsing it off with water, and polish dry. (This is a perfect use for that slightly moldy piece of lemon.)

Rub a little leftover tomato paste on copper to polish it. Rinse it off and wipe dry.

Another method is to put the copper item in a pot of water with 1 tablespoon salt and 1 cup white vinegar and bring to a boil. Let it cool, then wash the item with mild dish liquid and hot water, then rinse and dry.

Cast iron enamelware is nonreactive (unless the enamel is cracked or chipped). The cast iron absorbs and holds heat well. This type of cookware should only be washed by hand.

Remove stains and discoloration from enamelware with a paste made of equal amounts salt and vinegar. Scrub the stains with the paste, let it sit for fifteen minutes, then rinse off.

Plain cast iron cookware is wonderful to cook in, but the food should be removed as soon as it is cooked. Food cooked in cast iron absorbs a little iron, but food stored in cast iron may absorb too much. The little bit of iron that cookware adds to food is probably a good thing for growing children and women of childbearing age. Grown men are more likely to suffer from an overabundance of iron. This is an easily solved problem: Most healthy adult men benefit from donating blood.

Cast iron snobs never use soap on their cast iron cookware. A good way to clean cast iron skillets, roasters, Dutch ovens, spun steel woks, etc., is to use a bit of clean neutral-flavored oil (canola, for instance). Pretend the oil is soap (soap is, after all, made of oil or fat). Pour a little in the pan and scrub vigorously with a plastic scrubber. Use a rubber squeegee to scrape the dirty oil into your drippings can, then wipe the pan clean with a paper towel or old rag. Rinse the pan with hot water, shake it off, then heat it on the stove over a low flame until it's dry.

Tempered glass cookware must be protected from temperature shocks. My brother-in-law once took a large, beautiful Yorkshire pudding out of the oven and put it on the counter in a puddle of water. The glass baking dish immediately shattered, and that was the end of the pudding.

To prevent thermal shock, avoid putting hot glass cookware in water or on cold surfaces. Also put a metal spoon in your glass mug or measuring cup before pouring boiling water into it. The metal will absorb the heat and prevent the glass from breaking.

Unsafe at Any Heat

Aluminum pots and pans are very light, often very cheap, and are quite reactive. Acidic or salty foods will discolor the aluminum; so will boiling eggs. Aluminum exacerbates the smelly properties of the cabbage family. Storing salty or acidic food in an aluminum pot will pit the surface of the metal and contaminate the food with aluminum.

Even worse, aluminum melts at a relatively low temperature. The U.S. Consumer Product Safety Commission has received several reports of consumers who were burned by drips of molten aluminum after their cookware boiled dry.

The CPSC recommends that aluminum cookware should never be left unattended and should not be allowed to boil dry, especially over high heat. If you ever do encounter a red-, yellow-, or white-hot saucepan, frying pan, or teakettle, allow it to cool completely before you attempt to handle it, lest you spill molten aluminum on yourself.

I'd rather be safe than sorry, so I use stainless-steel and cast iron cookware.

Cooking Utensils, Good

Stainless-steel spatulas, wooden spatulas, bamboo spatulas, wooden spoons, stainless-steel spoons, stainless-steel ladles, glass or metal measuring cups.

Cooking Utensils, Bad

Anything plastic. It melts when it gets hot, and cooking often involves heat. The highest-quality silicone cookware and utensils can withstand heat up to about 550° Fahrenheit. The melting temperature of aluminum is 1220.666° Fahrenheit (see above for more details). A hot frying pan is an unsuitable location for a plastic spoon or spatula, as I have demonstrated on more than one occasion.

Silver Care

One of the best ways to protect your sterling and silver-plate tableware from damage is to *keep it out of the dishwasher!* The dishwasher's high temperatures and strong detergent are far too harsh for silver and will dull and ruin its finish. Silver and stainless steel can react during the wash cycle, leaving black spots on the silver wherever the two metals made contact. Worst of all, older hollow-handled knives that have been repaired may split open in the dishwasher.

The tarnish on silver is silver sulfide, which forms when the silver reacts with sulfur compounds in the air, or with sulfur-containing substances, such as eggs, onions, spinach, wool, felt, or rubber. Salt, chlorine, and acids will pit and damage silver surfaces.

The best way to keep silver gleaming is to use it often, wash it by hand in very hot water with a very mild dish liquid, then dry it thoroughly with a soft clean cloth. You can help slow tarnishing by storing your silver in Silver-cloth flannel bags or cloths that are impregnated with silver nitrate. There are many nontoxic, biodegradable silver polishes and polishing cloths on the market. Read the label and look for the words Biodegradable and Nontoxic.

If your valuable antique silver is extremely tarnished, you may want to have it professionally cleaned. Large pieces that have seams and joints, such as candlesticks, should never be immersed in liquid. But those of us who own inexpensive silver can use the following quick and easy method of tarnish removal:

Small Pieces

Fill an aluminum pan with a solution of 1 teaspoon baking soda and 1 teaspoon salt per cup of boiling water. If you don't own an aluminum pan, cover the bottom of a glass bowl with a piece of aluminum foil, then pour in the hot soda and salt solution.

Lower the silver into the hot solution and let it soak. An electrolytic reaction in the salty water will pull the tarnish off the silver and deposit it on the aluminum. Let the silver soak for a few minutes, then take it out of the pot, rinse it off, and rub it with a soft, dry cloth. If the silver is not quite clean, repeat the operation.

Large Pieces

Make a silver-cleaning bath by covering the bottom of your kitchen sink with a piece of aluminum foil. Pour in a couple tablespoons salt and a couple tablespoons baking soda and fill the sink with hot water.

Removing Wax from Silver Candlesticks

Use a hair dryer to heat the candle cup enough to melt the wax. Don't overheat the metal. Gently touch the candlestick to make sure it hasn't gotten too hot, then support the candle cup from underneath while you wipe the area with a paper towel. Cotton swabs work quite well to clean very small candle cups. Replace the paper towels or cotton swabs as they absorb wax.

Heavy Metal

Acidic foods such as tomatoes, sauerkraut, fruit, lemonade, fruit punches, carbonated beverages, tea, and wine can react with metal in containers and become poisonous. Here are the types of metal containers to avoid:

1. *Zinc:* Never store food or beverages in galvanized metal containers, which may leach toxic amounts of zinc into the food.
2. *Copper or brass:* Acidic foods such as lemonade, wine, tea, coffee, or tomato sauce will become toxic in copper containers.
3. *Lead:* Traditional pewter contains 25 percent lead and 75 percent tin; drinking or eating from pewter is not recommended.
   - Pewter should be used for purely decorative purposes, so you might as well keep it looking nice. Shine up your antique tankards by rubbing them with cabbage leaves, then buffing them dry.
   - Many antique ceramics have lead glazes; unless you have your great-grandmother's china tested for lead, you should probably avoid using it for serving food. Newer, decorative pieces with lead glazes usually have warnings on the bottom that say Not for Food Use. May Poison Food. But just in case, avoid storing food or beverages in ceramic containers that aren't specifically designed for food storage.
   - Lead crystal comes by its name honestly. Using a lead crystal wine decanter or lead crystal goblets for wine is not a good idea. The acidic wine may leach lead out of the glass, and you could end up as crazy as a Roman emperor.

Microwaveable Containers

A glass plate covered with an upside-down glass bowl, or vice versa, works very well in the microwave.

Never microwave metal, foil, plastic storage bags, grocery bags, newspapers, or plates or cups that are decorated with metallic glazes or enamels. These items may ignite in the microwave.

When subjected to high temperatures, some plastics may begin to break down and can contaminate food; never use containers in the microwave that are not labeled as microwave safe. I find it easiest to avoid putting any plastic items in the microwave at all.

Put your food on a plate rather than on a paper towel; many paper towels, especially recycled paper towels, contain toxins that may leach into food when microwaved.

Food Packaging

Dangerous Plastics

Many plastics start to break down as they age and when they are heated, scrubbed, or subjected to harsh detergents.

Plastics are also slightly fat soluble, which means that they are more likely to contaminate fatty foods rather than fat-free foods.

No plastic of any kind should ever be heated on the stove or in the conventional oven.

Some plastics are significantly more dangerous than others.

The Environmental Protection Agency (EPA) and the International Agency for Research on Cancer (IARC) have classified styrene, the main constituent of plastic foam, as a possible human carcinogen. Plastic foam begins to break down when it is heated and will contaminate hot beverages or food. Try to avoid drinking hot liquids out of plastic foam cups, and never put plastic foam containers in the microwave.

Bisphenol A (BPA) is a component of many common plastics. It is the main ingredient in polycarbonate plastic, which is commonly used to make baby bottles, reusable milk bottles, and reusable water bottles; it is also in the plastic resins that line food and beverage cans, in styrene (Styrofoam), and in polyvinyl chloride (PVC). Bisphenol is a hormone mimic that upsets natural hormone levels and causes genetic damage and miscarriages in laboratory mice.

At least one study has shown that bisphenol A can leach from plastic bottles in amounts that are harmful to laboratory mice, although other studies were less conclusive. The plastics industry claims that their products are safe, but the studies have led some experts to recommend that consumers avoid buying polycarbonate or Nalgene water bottles, milk or juice in returnable polycarbonate bottles, and polycarbonate baby bottles. Choose polyethylene or polypropylene baby bottles and reusable water bottles.

Single-use plastic beverage bottles are not designed to be refilled. If they are reused, their plastic may begin to break down and contaminate liquids.

 Polycarbonate plastic was invented in 1953. Though researchers had reported in 1938 that BPA mimicked the hormone estrogen, no one seems to have worried about the possible health effects of the chemical.

In 2003, Patricia A. Hunt, a reproductive biologist at Case Western Reserve University in Cleveland, and her colleagues were trying to crack the mystery of why up to a quarter of all fertilized human eggs have the wrong number of chromosomes (aneuploidy). Aneuploidy causes spontaneous miscarriages and 10 to 20 percent of all birth defects, including Down's syndrome. Previous studies had failed to link smoking and alcohol to these genetic birth defects.

When the scientists began examining the eggs of their lab mice, they were bewildered by wildly fluctuating rates of aneuploidy in lab mice that had not been purposefully exposed to any chemicals. The percentage of abnormal mouse eggs ranged from a low of 2 percent to a high of 40 percent. "It was a big disaster," Hunt said.

Eventually the scientists solved the mystery: An inexperienced and overzealous animal technician had washed the polycarbonate cages and water bottles with a harsh detergent, and BPA was leaching into the animals' water. Further experiments revealed a link between BPA exposure and damaged egg cells. Many other animal studies have shown that very low levels of BPA disrupt fetal development. Animals exposed in utero have damaged long-term memories, the males have lowered sperm production and an increased risk of prostate cancer, the females have an increased risk of breast cancer, and both genders are more likely to become obese due to an overabundance of fat cells.

As plastics get reused, they begin to leach BPA into the liquids stored in them. Studies of human mothers and their babies showed that BPA readily passes from the mother to her developing child. Though adults quickly metabolize and inactivate BPA, fetuses and infants lack the enzymes to break it down.

The good news is that, like alcohol, BPA only harms fetuses whose mothers ingest it while they are pregnant.

Plastic Wrap

Though all plastic wrap is not alike, I have better things to do than try to ferret out exactly which plasticizers are in each bit of food wrapping that is carried through my door. Fatty foods such as cheeses and meats will absorb some of the plasticizers from plastic wrap and plastic bags. If you want to minimize your exposure to these chemicals, when you bring groceries home, remove the plastic packaging and wrap all your cheeses and meats in freezer paper or waxed paper before putting them in a plastic bag or container.

Unbleached waxed paper is an excellent alternative to plastic wrap. It is nontoxic and biodegradable, so after it is used it can be thrown in the compost pile.

Safely Contained

1. Glass is the most chemically inert packaging material. (Lead crystal is the big exception to this rule. See page 126.)

   As much as possible, try to buy food, especially acidic or fatty foods such as milk, juice, tomato sauce, and condiments, in glass containers rather than in plastic-lined tin cans or plastic containers. Try to use glass food storage containers whenever possible. Avoid buying oil in plastic bottles.

2. Aluminum foil is a safe, reusable food covering. Just don't put it in the microwave.

3. Polypropylene and polyethylene are relatively safe, inert plastics that don't contain either chlorine or plasticizers. If you are buying plastic food storage containers, look for containers labeled HDPE (high density polyethylene) or PP (polypropylene).

If you are truly serious about reducing your exposure to toxic chemicals, cleaning them out of your kitchen is a huge step in the right direction. Following the rules of safe food handling is equally important, since there is nothing nontoxic about the prescription medicines that are required to kill off virulent food-borne diseases.

Once the kitchen is clean, we can move on to other areas of the house.

CHAPTER 3

The Low-Maintenance Bathroom

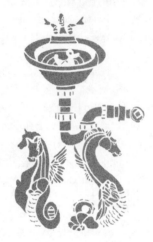

While I suppose it is possible that some people enjoy cleaning their bathrooms and want to fully savor the experience, I would rather cultivate a low-maintenance bathroom that requires a bare minimum of upkeep. I realize that everyone has different ideas of fun, but I find it much more diverting to soak myself in a tub of hot water than to scrub out a grubby shower stall.

A low-maintenance bathroom, like a low-maintenance garden, begins with materials that are well adapted to local conditions so they don't require a lot of fussing in order to stay in good shape. (Low maintenance is also a state of mind. The highest maintenance bathroom I have ever heard of was in a mansion where a friend of mine was the housekeeper. The bathrooms had to be completely cleaned after each use and every detail had to be perfect, right down to the elaborately folded toilet paper ends.)

Designing a low-maintenance bathroom requires a bit of forethought and planning, but the time savings can be substantial. If a bathroom is badly designed, even the most diligent housekeeper will have trouble keeping it clean.

Cleaning the bathroom does not have to be time-consuming and toxic. It isn't difficult or expensive to design a low-maintenance bathroom that features easy-to-clean wall surfaces, flooring, and fixtures, yet remains an attractive location to perform one's ablutions. Once you know the techniques, about ten minutes of cleaning per week should be sufficient to keep this bathroom clean, sanitary, and sparkling. This adds up to less than nine hours per year of bathroom cleaning. Unfortunately, the no-maintenance bathroom does not exist.

If you are cursed with a high-maintenance bathroom, be gentle; there is no point in wearing yourself out trying to perfect a bathroom that is either so old and worn out that it has permanently lost its shine, or a designer bathroom that is composed of high-maintenance materials such as glass, stainless steel, and dark-colored tiles and bathroom fixtures.

Designing a Low-Maintenance Bathroom from the Bottom Up

Floors

Bathroom carpeting is a really bad idea, especially in households with young boys, or older boys, or men, or people who take baths or showers. Because carpeting tends to stay damp, it is a breeding ground for mold and mildew. If you are unfortunate enough to have bathroom carpeting, try to replace it with nonporous flooring as soon as possible. The only rugs that belong in a bathroom are the kind that can be thrown in the washing machine and dryer.

Though many modern or remodeled bathrooms have resilient vinyl flooring, it is a problematic material that may emit poisonous fumes for several years after it is installed, is very difficult to dispose of, produces deadly smoke if it catches fire, and is not very durable. If your house was built before the 1950s and the bathroom has sheet flooring, there is a good possibility that there is an intact ceramic tile floor underneath the vinyl or linoleum flooring. In contrast to vinyl, ceramic tiles are durable, waterproof, easy to keep clean, completely nontoxic, and are made of abundant natural materials (clay and sand). A tiled floor is even easier to keep clean if you take advantage of a really high tech invention: colored grout. Old-fashioned white grout is very easily stained, so fastidious housekeepers used to spend a lot of time on their hands and knees scrubbing the joints between their bathroom tiles; you can save yourself a lot of work by choosing very dark or black grout that won't show stains. (Remember, a stain is simply a permanent change in color. A newly washed T-shirt can sport a rust stain; so can perfectly clean grout. The presence of a stain does not mean that a surface is dirty; the absence of stains does not mean that a surface is clean.)

If your tiles have already been grouted, do not despair: White or light-colored grout can be stained a darker color with special grout-stains that are available at many home improvement, flooring, and tile stores.

Other nontoxic flooring, such as well-sealed stone, hardwood, or concrete, can also be used in bathrooms, though they aren't as easy to keep clean as a glazed tile floor. Real linoleum, which is biodegradable because it is made of organic materials (linseed oil, wood byproducts, limestone dust, and natural pigments baked onto a natural jute backing), must be very well sealed and caulked where it meets the walls and fixtures to prevent water from seeping into its edges and ruining it.

Walls and Ceiling

Dark discoloration caused by mildew, which is the common name for a very shallow growth of mold, is often found on bathroom surfaces. The amount of steam created by a long, hot shower or bath can leave the walls dripping. Unless you want to cultivate a mildew garden, the bathroom is not the right venue for elegant matte painted finishes or flocked or textured wallpaper. The only absorbent materials that belong in a bathroom are towels, washcloths, and bath mats. Bathroom walls should be finished with washable gloss or semigloss paint, or another very smooth surface such as ceramic tile, or wood paneling sealed with a nontoxic water-based finish (see sources at the back of the book).

Since mold and mildew cannot grow on dry surfaces, keeping the bathroom walls clean is largely a matter of keeping them dry. If the bathroom is allowed and encouraged to dry out completely at least once a day, bacteria, fungi, mold, and mildew will be unable to survive.

An efficient bathroom exhaust fan is one of the best antifungal devices ever invented. In order to prevent excess condensation, especially in a cold climate, choose an exhaust fan that is capable of venting twice the air volume of your bathroom per minute. Running the fan while you bathe or shower and leaving it on for ten or fifteen minutes afterward will go a long way toward keeping your bathroom mildew free. If the walls are still wet after you turn off the fan, wipe them dry with a towel. If you are less than seven feet tall, try putting a towel over a mop head or Dutch Rubber Broom (see page 67) and use it to dry the top of the walls and the ceiling. (For more information on preventing mold and mildew, see "Preventing Fungi, Mold, and Mildew," page 290.)

Storage

Adequate storage is an essential feature of a low-maintenance bathroom. Remember: moving the clutter off a surface so you can clean it usually takes longer than the actual cleaning process. If you have to move twenty-nine separate items off the countertop in order to wipe it down, you will probably clean it far less often than if those twenty-nine items were stored in a couple of decorative bowls or baskets.

You can also greatly increase the capacity of your bathroom cupboards and cabinets by cutting up square plastic bottles to make stackable cubbyholes to hold small grooming items, such as fingernail clippers and dental floss. (For more storage ideas, see "Grace's Box Tricks," page 17.)

Soft vs. Hard Water

Well-chosen bathroom fixtures can help speed the cleaning process, thus encouraging more frequent cleaning. The lowest-maintenance bathroom is one that is cleaned often enough to prevent mineral deposits from hardening.

Hardened mineral deposits are generally the biggest challenge one faces when cleaning a bathroom. When hard water evaporates from a surface, it deposits a layer of minerals such as calcium, magnesium, or iron. When these same minerals react with dissolved soap, they transform the water-soluble soap into an insoluble scum that sticks to tub and shower walls.

Though installing a water softening system would lighten all your cleaning chores—from laundering clothes to washing dishes to shampooing your hair—softened water is a health hazard and adds pollutants to wastewater. Water softeners add either washing soda (sodium carbonate), borax, phosphates, or sodium to the water, rendering it less than ideal for consumption by man, beast, or leafy green plants.

Hard water is not a health hazard. In fact, the extra minerals it contains, especially calcium and magnesium, may actually improve one's health. It is therefore much healthier to remove the mineral deposits from your appliances and fixtures rather than to add pollutants to your water. Luckily, there are many simple, nontoxic methods for dealing with the deposits left behind by healthy, mineral-enhanced water (see page 82).

Hot Water

Though the water heater is generally not located in the bathroom, it is an essential piece of bathing equipment. The most durable and efficient standard water heaters have the thickest insulation, the biggest heating elements and burners, and the longest warranties (up to twelve years).

Tankless water heaters, which are also known as "on demand heaters," are more efficient and more expensive than standard water heaters. Tankless heaters do not store hot water—they heat it only as needed.

The most environmentally friendly water heating devices are solar hot water heaters, which are expensive to install but cost nothing to operate.

No matter what type of water heater you choose, you should keep it set no hotter than 120° Fahrenheit in order to prevent scalding mishaps.

Materials

Though standard residential toilets are generally made of vitrified porcelain—which is a very hard, smooth, and easily cleaned material—many sinks, bathtubs, and showers are made of synthetic materials such as acrylic or fiberglass—which are easily scratched and damaged. The roughened, damaged surfaces can be very difficult to keep clean. Maintaining enameled steel or cast iron bathtubs and porcelain sinks is much easier.

Smooth glass and mirrored surfaces are also high-maintenance materials because only constant polishing will keep them free of water spots.

Colors and Finishes

My friend Lynda, who is one of my chemical consultants, is also my soap scum researcher because she is the dissatisfied owner of a dark brown fiberglass bathtub. Her tub is the perfect venue for testing soap scum removal techniques because the white scum shows up so clearly against the dark background of the scum-attracting fiberglass.

Lynda did some very fine research and developed some effective nontoxic soap scum removal methods for fiberglass fixtures. But if you're in the market for new fiberglass fixtures, take her advice: Buy white ones that won't show soap scum. If you must have colored fixtures, buy porcelain or enameled ones.

My friend Susie, whose well water has a high iron content, informs me that tan or beige ceramic or enameled fixtures will hide the rusty stains that the water leaves behind. If you can't see the stain, there will be nothing to remove.

Choosing Hardware

Leaking faucets, shower heads, and toilets can waste many gallons of water in a very short period of time. When hot faucets leak, they also waste large amounts of energy in the form of heated water. You can conserve water and energy by fixing leaks and installing low-flow faucet aerators and low-flow shower heads with shut-off valves. Water-saving toilets are required in most parts of the country.

Most faucets that leak have worn out washers that can no longer form a watertight seal when the faucet valve is screwed against them. The easiest way to prevent faucet leaks is to buy the highest quality washerless faucets you can afford. The best washerless faucets are elegantly engineered and very durable; water flows through them only when the hole in a stainless-steel ball or ceramic plate in the handle aligns with an opening in the body of the faucet. When washerless faucets are turned off, there is nowhere for the water to flow.

If you don't enjoy polishing metal, choose faucets that have a brushed metal or gun metal finish. These matte metal finishes disguise water spots.

Try to avoid buying faucets with hollow, clear plastic handles. Given enough light, these handles make dandy little terrariums for growing algae. Cleaning the algae out of faucet handles is an unrewarding job that no one should have to do.

Grime Prevention and Cleaning Techniques

Preventing bathroom grime is usually preferable to cleaning it up. Many bathroom cleaning chores can mostly be avoided simply by keeping bathroom surfaces dry. Though doing little bits of cleaning every day may seem monotonous, I would much rather spend a few minutes doing daily bathroom maintenance than wait until the job takes three hours or more.

Tools

The following equipment should be kept in the bathroom. Supplies for more specialized, infrequent cleaning can be gathered from other parts of the house when necessary.

1. A spray bottle filled with distilled white vinegar made from grain.
2. An assortment of cleaning rags: worn-out bath towels that have been cut down to a convenient size, old washcloths, and cut up old T-shirts. Store them under the sink, in a cabinet, or in a bathroom drawer.
3. A few worn-out toothbrushes to be used to clean difficult areas.
4. A couple of plastic scrub brushes: one for the sink and one to be kept in the shower.
5. A sturdy toilet brush with a holder.

6. Optional: A plastic shower squeegee that can be hung in the shower. (This is optional because some people prefer drying their showers with a bath towel before they throw it in the laundry.)
7. Also optional: A bottle of extremely cheap vodka for cleaning.

REMEMBER: NEVER MIX PRODUCTS THAT CONTAIN CHLORINE WITH ANY OTHER PRODUCTS! *Many scouring powders contain chlorine. If these products make contact with ammonia-based products, such as glass cleaner, dishwashing liquid, metal cleaner, toilet bowl cleaner, or rust remover, deadly chlorine gas can be produced.*

Bath Towels

If damp towels are hung up and allowed to dry every day, they should still be relatively clean by the end of the week, since in a perfect, childless world, towels are only used to dry freshly washed bodies. Before you throw them in the laundry, use these towels to dry and polish damp but clean bathroom walls, mirrors, sinks, counters, shower stalls, and bathtubs. If your youngsters' towels are clean enough, you can use them to dry the floor.

Now may be the appropriate time to mention that white bathroom towels are not a particularly good idea for the average household. It is quite common for youngish family members to misunderstand a towel's expected role and use it to remove dirt rather than to wipe various body parts dry after all the dirt has already been washed off. If your family cannot be persuaded to wash before toweling, you might want to match your towels to your local earth tones. "Natural" colored cotton towels (light tan) are also a very nice alternative to white ones.

Choosing a Scum Free Soap

Since hard water spots and soap scum develop when water evaporates, leaving minerals and soap residue behind, if you let the water dry on your shower walls, they will get dirty rather quickly. If you dry the shower walls with a towel or a shower squeegee before you exit, however, you will greatly reduce the amount of cleaning you have to do.

Regular soap is produced by combining animal fat with lye; when this type of soap is used in hard water, it produces soap scum. (See page 150 for more information on soap scum.) Detergents, which are petroleum products, were invented to prevent soap scum. Because detergents do not combine with water-soluble minerals, they don't leave a residue. Detergent has become so common that most bath soaps, both solid and liquid, are actually detergents.

If you don't like the idea of scrubbing yourself clean with petroleum, but you want to prevent soap scum, castile soap is a wonderful alternative.

Castile soap is a very gentle natural product made from vegetable oil; no matter how hard the water, castile soap does not form soap scum. For a couple of decades now, my husband and I have been using Dr. Bronner's Magic Soaps. These well-known natural castile soaps have been made from olive and coconut oils by the same family-owned company since 1929. Dr. Bronner's is available at most health food stores, or you can contact the company at www.drbronner.com.

Cleaning the Shower While Showering

Preventing grime from settling is far easier than removing it after it has built up.

I never realized how much easier it is to clean a bathroom when one is only using castile soap until we moved and my cleaning routine went out the window for much, much longer than I like to admit. When I finally got around to scrubbing our shower, it was nearly the anniversary of the last time I had scrubbed it. I thought I was in for a day-long struggle that might perhaps involve a jack hammer. I brought a scrub brush into the shower with me and, after I was clean, I addressed my attention to the shower walls. Much to my astonishment, the residues surrendered at the first touch of my brush, and I wasn't even using any cleanser.

Now I keep a shower squeegee, a scrub brush, and an old toothbrush in the shower. After each shower I squeegee the walls dry, and once every couple of weeks I scrub the shower walls and door. I rarely have to resort even to a spray of vinegar to clean my shower.

Bathtubs generally should be scrubbed, rinsed, and dried after each use because humans steeped in hot soapy water produce a particularly tenacious scum. Using castile soap will make the frothy scum much less likely to cling to the bathtub walls, but you will still have to wipe or scrub the bathtub and rinse out the residue after each bath, or your bathtub will quickly become grimy.

Toilet Grime Prevention

Because toilet bowls hold water all the time, algae tends to grow in them unless it is regularly discouraged. Minerals can also precipitate out of hard water and form deposits below the water line. Simply scrubbing the toilet bowl with a toilet brush, if done often enough, can remove the algae as well as the mineral deposits. But if you wait long enough between cleanings, the mineralized layers will grow deep enough and hard enough that they can't be scrubbed off. This is when many people turn to dangerous chemical toilet bowl cleaners.

Here is a really easy, nontoxic way to clean the mineralized deposits out of your toilet bowl:

Materials: Toilet bowl plunger, jug of distilled white vinegar

TECHNIQUE

1. If you have any type of "automatic toilet cleaner" or deodorizer installed in your toilet bowl or tank, remove it. Flush the toilet to get rid of the chlorine; you will be pouring vinegar into the toilet and you don't want to produce chlorine gas. Send the "automatic toilet cleaner" to the hazardous waste facility where it belongs.
2. Put the working end of the toilet plunger over the hole in the bottom of the toilet bowl and gently force out the water by slowly pushing the plunger down, releasing it, then pushing again. Keep pumping until the bowl is nearly empty.
3. Pour enough white vinegar into the toilet bowl to fill it to its normal level. (This should take between one half and one gallon of vinegar.) Let the vinegar sit in the toilet bowl as long as possible, preferably overnight or while you are at work.

4. After the vinegar has been softening the mineral deposits for several hours, scrub them off with a toilet brush. (If you have waited a few years between cleanings, you may need to invest in a few gallons of vinegar because it may take several vinegar soakings to completely dissolve all the deposits.)
5. Flush.

Proper Toilet Etiquette

Our friend Al Parella, who runs the sewage treatment plant in Duluth, Minnesota, has a request: "Don't use the toilet as a garbage can. If it's not water soluble, don't put it in the toilet." Sewage treatment plants are completely dependent on microbes to digest the sewage and kill pathogens. Al refers to these microbes as his "little friends." If enough chemicals, such as paint thinners, solvents, petroleum products, pesticides, chlorine, and even toilet cleaners, are flushed down toilets or poured down drains, large numbers of these necessary microbes can die off, leaving a stinking mess at the treatment plant. Antibiotics and antimicrobials, which are designed to kill bacteria, can also damage these helpful microbes.

When you need to dispose of chemicals or pharmaceuticals, bring them to your local hazardous waste facility (see page 303).

Flushed

Purposefully flushing trash or food down the toilet is a waste of water, and even if the debris successfully navigates your sewage line, it may still cause trouble at the other end. Panty hose, for instance, have very high tensile strength and can catch and snag on the sewage treatment equipment and burn out the motors. Plastic bags and other plastic packaging do not break down in the plant and must be skimmed out of the wastewater. A smoothly functioning sewage treatment plant helps protect water quality. Keeping the local sewage treatment facility working efficiently should be a high priority for everyone.

Feminine hygiene products, even the varieties that are supposed to be flushable, should never be flushed down any toilet that is connected to a septic system because tampons and sanitary napkins don't break down quickly enough to prevent premature clogging of the holding tanks. Plastic applicators are not biodegradable and should never be flushed down any toilet. There is no such thing as a flushable sanitary napkin. Tampons and flushable cardboard applicators tend to clog all but the most vigorous of toilets. The simplest way to deal with these wastes is to put a plastic container with a very secure lid (such as a large yogurt container) in the bathroom as a receptacle for used feminine hygiene items. When the container is full, throw it in the garbage.

Oops!

Solid objects that are flushed down the toilet either by accident or by toddlers can cause great inconvenience. If you cannot keep track of your toddler well enough to prevent rubber ducky flushings, you might want to consider putting a lock near the top of your bathroom door; the bathroom is simply not a safe place for unsupervised toddlers.

My children have never flushed inappropriate objects down the toilet, but I have, repeatedly. While I was in college, I learned that if the lid was up when I flushed, something would inevitably fly into the toilet, sometimes from all the way across the room, and that object would inevitably be one that was perfectly shaped to clog a toilet, such as swim goggles or a toothbrush. Also, if I stood near an open toilet, even if it wasn't flushing, anything that wasn't actually attached to my body would fall in. This category unfortunately included all items in pockets, overall straps, etc. My current technique is to sneak up on the toilet with all my loose items already lowered beneath the elevation of the bowl.

Because of my own sorry history with commodes, I was amused by the news item about the man who dropped his cell phone into the toilet on a Metro-North train into New York City, then got his arm stuck while trying to retrieve the phone, causing long delays during the evening commute while rescue workers demolished the toilet in order to release his arm. My immediate reaction was that here was a forty-one-year-old man who had previously led a charmed life, and who had obviously only associated with others who led similarly charmed lives. I—who have not led a charmed life—would have been expecting a loose phone to fall into the toilet, and I would have known that no object is ever easily retrievable after it has fallen prey to a flushing toilet.

Closing the lid before flushing the toilet may prevent more than just clogged toilets: The ever curious Professor Gerba, whom we last encountered in the Kitchen chapter, discovered that the flushing action of toilets propels tiny droplets of bacteria-laden toilet water into the air. These droplets can stay aloft for up to two hours before descending to contaminate bathroom surfaces.

Close that lid, then flush!

Water Conservation

It is possible to misuse a toilet even when you are using it for its appointed purposes. Unnecessary flushing is a terrible waste of water. Anyone who has lived through a severe drought or who owns a well is likely to have learned that it is not necessary to flush the toilet unless there is solid material in it. This philosophy is succinctly summed up by this charming folk rhyme: "If it's yellow, it's mellow, if it's brown, flush it down." Though this water-use philosophy can cause intense culture clashes when the People of the Drought meet the People of the Piped-In Water, most urine is sterile and is very unlikely to cause disease.

Clog Busting

Though there are the occasional worst-case clogged toilet scenarios involving tree roots and sewer lines, which require professional intervention from the Roto Rooter man, most toilet clogs can be dealt with by the homeowner.

There are three different ways to unclog a toilet: Dissolve the clog with chemicals; dislodge it with a plunger; or drill through it with a snake (auger). Chemical drain cleaners are extremely corrosive and can burn unprotected skin; they can also react with chlorine to form deadly chlorine gas. (And Al at the treatment plant does not appreciate what chlorine does to his little microbial friends.)

A metal auger is rather tricky to use and can damage the toilet. Toilet design includes a sharp bend (a trap) that holds water in the bowl and prevents sewer gases from wafting into the bathroom; the waste pipe below the toilet is perfectly straight. Clogs occur inside the toilet, not in the waste pipe. Plungers are designed to produce enough water pressure to push the clog past the bend in the toilet. A plunger is really the best tool for dealing with the average clogged toilet without damaging either the toilet or one's self. The most effective toilet plungers are made of flexible rubber and have a double cup, like a small bell inside a larger one.

Proper Plunger Technique

1. Prevent the water from overflowing by turning off the oval valve behind the toilet. If there is no shut-off valve, take the lid off the water tank and lift the float in order to stop the water flow. Prop up the float, then go get your plunger.
2. Submerge the bell of the plunger in the toilet bowl and, without trying to form a seal against the toilet bowl, slowly push on the handle a few times until you have burped all the trapped air out of the plunger. If the water level in the toilet bowl is not high enough to completely submerge the plunger, pour more water into the bowl. Plungers are most efficient when their bells are full of water rather than air.
3. Once the air has been expelled, cover the hole in the bottom of the toilet bowl with the bell of the plunger and angle the plunger so it can form a good tight seal. Push the plunger hard against the toilet outlet, but be careful to maintain the seal. You should be able to develop a lot of water pressure using this technique. Release the pressure but don't lift the plunger off the outlet hole. Repeat until the toilet flushes and empties completely. The toilet will make a loud burping sound when the clog is released.
4. Turn the water back on using the valve behind the toilet.
5. Flush the toilet and swish the plunger around to wash it off in the clean water. Flush the toilet again.
6. Put the plunger back in its storage bucket.

Clogged Sink or Bathtub Drains

The most common cause of clogged bathroom drains is hair, especially long hair. Install sink strainers in your bathroom drains and try to train your family members to clean their hair out of the shower rather than attempt to wash it down the drain. Hair is not water soluble and will eventually prevent water from draining out of the sink or shower.

~ SEWER RATS

There is probably no more effective illustration of the interconnectedness of life than finding a rat in a toilet. This charming phenomenon usually occurs because a trail of food from a garbage disposal has attracted a sewer rat, which has taken a wrong turn and surfaced in the toilet. Many municipal websites contain information about dealing with rats in toilets.

The general advice on commode rats begins with kitchen practices designed to make waste pipes less attractive to rats by keeping the kitchen drain free of food:

1. Use garbage disposals as little as possible.
2. Keep your sink rinsed clean.
3. Never throw grease down the drain.
4. Clean out your kitchen drain once a month by pouring in half a cup of baking soda followed by a cup of vinegar. When the fizzing stops, pour in a kettleful of boiling water.

   If you are not willing to forgo using your garbage disposal and sewer rats are a problem in your area, you will need to practice preventive measures:

   1. Keep the toilet lid down whenever the toilet is not in use.
   2. If you discover a live rat in your toilet, shut the lid, then flush. (Don't worry about the rat, it won't drown. Rats can, in fact, tread water for three days!)

Everett, Washington's website recommends that you flush the toilet at least five times. If the rat is still in the toilet after the fifth flush, call Animal Control.

There is a very effective little tool that pulls hair out of shower and sink drains. Available at hardware stores, it looks like a giant pipe cleaner with a plastic handle on one end. If your drain is slow, push the giant pipe cleaner down the drain and slowly pull it up again. Astonishing amounts of hair will stick to the nylon bristles. Remove the hair and shove the pipe cleaner down the drain again. Repeat until the drain is free of hair.

If hair is not the cause of your clog, you can try a plunger, which is most effective when it works with the maximum water pressure possible:

1. In order to maximize the plunger's effectiveness, you will need to remove the pop-up drain plug from the sink or bathtub so the plunger can make an effective seal over the drain hole. Stuff a wet

rag into the sink or bathtub overflow hole (this is the hole at the back of the sink right below the faucet). Plugging the overflow hole will prevent it from leaking air and reducing the plunger-pressure.

2. Run the water until the sink, bathtub, or shower is holding enough water to cover the plunger bell.

3. Put the plunger in the water and pump it up and down a few times to burp out all the trapped air. Place the cup of the plunger over the drain and pump it up and down a few times without breaking the seal between the plunger and the sink. You should feel a lot of water pressure when you do this. Yank the plunger off the drain. Repeat several times, making sure to burp all the air out of the plunger before you pump.

4. If your drain is still too slow, pour in half a cup baking soda, then a cup of white distilled vinegar. When the fizzing stops, pour in a kettleful of boiling water.

5. If the sink drain is still clogged, try removing the J trap and cleaning the gunk and hair out of it. If you don't know what a J trap is or you don't own any tools anyway, you probably need to call an expert.

Nontoxic, Timesaving Cleaning Techniques

Rapid bathroom cleaning depends on a combination of factors: The bathroom must be composed entirely of smooth, easily cleaned surfaces; it must be cleaned frequently enough to prevent grime from hardening; and the cleaning products must not leave a residue that needs to be rinsed off.

It is completely unnecessary to clean a home bathroom every day, though there are minor things that can be done daily to reduce your total cleaning load. For instance: If you use regular soap, you can prevent the formation of soap scum by wiping the sink dry each day with a lightly used hand towel before you drop it in the hamper. Better yet, if you switch to castile soap, you will find that there is no need to scrub your sink with any type of abrasive, since the residue from castile soap never hardens.

❧ DRAIN DANGERS

All chemical drain cleaners are extremely dangerous. If you spill drain cleaner, it will eat through *everything*. Spattered drain cleaner or toilet bowl cleaner is a hazard to health, happiness, and eyesight. A drop of water landing in a container of liquid drain cleaner or toilet bowl cleaner will react and cause instant and disastrous spattering akin to the spattering that occurs when a drop of water lands in a skillet of hot grease, but spattering drain cleaner will cause far more damage: A single drop of a strong acid or base can ruin an eye. (If you do get splashed by a corrosive material, you need to flush the affected area with a lot of water for a long time.)

ACID DOWN THE DRAIN

Some liquid drain cleaners utilize very strong acids, such as sulfuric acid; liquid toilet bowl cleaners often contain hydrochloric acid; solid toilet bowl cleaners often contain sodium bisulfate. If these strong acids are spilled on a vinyl bathroom floor they will yellow the vinyl, and if not neutralized, they will eat through the mastic. If the acid gets to the wood underlayment, it may start a fire. Even if there are no flames, the acid will gradually char and blacken the wood.

Sulfuric acid is known to the chemical industry as oil of vitriol. It is so infamously corrosive that in the 1800s it was used as a weapon of vengeance to disfigure enemies, hence the word "vitriolic."

Oil of vitriol is extremely slippery and is quite hazardous when spilled on a floor because it is impossible to step on it and remain upright. I won't delve further into the gory details of this type of accident.

ALKALI DOWN THE DRAIN

Some liquid drain cleaners contain potassium hydroxide, sodium hypochlorite, or sodium hydroxide, all of which are very strong and very dangerous bases (alkalies). If these alkaline drain cleaners are mixed with other products, toxic or flammable gases can be produced.

NEUTRALIZE

If despite the warnings, you decide to use strongly corrosive chemicals anyway and you happen to spill some, here's what you must do:

Spilled corrosive substances must be neutralized, or they will remain dangerous indefinitely.

Read the label before using a chemical product. If an accident occurs, you will know what the recommended neutralizer is.

Neutralizing must be done very carefully, or disaster may result. Safely neutralizing a strong acid or base involves slowly and carefully adding a little bit of the corrosive chemical to a lot of the neutralizer. The neutralizer must be relatively weak because neutralization creates heat; if the chemical neutralization is too fast, it can create enough heat to cause popping and spattering. Just diluting these strong chemicals also produces heat. For instance, when drain cleaning crystals are poured into a drain filled with water, the water boils.

Neutralizing Acids

Toilet bowl cleaners, some drain cleaners, kitchen/bathroom cleaners that remove hard water deposits, metal cleaners, and rust removers are strongly acidic. They can burn skin and cause blindness. Here are directions for safely neutralizing a strong acid:

1. Read the label. Make sure that you really are dealing with an acid. If you have a medical emergency, call 911 and follow the instructions on the label. Open a window; the vapors can be harmful.
2. If you have spilled a strong acid such as toilet bowl cleaner on the floor, remain calm. Remember that you need to neutralize the acid slowly in order to prevent spattering.
3. This occasion demands that you wear rubber or plastic gloves and a pair of chemical safety goggles.
4. Pour a lot of *baking soda* on the *dry* part of the floor, then use a rubber squeegee or rubber spatula to move a little bit of the acid at a time over to the baking soda. (Do not use metal tools to move the acid. Hydrochloric acid can react with metal to form flammable hydrogen gas.) See optional step below.
5. Slowly and gradually add the acid to the baking soda until all the acid is neutralized. You can tell that the neutralization is complete when there is no fizzing and no heat is being released.
6. Optional step: Before you add the baking soda, plain dry sand can be very gently poured onto the puddle of acid to make it easier to work with and to prevent splashing. Sand is inert and will not react with the acid.

(Note: *Never* use sawdust, flour, sugar, or other granular or powdered combustible materials for sopping up chemical spills, lest you end up with a chemical spill *and* a fire!)

(continued on next page)

(continued from previous page)

Neutralizing Bases (Alkalis)

Strong bases can burn skin and cause blindness.

Powdered drain cleaner and oven cleaner may both contain sodium hydroxide (lye). But read the label: Some drain cleaners are acidic and contain sulfuric acid.

Here is the safe way to neutralize a strong base:

1. Read the label. Make sure that you really are dealing with a base. If you have a medical emergency, call 911 and follow the instructions on the label. Open a window; the vapors can be harmful.
2. If you have spilled a strong base such as oven cleaner on the floor, remain calm. In order to protect your skin and your eyesight, you need to neutralize the base slowly and gently.
3. If you have spilled a dry product or a very thick paste:
    a. Don't add water! Contact with water will produce heat, and there will be popping and spattering.
    b. Avoid all contact with the chemical, and wear rubber or plastic gloves, a dust mask, and safety goggles.
    c. Use a rubber squeegee or rubber or plastic spatula to sweep the dry material into a plastic dustpan, and put the chemical in a plastic container with a well-fitted lid for later transport to the Hazardous Materials disposal site.
        Do not put the chemical in the garbage or trash! Contact with moisture will start a fire!
    d. An alternative disposal method is to don goggles and rubber gloves, then put 2 to 3 gallons of water in a clean, empty 5-gallon bucket. Gradually add the caustic material, a tiny bit at a time, to the water in the bucket. When the caustic material is diluted, it can be poured down the drain.

Abrasive cleansers tend to be counterproductive. Fiberglass and acrylic are relatively soft materials that are easily damaged by abrasives. Once these synthetic surfaces lose their shine, they become much more difficult to keep clean. Abrasive cleansers can also damage glass and highly polished metals.

Even if your fixtures are made of durable porcelain, which is not readily damaged by gentle abrasives such as Bon Ami, you may still want to forgo abrasive cleansers. These products leave a gritty residue behind that must be rinsed off if you don't want to end up with a gritty residue on your

    e. When all the powder or paste is swept up, wash the floor with a large amount of *undiluted vinegar.*
4. If you have spilled a liquid base, plain dry sand can be poured very gently on the puddle to make it easier to sweep up. After it is swept up and put in a plastic container, wash the floor with *undiluted vinegar.*

A MESSAGE FROM THE OTHER END OF THE DRAIN

Our friend Al, who runs the sewage treatment plant, is not fond of corrosive chemicals. He told me that "Once you've got this type of chemical in your house, it's a liability until it's gone. I don't use this stuff. Ninety percent of the time, a plunger will take care of the clog; an auger or snake will fix the other ten percent of clogs." He added that if you do use a chemical in your drain and it doesn't work, the next person who works on the drain will be endangered, either because the chemical will splash up when a plunger is used, or when the pipes are opened up and the drain cleaner spills out.

The Low-Down at the Water Line

Very strong acids and bases are a hazard to the life, health, and welfare of both macroscopic and microscopic life forms. Drain cleaner or toilet bowl cleaner should never be poured down any drain that ends in a septic system. These strong chemicals will kill the bacteria that make the septic system work, causing a much bigger problem than a slow drain.

In the inimitable words of John W. Hill and Doris K. Kolb, who wrote *Chemistry for Changing Times,* "The best drain cleaner is prevention: Don't pour grease down the kitchen sink and try to keep hair out of the drain. If a drain does get clogged, a mechanical device such as a plumber's snake is often a better choice than a chemical drain cleaner."

behind. The cleanser grit on bathroom fixtures may actually be thicker and harder to rinse off than a week's accumulation of soap scum and grime.

Cleaning Methods

Deep Cleaning

Before you can begin to use weekly quick-cleaning methods, you need to prepare by doing a deep cleaning to remove all the built-up grime. The most difficult cleaning challenges are likely to come from fiberglass and acrylic (plastic) sinks, showers, and bathtubs that have a heavy build-up of soap scum, toilets that have not been cleaned in a long time, and faucets and showers that have acquired a crust of hardened mineral deposits.

Removing Soap Scum

It is always easier to clean a tub or shower immediately after it has been used. The moister the soap deposits, the easier they are to remove. But let's address the possibility that you have inherited or accumulated a good, solid layer of soap scum or hardened mineral deposits on your bathroom fittings:

Borax, a naturally occurring mineral that is sold as a water softener and laundry aid, is a very effective nonabrasive cleanser. You can use it to scrub built-up soap scum off fiberglass, porcelain, or enameled finishes; just wet the scummy surface, sprinkle a little borax on a stiff scrub brush, and apply with a lot of elbow grease. Borax is water soluble, so it rinses off surfaces easily without leaving grit behind.

Clean soap scum off a tub or shower stall by applying hot vinegar with a sponge or rag, then scrubbing hard with a stiff-bristled scrub brush. (If you boil the vinegar in the microwave you can end up with a clean microwave as well as a clean shower. See chapter two, "The Kitchen," page 95, for further details.)

Heated Murphy's Oil Soap, applied with a stiff scrubbing brush and a lot of elbow grease to a scummy fiberglass bathtub, will remove large quantities of hardened soap scum. (Extremely thick soap scum may need to be scraped off with a plastic spatula or credit card.) Tests conducted by Lynda, my soap scum investigator, showed that, unlike all the other products she tested, Murphy's Oil Soap also prevented scum recurrence for up to three weeks. (The same method will of course work on scummy sinks and showers.)

Wipe the sides of a freshly cleaned tub or shower stall with a soft cloth dampened with Murphy's Oil Soap and water; this significantly slows down further soap scum development. (Murphy's Soap is quite slippery, however, so it needs to be rinsed off very thoroughly, and you should not apply it directly to the shower or bathtub floor.)

Remedial cleaning is extremely time consuming; Lynda now swears by scum prevention and rinses and wipes her bathtub dry after she bathes.

Removing Mineral Deposits

The minerals from hard water can form rock-hard deposits capable of clogging faucet filters and shower heads.

To unclog a shower head, first remove it from its pipe by holding the incoming pipe stationary with a pliers held in your less dexterous hand, while using your dominant hand to unscrew the shower head with either a channel-lock pliers or a wrench. (One-handed attempts at shower head removal may result in broken or bent pipes.) Then heat a quart of distilled white vinegar in a saucepan, remove the saucepan from the heat, and submerge the shower head in the hot vinegar. Let the shower head soak for at least an hour, or until the deposits have dissolved and water runs freely when poured through the shower head. Rinse the shower head well before reinstalling it.

Clean mineral deposits off of faucets by wrapping them in rags that have been soaked in hot vinegar. Use string or rubber bands to hold the rags in place, then cover the whole mess with a plastic bag to keep it moist. Wait a couple of hours, then remove the rags and scrub the softened deposits off with an old toothbrush.

The wet vinegary rag treatment will also remove rust stains from porcelain.

Cleaning Glass Surfaces

Commercial glass cleaners contain ammonia, which, though it emits potentially irritating fumes, breaks down into pure water and does not leave a residue. Unfortunately, most glass cleaners also contain waxes, which do leave a residue.

Plain vinegar does a wonderful job of cleaning mirrors and other glass, unless that glass is coated with wax. Unless the wax is removed, attempts to clean the glass with plain vinegar will simply smear the wax coating. Here is how to remove the waxy residue left behind by commercial glass cleaners: Pour two cups water and a half cup distilled white vinegar into a spray bottle. Add a half teaspoon dish liquid. Spray on the glass surface, wait half a minute, then polish the glass dry with a clean rag.

After the waxy buildup has been removed, the glass can be cleaned with plain white vinegar.

Nontoxic Mildew Killer

Sometimes, despite your best efforts, a crop of mildew will appear in the bathroom.

- Surface mildew is quite easy to eradicate with full strength white vinegar. If your bathroom walls are growing mildew, wipe the mildewed spot with a vinegary rag. You could also spray on the vinegar, let it sit for a few minutes, then wipe it dry. If the mildew has left a stain, try spraying hydrogen peroxide on the spot, waiting a few minutes, then rubbing the area dry with a clean cloth. Repeat as needed. (Hydrogen peroxide is a bleach, however, and it may change the color of the paint. Test the peroxide on an out-of-the-way area if you are worried about a color change.)
- If you have very persistent patches of mildew, try this: Put some white vinegar in a glass jar and add an inch-long section of copper wire. Let it sit for a few days, then pour the vinegar into a spray bottle, leaving the copper wire behind. (Do not leave the copper in the vinegar longer than a couple of days, or too much copper will dissolve into the vinegar, and you will end up with a solution that will dye your walls a bluish-green.)

  Use the coppery vinegar to clean off the patches of mildew. Copper kills fungi, and the tiny bit of copper that has dissolved into the vinegar will help prevent the mildew from returning. Wipe the walls dry; rinsing is unnecessary.
- Well-established patches of mildew can be scoured off a wall or out of grout with a scrub brush or an old toothbrush dipped in a paste of borax and water. If the mold has penetrated the wall, leave the borax paste on the wall for a couple of days before vacuuming it off. If you allow mildew to grow unmolested for a very long time (years, perhaps), it will penetrate the wall quite deeply. If a coat of stain-sealing paint cannot solve the problem, you may need to replace the wallboard.

Floors

Please read chapter two, "The Kitchen: Mopping Up," page 67, for detailed information on cleaning floors.

Routine Cleaning

Once you have deep-cleaned your bathroom surfaces until they squeak, keeping them clean is quite easy. There is no need to use dangerous disinfectants, antimicrobials, or chlorine cleansers in the bathroom—the same disinfecting techniques that work in the kitchen also work magnificently in the bathroom.

A very good time to clean the bathroom is on a weekend right before you take a bath or shower. If you wash the sink, toilet, and bathroom floor before you bathe, then clean yourself and the shower, you will be able to emerge gleaming and triumphant into a clean bathroom, like Venus on her half shell.

The following steps take about three minutes:

1. Clear everything off the bathroom counter.
2. Sweep the dust and hair off the floor.
3. Use a clean rag, a piece of toilet paper, or a washcloth to wipe the hair off the counter and out of the sink.
4. Spray white vinegar on all the surfaces of the toilet: the lid, front and sides of the tank, the top and bottom of the lid, top and bottom of the seat, and inside and outside the toilet. Pour a little white vinegar in the toilet bowl.
5. Wet a clean rag with warm water and wring it out well, then use it to wipe down the vinegary toilet. If you are squeamish about cleaning toilets, use disposable rags for this job. Waste is ignoble; there is no more honorable end for a clean but holey sock than to be used to clean a toilet, then laid to rest in the garbage can or compost heap.
6. Scrub the toilet bowl with a toilet brush. Flush the toilet, then swish the brush around in the fresh water to clean it off. Replace the brush in its holder.
7. Spray the sink, counter, and faucets with white vinegar. Scrub the sprayed surfaces with the sink scrub brush. Spray the mirror with white vinegar.
8. Wipe the mirror dry with a slightly used towel, then use it to dry

the sink, counter, faucets, and, last of all, the floor, before throwing the well-used towel in the hamper. Put out a fresh towel.

9. Spray the floor with white vinegar, then wipe it dry with another towel. Throw the towel in the hamper. (The official hotel-maid technique is to move the towel around with one foot. Using a Dutch Rubber Broom works just as well.) After the bathroom surfaces dry, all the vinegar smell will disappear, leaving lovely clean air behind.

The Shower

After three minutes of hard cleaning, it will be time to take your shower or bath. Bring the spray bottle of white vinegar into the shower with you. Turn on the water and get the walls and shower door or shower curtain completely wet. Turn off the water and spray all the surfaces with white vinegar, then scrub the surfaces with your shower scrub brush or an old washcloth. Use an old toothbrush to scrub the more inaccessible areas. Turn the water back on and rinse off the walls and door or curtain. Shower as usual, making sure to rinse the blobs of shampoo and hair conditioner or cream rinse off the shower walls and door or curtain. Either squeegee the water off the shower stall or wait until after you have dried yourself, then use your towel to dry off the entire shower. Throw your towel in the hamper, and put out a fresh one.

The Shower Curtain

Vinyl shower curtains and curtain liners are so flimsy and prone to mildew that they really should be considered disposable products.

Woven polyester/nylon shower curtains, which are available at many department stores, are less likely to mildew because they dry very quickly; they are also durable, machine washable, and far more environmentally friendly than the chlorine-based vinyl shower curtains. Throw your nylon shower curtain in the washing machine when it starts to look dingy. Let it drip dry by hanging it back up on the shower curtain rod.

The Tub

It is much easier to clean a tub immediately after someone has taken a bath and softened up the bathtub ring.

Spray white vinegar all over the tub's interior. Scrub the surfaces with a scrub brush. Rinse the tub then dry it off with a towel.

Special Circumstances Cleaning

If you are extremely worried about bathroom sanitation because, for instance, a family member has caught the plague, there is no need to resort to toxic disinfectants or chlorine bleach. The same one-two punch that kills dangerous bacteria in the kitchen (see page 115) will kill them in the bathroom: After you spray your bathroom surfaces with vinegar, follow it with a spray of hydrogen peroxide, then scrub and wipe dry.

If you are expecting a visit from the queen or your in-laws, or you are trying to gussy up your house in order to sell it, here's how you can give your metallic and glass surfaces a high shine: clean the surfaces with vinegar, and dry them thoroughly. Put a little dab of cleaning vodka on a soft, clean, lintless cloth (an old diaper or piece of T-shirt is perfect for this) and polish up the mirrors, faucets, and other shiny surfaces.

Alcohol works wonderfully for polishing purposes, but unfortunately, rubbing alcohol and denatured alcohol are extremely toxic. Cheap vodka is a wonderful substitute because all vodka is high-proof (about 80 proof or 40 percent alcohol), colorless, and has a neutral smell. Though there are alcoholic substances with higher proofs than vodka, most of them are not suitable for cleaning purposes. Cleaning your bathroom with Bacardi Rum or Jack Daniel's Tennessee Whisky is not recommended because they smell like booze and would leave colored stains behind.

Smells

The inevitable stench that periodically fills our bathrooms is a source of great embarrassment for many and a source of great revenue for the manufacturers of air "fresheners" and "deodorizers." Unfortunately, these products are sadly mislabeled. They do not remove odors, nor do they make the air fresh; they simply fill the air with chemicals that overwhelm and desensitize our olfactory cells.

Propane, butane, ethanol, benzene, formaldehyde, acetone, and methanol are just a few of the thousands of volatile, flammable ingredients that are commonly used to help us and our bathrooms look and smell pretty (unless we catch fire!).

Solid air fresheners and deodorizing cakes for urinals, toilet tanks, and toilet bowls may be exceptionally dangerous. Many of these products are essentially solid cakes of mothballs that have been impregnated with fragrance.

Nontoxic Air Freshening

A six-year study conducted by EPA researchers showed that, even in the most heavily industrialized areas, indoor air is far more contaminated than outdoor air. The average resident of industrial Jersey City who is respiring indoors is inhaling between two and five times more hazardous chemicals than he would if he were sitting in a rocking chair on his front porch. The air in an average rural home is between five and ten times more polluted than the air outside. (For more information, please read chapter seven, "Indoor Air Quality," page 278.)

To truly freshen your bathroom, you need to vent the odoriferous air outside. If the weather is warm, open a window and turn on the bathroom exhaust fan.

If you can't open a window, here is a simple, inexpensive, time-honored method for deodorizing bathroom air: Light a match. A lit match will completely consume the odor.

Define Clean

The common conception of personal cleanliness may not coincide well with reality. Though hand washing has been proven to reduce the transmission of communicable diseases and infections, there is no scientific evidence that shows that frequent bathing prevents infections.

Many studies have shown that each of us hosts a unique population of skin-dwelling bacteria. Astonishingly, the type and number of these microbes is not changed by bathing or by abstaining from bathing. In other words, when you return home from a two-week camping trip in the desert, you will have the same number of bacteria on your skin before and after you take your much-needed bath.

Though bathing does not change the number of skin-dwelling bacteria, frequent and vigorous hand washing can cause chapping and actually encourage the growth of dangerous bacteria on the skin. Researchers have shown that frequent washing and harsh detergents can double the number of pathogenic bacteria that live on the skin of the hands.

Normal healthy skin is naturally acidic and is resistant to pathogenic bacteria. Soap is alkaline and tends to reduce the acidity of the skin, leaving it open to colonization by foreign bacteria. Be gentle with your skin! Wash thoroughly but gently after you get your hands dirty.

Try to avoid harsh detergents. Wear rubber gloves when you wash dishes, and use moisturizing lotions and oils frequently.

Personal Care Products

It is not just mechanical damage to the skin that can cause health problems. Many of the common ingredients in skin and hair care products, cosmetics, and toiletries are quite dangerous when absorbed through the skin.

We live in a chemical world and, as a chemist once said to me, "We are chemicals; chemicals are us." Choosing personal care products can be quite confusing, especially since there really is no such thing as a perfectly safe ingredient. The scientific terminology for ordinary substances, such as table salt (sodium chloride, or NaCl), the glycerin that forms when soap is made from natural vegetable oils or animal fats (glyceryl monostearate), and vitamin E (tocopherol), can sound intimidating. Some ingredients that are found in very small amounts in personal care products, such as sodium laureth sulfate, though considered safe when used in diluted form, may cause skin damage if used undiluted. As the label on Dr. Bronner's says: Dilute! Dilute!

Unfortunately, there are so many synthetic chemicals on the market that not even the most brilliant chemist in the world could possibly keep track of them all. Chemical compounds are often given more than one name, and laws protecting "proprietary information" allow manufacturers to keep many of their ingredients secret. This obfuscation means that unless you are buying products that disclose *all* of their ingredients, you have no way of knowing what you are really using. Products with lists of vague ingredients such as "fragrance," "parfum," or "emollients," rather than the individual ingredients, or with lists of active but not inactive ingredients, may have something to hide.

Some Dangerous Common Ingredients in Synthetic Beauty Products

Acetone is a perfect example of a substance that is found in nature, yet is quite dangerous. It is a very volatile chemical that is produced by plants and during forest fires and volcanic eruptions; it is also a byproduct of body fat metabolism. Acetone is a very strong solvent that is commonly used as nail polish remover. It may be acutely toxic if large amounts are swallowed, inhaled, or absorbed through the skin. Acetone exposure can damage the central nervous system and irritate the skin, eyes, and respiratory tract. Animal studies have shown that long-term exposure can cause birth defects; kidney, liver, and nerve damage; and damage to the reproductive system.

Isopropyl alcohol (sometimes known as rubbing alcohol) is sold by the bottle for use as a topical disinfectant and skin rub; it is also a common ingredient in many personal care products. Isopropyl alcohol can cause dermatitis and skin damage; the fumes can cause dizziness, weakness, fatigue, and nausea; and it can cause nausea, vomiting, and diarrhea if swallowed. Chronic overexposure to isopropyl alcohol can cause kidney, liver, and brain damage.

Denatured alcohol is commonly used as a skin disinfectant and for alcohol skin rubs. Denatured alcohol is ethyl alcohol, the same type of alcohol that is found in alcoholic beverages, but law requires that a noxious substance be added to this alcohol to prevent people from drinking it. Most denatured alcohol labels do not identify the denaturing agent. The last bottle of denatured alcohol that we ever bought was cut with acetone. We discovered this through an incendiary accident involving our then-nine-year-old boy, a Waterpik, and a match. Acetone not only has a very characteristic sweet, solvent smell, it also burns much more furiously than does ethyl alcohol.

Glycol ethers such as propylene glycol are found in moisturizers, lotions, perfumes, soaps, shampoos, cream rinses, cosmetics, deodorants, and tooth-paste. It is also used as an antifreeze, in brake and hydraulic fluid, and as a de-icer. It can cause contact dermatitis and kidney and liver damage. If taken internally, it can cause intestinal distress and damage the nervous sys-tem. Would you purposefully put antifreeze under your arms or on your toothbrush?

Formaldehyde is commonly used as a preservative in shampoos, cosmet-ics, nail polish, and embalmed corpses. It is a known carcinogen and causes birth defects in laboratory animals.

Triclosan is the most commonly used antimicrobial. It is found in antimi-crobial toothpaste, deodorant soaps, deodorants, antiperspirants, body washes, detergents, cosmetics, lotions, and hand soaps. It is also found in a large percentage of our surface waters (see page 73).

Some Discouraging Words about Nail Polish and Hair Spray

A study headed by Ruthann Rudel of the Silent Spring Institute, a non-profit organization in Boston, Massachusetts, tested the air and the dust in 120 homes on Cape Cod. The study focused on Cape Cod because the area has elevated rates of breast, colorectal, lung, and prostate cancers.

The researchers found very high levels of eight different phthalates in the dust of all 120 homes. Phthalates are hormonal mimics that confuse the body, which can wreak havoc with the endocrine system and cause cancers and birth defects in animals.

One of these common phthalates [bis(2-ethylhexyl) phthalate (DEHP)] is used in the manufacture of flexible polyvinyl chloride products (PVC), such as shower curtains, shoes, and floor tiles. It is no longer used to manu-facture children's toys because it is considered too dangerous.

Other very common phthalates [dibutylphthalate (DBP), dimethylph-thalate (DMP), and diethylphthalate (DEP)] are used as solvents for fra-grances in perfumes, soaps, shampoos, cream rinses, and lotions, and as plasticizers in nail polish, hair spray, and cosmetics. The researchers also found very high levels of nonylphenols and nonylphenol ethoxylates in the air in these homes. These chemicals are found in some laundry detergents, disinfecting cleaners, all-purpose cleaners, hair dyes, and other hair care products.

The Centers for Disease Control released a report in March 2001 entitled "National Report on Human Exposure to Environmental Chemicals." Through urine testing, researchers determined that young women of reproductive age have very high levels of phthalate contamination. This is not surprising when one looks at the types of products that contain phthalates, but it is frightening news nevertheless because many studies dating back as far as 1985 have shown that phthalates cause birth defects, low sperm counts, and other reproductive damage in laboratory animals.

Phthalates are easily absorbed through the skin when they are applied in the form of nail polish, cosmetics, perfumes, and perfumed products. They are also extremely volatile; the fumes from nail polish, perfumes, and hair sprays are all easily absorbed into the system after they are inhaled. The law does not require ingredient labeling of fragrances and perfumes, so the only personal care products that generally list phthalates as ingredients are nail polishes.

There is no reason to make yourself sick in order to make yourself beautiful.

Homegrown Beauty

Before the advent of modern manufacturing, most householders made their own soap out of animal fat and lye, then they had to soothe their dry, cracked, red hands with vegetable oil, milk, or butter.

If you don't mind the mess, quite a few ordinary food items can be used on the skin and hair to great effect.

Feed Your Skin

There are many foods that can help moisturize your skin. But it is not necessary to sacrifice large amounts of food to the goddess Aphrodite; the leftovers from food preparation will do. Once you know which foods to smear on your face or hands, you will be able to cook and beautify at the same time.

- Plain, unflavored yogurt helps restore the normal acidity to skin, and it makes a good cleanser for oily, acne-prone skin.

- Lemon juice diluted with water makes a good astringent rinse for oily skin.
- Remember Cleopatra in her milk bath? Whole milk makes a good facial cleanser for dry skin. Apply it with a cotton ball, then rinse it off with warm water.
- When you are cooking, moisturize your hands with leftover cooking oil or the residue from the inside of avocado skins.
- Egg white tightens the skin and shrinks the pores. After you break eggs into a frying pan, smooth the slime from the inside of the eggshells on your face. Let the egg white dry, then rinse the dried egg off your face with warm water. Your face will feel remarkably smooth afterward.
- Leftover cooked oatmeal makes a great cleansing mask, and wearing it is certainly more pleasant than eating the stuff!
- Vinegar may be the best all-purpose beauty potion:
  - Wipe or spray your skin with distilled white vinegar or apple cider vinegar to restore its natural acid mantle after dishwashing or bathing.
  - Rinse your hair with vinegar to remove the alkaline deposits left behind by shampoo. The vinegar will smooth your hair and help prevent frizziness.
  - If your skin tends to be dry, try washing yourself with half vinegar and half warm water rather than with soap. The vinegar will help cut body oils and will not dry out your skin. And, no, you will not walk around smelling like a pickle all day. Dried vinegar has no smell.
- Epsom salts and kosher salt are healthy alternatives to commercial bath salts or beads.

There are many excellent books about making your own beauty products. *Natural Beauty at Home* by Janice Cox comes highly recommended.

Beeswax, oils, and other ingredients that can be used in homemade toiletries and cleaning products are available online through www.fromnaturewithlove.com or www.snowdriftfarm.com.

If you prefer your natural beauty products in a bottle rather than in the shell, there are many possibilities:

Organic food markets and health food stores are good places to start looking for more natural and less toxic products. Whenever possible, choose products whose entire list of ingredients is easily comprehensible to you. For instance, here are the ingredients for Dr. Bronner's peppermint castile soap: water, saponified coconut-hemp-olive oils (with retained glycerin), olive fatty acids, peppermint oil, rosemary extract. Website: www.drbronner.com.

Burt's Bees is another company whose products contain all natural ingredients, such as botanical oils and extracts, natural pigments, and beeswax. They manufacture toothpaste, soaps, skin care products, shampoos, hair conditioners, cosmetics, toothpaste, and deodorants. I can easily comprehend all the labels on all their products. In fact, most of their products are composed entirely of edible organic ingredients. Website: www.burtsbees.com.

Tom's of Maine is another environmentally responsible company that manufactures all-natural grooming products such as soap, toothpaste, deodorant, and shampoo. Their products contain botanical extracts as well as natural minerals. Website: www.tomsofmaine.com.

Less Is More

I am not willing to spend all my time searching for the perfectly safe version of every single product I use, nor am I willing to devote my life to concocting these products for myself. Fortunately, one can save a lot of time and footwork by using the Internet to do a little research; many companies

---

❧ VICTORY!

The Organic Consumers Association (OCA) and Dr. Bronner's filed a lawsuit in June 2005, seeking to force the USDA to allow certification of organic body care products. In August 2005, after intense pressure from consumers and businesses who wanted truthful labeling, the USDA agreed to allow certification and labeling of nonfood products that contain no synthetic ingredients and whose natural ingredients meet all national organic standards. Look for personal care products that sport a seal that says USDA Organic. Products without this seal are not made of organic ingredients, no matter how pure and natural their labeling makes them seem.

that produce natural care products have very informative websites that explain their philosophy of business and how they choose ingredients for their products.

Less is more. Most of us tend to use much larger amounts of all our grooming and cleaning products than is necessary. As an old ad used to say: "A little dab'll do ya!" Everything is dangerous when used immoderately: If you eat too much salt, you die; if you drink too much water, you die. Moderation is the key. Read the labels, then choose the products that make you comfortable. Remember that anything other than pure water becomes a pollutant when it goes down the drain.

CHAPTER 4

The Bedroom

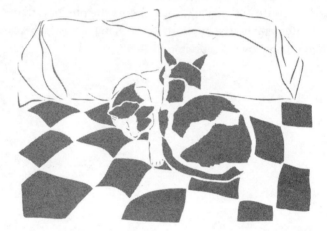

Since the truly interesting things that happen in our bedrooms are well outside the scope of this book, I shall limit myself to writing about keeping the bedroom clean and wholesome.

We spend about a third of our lives asleep, pressing our noses into the bedding and drooling into the pillows. This long and close contact assures that contaminants in the bedding can have profound effects on our lives. Dust mite droppings make allergy sufferers miserable, and fumes from volatile organic compounds (VOCs) in bedroom furniture and carpeting degrade the air quality in our bedrooms. Indoor pollution levels can skyrocket when the windows are kept closed at night due to inclement weather. Even our houseplants, which can greatly improve the indoor air quality during the day, are relatively inactive at night. (No light means no photosynthesis, reduced metabolic rates, and no oxygen production.)

Cleaning Pillows

Down-filled items sustain damage each time they are washed. Zippered slip-cases and pillowcases protect pillows and make them last longer. When, despite your best efforts, your pillows get dirty, they can be machine washed in cold water: Set the machine on the gentle cycle and use a small amount of Woolite or other very gentle detergent.

Old and delicate feather or down pillows may give up the ghost and spew feathers inside the washing machine. Before washing an aged feather or down pillow, zip or tie it securely inside a pillowcase.

If, like me, you sleep best on a pillow that is so ancient and emaciated that you fear for its life if it is subjected to the rigors of the wash cycle, try putting it out in a hard rain, then let it dry in the sun. After its initial rain-washing, put it outside in the daytime and bring it inside at night and during inclement weather until it is fully dry and fluffed and ready to resume service.

Maintaining Down-Filled Comforters, Quilts, and Featherbeds

Tossing these feathery items in the air a couple of times each morning will help maintain their loft. Regular airings outdoors keep down-filled comforters, quilts, and featherbeds fresh-smelling and fluffy: Shake them vigorously, then drape them over a pair of parallel clotheslines, railing, fence, or picnic table (cover the table with a clean sheet or towels) to air them out in the sun. The fresh air and sunshine will make the bedding smell wonderful and the heat of the sun will make the feathers expand. Shake the bedding hard before you bring it back inside.

How Often Should the Bed Linens Be Changed?

In order to inhibit the dust mite population and protect those who suffer from dust mite allergies, bed linens should be changed at least weekly. (Ask your allergist for guidelines.) But if you belong to the allergy-free crowd, your bed linen options are much more flexible. Healthy people generally survive even if their bed linens are changed infrequently. If you are healthy and

---

✎ SOFT AND DUSTY

Researchers have confirmed that the bulk of all inhaled allergens originate in the bed. House dust mite allergens have been linked to the development of asthma in infants, and certainly exacerbate the problem. So, for many years, health professionals advised asthmatics to use safe, hygienic, synthetic-stuffed pillows and comforters rather than down- or feather-filled bedding. Feathers and down, after all, come from birds, and birds are dusty.

The idea seems logical, but unfortunately, it has been proven false: Studies conducted by the Wellington Asthma Research Group in New Zealand have shown that synthetic-filled bedding is more likely to cause or aggravate asthma than feather-filled and down-filled bedding.

The sufferers are probably reacting to the huge numbers of dust mites that dwell in the synthetic stuffing: When researchers measured the concentrations of house dust mite allergens in synthetic-filled versus feather-filled duvets in homes in Wellington, they found that the synthetic bedding contained ten times as much house dust mite allergens as did the feather bedding.

Another study, published in *The New Zealand Medical Journal* in April 2002, showed that synthetic pillows contained about seven times more dust mite allergens than feather pillows.

After these studies, the Wellington Asthma Research Group concentrated on the question of why the synthetic bedding was harboring greater numbers of dust mites, and they discovered that the coverings of synthetic pillows and bed coverings are made of coarser material than are the pillows and comforters stuffed with feathers or down. (Feathers and down are escape artists that can only be contained by finely woven fabric. Synthetic fillings are less active and therefore can be contained within cheaper, more coarsely woven material.) The researchers measured the weave of the materials and found that the average synthetic pillow was covered with fabric that had 57-millimeter-wide spaces between the threads, while the average feather pillow sported fabric with 18-millimeter spaces. The average width of a larval house dust mite is 20 millimeters. So the same fabric that keeps the feathers *in* also keeps the dust mites *out*.

Rob Siebers, a senior research fellow with the Wellington Asthma Research Group, recommended that asthmatics "replace all synthetic bedding with feather bedding."

---

comfortable on sheets that are changed biweekly, monthly, or even yearly, there is no compelling reason to change your practices.

Of course, if some untoward accident has besmirched your snowy linens, it is time to change them. And while we are on the subject of messy bed linens, if you have trouble sleeping when you have a cold and a runny nose,

---

✦ SHEET MANAGEMENT

IDENTIFYING THE SHEETS

If your household goods encompass several different sheet sizes and you have trouble distinguishing between them, here are a couple of suggestions:

1. Choose a single color for each sheet size. For example, blue for king, green for queen, pink for twin, yellow for double. Such color-coding works well if you can remember which color you have chosen for each size. I can stare at newly laundered, gaily patterned sheets that we've owned for the past ten years and be completely unable to remember whether they fit our queen-size bed or our daughter's double bed.
2. Use a laundry-marking pen or permanent marker to mark each corner of each sheet with its size: "T" for twin; "F" for full; "Q" for queen; and "K" for king. This will free you from the ever-annoying game of "Find the Label."

STORING THE SHEETS

If you have been cursed with an inadequate linen closet, try rolling your sheets and towels rather than folding them. Rolled linens require less than half as much storage space as they would need if folded. Rolling the sheets is a rather pleasant two-person operation that looks rather like dancing the minuet: Each partner holds a corner of the short side of the sheet in each hand; each partner closes his/her hands together to fold the sheet in half lengthwise, then grasps one folded corner in each hand and repeats the step. The sheet is now folded twice lengthwise. Now one partner stands still and keeps the sheet taut while the other partner rolls the sheet as tightly as possible.

If your linen closet is still inadequate even for rolled linens, try storing the bedclothes in the room where they will be used. If you have absolutely no closet space, shelf space, or room for an under-the-bed drawer or storage box, try storing extra blankets and linens by laying them out flat between the mattress and box spring.

try folding a clean terrycloth towel around your pillow; the absorbent terrycloth will wick the wetness away from your nose and may make you comfortable enough to sleep.

Blankets and Comforters

Woolen blankets are naturally flame-resistant and nontoxic, and down or feather comforters have been proven more wholesome than synthetic bedding for those with dust allergies. Both of these natural choices will stay cleaner and more dust-free if you cover them with a duvet cover. It is easy to make a duvet cover out of two flat sheets that are one size bigger than your bed (for example, if you have a full-size bed, buy two queen-size flat sheets). Pin the top and both sides of the sheets together, right sides together. Stop pinning the sides of the sheets four inches above the bottom hem. Two inches above the bottom hem, fold up the bottom of one of the sheets, wrong sides together, and pin the new hem at the sides of the sheets so the folded sheet forms a pocket and the unfolded sheet hangs down two inches below it. Sew the sheets together at the top and sides. Turn the new duvet cover right side out, and attach the fasteners of your choice (ribbon ties, Velcro, or buttons and buttonholes) to the top and bottom sheets at the bottom of the duvet so that after the blanket is inserted into the duvet cover, the cover can be closed like an envelope.

You can impress your family with your prowess at inserting a blanket or comforter into a duvet cover with this nifty little trick: Lay the blanket or comforter down across the bed, turn the duvet cover inside out, and lay it out over the blanket or comforter. Reach inside the duvet cover until you can grasp both top corners of the blanket or comforter so you are holding one pair of corners in each hand. Grip hard and, with a graceful swishing motion, invert the duvet cover so it lands right-side out. Arrange the bottom of the blanket or comforter so it is nestled inside the bottom pocket of the duvet cover, flap the longer side of the cover across the bottom opening, then tie, snap, or button the fasteners.

Blanket Maintenance

Blankets should be aired out at least twice a year: before you put them on the bed for the season and after you take them off for the season. If you are a city dweller who cannot air your woolen blankets outdoors, you may need to bring them to a Green cleaner once a year.

Mattresses

Fire "Safe" but Still Dangerous

Most mattresses contain polyurethane foam that must be treated with flame retardants in order to meet stringent fire-safety codes. The most common flame retardants are PBDEs (polybrominated diphenyl ethers), which have been classified as persistent organic pollutants (POPs). This classification puts them in the same category as the already banned PCBs (polychlorinated biphenyls), and DDT (dichlorodiphenyltrichloroethane). When ingested or absorbed, the flame-slowing PBDEs, like all other POPs, build up in fatty tissue and can cause birth defects and reproductive damage.

PBDEs also have a nasty tendency to migrate, and they have been detected in ever increasing concentrations in remote Arctic lakes as well as in mothers' milk. Arnold Schecter, an environmental sciences professor at the University of Texas School of Public Health in Dallas, coauthored a study of PBDE contamination in supermarket foods. Schecter and his colleagues analyzed food samples from major supermarkets in Dallas and found that *all* the food that contained animal fats was contaminated with PBDE. Schecter said: "Although these findings are preliminary, they suggest that food is a major route of intake for PBDEs."

The current theory about how PBDEs get into our food is that particles (also known as dust) escape from the flame-resistant mattresses, furniture, electrical equipment, computers, and televisions. These pesky particles fall to the ground and into the water, where animals ingest them.

The levels of PBDEs found in U.S. groceries were nine to twenty times higher than levels found in Spanish or Japanese groceries. This is not surprising, since the United States uses more PBDEs than do other countries. PBDEs were banned in Europe in 2004.

Unstained Yet Unhealthy

Most mattresses are also chemically treated for stain and water repellence. Slick, durable chemicals—such as Teflon and Scotchgard (and PCBs, those hardy, fire-resistant lubricants and insulators that were so admirably useful until they were banned in 1977)—are environmentally dangerous because of the very properties that make them so useful: They don't biodegrade.

Choosing a Mattress

Natural mattresses and box springs made with organic cotton, wool, or natural latex padding tend to be rather expensive compared to standard mattress sets. A pure wool– or pure cotton–stuffed futon is probably the only inexpensive, nontoxic alternative. Futons, and the people who sleep on top of them, benefit greatly if the futon is dragged out into the fresh air and beaten on a regular basis.

If a futon mattress is too hard, put a feather bed or a washable shearling-wool mattress pad on top of it to add an extra layer of give. It is much easier to wash these mattress-toppers than it is to wash a futon.

Eventually your aged futon, like all its cottony predecessors, will become so thoroughly flattened that it must be allowed to return to the earth from whence it came. This is the true beauty of a futon: Since it is made entirely of cotton, it can be safely disposed of in a compost pile, whereas regular mattresses must be sent to the landfill.

If you need a regular mattress and box spring in order to sleep soundly, learn to say no to mattress salesmen who are trying to sell you extra protection against dust mites, spills, and stains. These additional treatments will only add to the contaminants wafting out of your new mattress.

If you have a dust mite allergy, you might want to replace your innerspring mattress, which harbors significantly more dust mites than do solid, natural-rubber (latex) foam mattresses.

The recent spate of negative publicity about dust mites has encouraged a thriving industry that revolves around discouraging dust mites; toward this end, many mattresses are treated with a miticide in order to kill the dreaded dust mite. Human beings have coexisted quite happily and healthily with dust mites for millennia. Unless you are severely allergic to dust mites, there is no reason to worry about the minuscule creatures at all.

Keeping It Covered

A high-quality mattress cover made of high-thread-count cotton will protect your mattress from stains and from allergies caused by dust mites.

The thread count refers to the number of horizontal and vertical threads per square inch of fabric. The higher the thread count, the more threads there are and the smaller the gaps are between the threads; a thread count of 260 or higher is necessary for feather- and dust-proof mattress and pillow covers.

Choose 100 percent cotton covers; cotton/polyester blends are almost inevitably treated with permanent-press resins. To help make these items more affordable, look for sales on discontinued or slightly irregular luxury cotton covers.

Keep It Dry

House dust mites thrive in humid conditions. If someone in your family is suffering from dust mite allergies, give away the humidifier and use a dehumidifier during the humid season.

Mattress Flipping

Mattress flipping and mattress rotating are parts of a mattress-maintenance routine that prolong the lives of mattresses and help prevent the mattress from forming permanent impressions of your and your beloved's bodies.

Here's how:

1. Follow the manufacturer's recommendations about flipping frequency.
2. Don't bend, fold, drag, or drop your mattress. Most mattresses that are not made entirely of foam, cotton, or wool are framed by a border wire that can get permanently bent out of shape.

3. Remove the mattress cover and vacuum the top and sides of the mattress before you flip or rotate it. Launder the mattress cover.
4. Those handles on the sides of your mattress are there for a reason; use them whenever you are moving your mattress. Mattresses can be extremely unwieldy, and mattress flipping is generally a job that requires two people. (Flipping and fluffing a futon can be quite strenuous, and may require more than two people.)
5. Rotate the mattress by grasping its handles and moving it until the head section is over the foot of the box spring or platform. Realign the sides of the mattress with the box spring or bed frame.
6. Flip the mattress by grasping the handles and pulling the mattress so it is hanging halfway off the box spring or platform. Stand the mattress up on its edge in the middle of the box spring or platform, then lower it to expose the underside. Center the flipped mattress back into position.

Note: If you like sleeping in a nest that conforms perfectly to your body, don't flip your mattress. I never flip mine. If you like a really soft nest, try a featherbed.

BABY BEDS

Bedtime can be quite hazardous for very young babies. Sudden Infant Death Syndrome (SIDS) is the most common cause of death for infants between the ages of one month and one year. Research has shown that soft mattresses, washable sheepskins, waterbeds, cushions, pillows, loose or fluffy bed coverings, and stuffed toys can cover a baby's face and impede her breathing.

Here is a list of recommended infant bedding: The bottom layer should be a firm mattress in a safety approved crib. The middle layer should be a waterproof mattress pad, preferably a nontoxic one made of rubber or wool. The top layer should be a tightly fitted sheet. That's all, folks!

All the warmth the baby needs should be provided by her seasonally appropriate, sleekly fitted sleepwear.

Visit the Consumer Product Safety Commission's website for the most recent information on crib safety: www.cpsc.gov.

Stain Prevention

A washable mattress pad puts an absorbent extra layer between an expensive mattress and the moist and messy humans who sleep on top of it. Since young humans are often excessively moist, it is a good idea to cover a toddler's mattress with a waterproof cover, then put the mattress pad on top of it. Cotton-covered rubber mats are the most comfortable, durable, and easily washed.

Odor Eradication

Here are some useful stench- and stain-eradication techniques for the accident-prone mattress:

Urine
- If your toddler or puppy has marked your mattress with urine, dampen the offending spot with water, then sprinkle borax over it. Rub the borax into the spot, let it dry, then vacuum up the dried borax.
- Or dampen the spot with vinegar and water, then pour on baking soda and rub it in well. Let the spot dry, then vacuum up the dried baking soda.
- Or use a bioenzymatic pet odor neutralizer. Follow the directions on the label. The enzymes in these products actually digest and eliminate animal-based stains and odors. Enzyme-based pet odor eliminators are available at pet stores as well as at do-it-yourself building centers.

Enzyme odor eliminators are the safest and most effective odor neutralizers on the market. Chemically based "odor neutralizers" do nothing to actually break down and eliminate odoriferous molecules.

Vomit or Feces
- Scrape off the solids, then treat the spot with a bioenzymatic odor neutralizer. Follow the directions on the package label.

- Or scrape off the solids, then treat the spot with vinegar and baking soda. Wait until the fizzing stops, then blot the liquid up with a clean, dry, absorbent rag. Repeat as necessary.

Blood
- Sponge off as much of the stain as possible with cold water and a little bit of castile soap, wiping from the outside of the stain toward the inside. Soak up the excess moisture with a clean, dry cloth. Repeat as necessary.
- Or after you have sponged off as much of the blood as possible, pour a capful of straight 3 percent hydrogen peroxide on the stain and let dry.
- Or after you have sponged up the blood, use a bioenzymatic cleaner to eradicate the blood stain.

Well-Preserved but Unhealthy

Formaldehyde is useful for preserving the dead, but it is not so good for those of us who are still breathing. Unfortunately, many modern materials emit formaldehyde fumes for several years after they are installed . . .

Sheets and Pillowcases

Permanent-press, wrinkle free, or easy care cotton or cotton blend sheets are treated with resins that contain formaldehyde. Until these sheets have been washed enough times that they are capable of wrinkling, they can emit formaldehyde fumes. This makes old sheets preferable to the vast majority of new sheets.

Natural cotton sheets are usually more expensive than the permanent-press variety, but there are two inexpensive exceptions: cotton flannel sheets and those made of cotton knit T-shirt material. These fabrics are not treated with resins because they are meant to be soft, not crisp.

Linen sheets are organic, and though they may need ironing and can be quite expensive, they are so durable that they may outlast their owners. (I like to think of linen sheets as the parrots of the bedding world; parrots are far more expensive than parakeets, but parrots can live for 150 years, while parakeets fall off the perch at age ten.)

Clean Air Choices

If weather permits, keep a couple of bedroom windows open at night in order to prevent the build-up of toxins in your bedroom. Reducing these toxic vapors (No, I'm not talking about the vapors emitted by bean-eaters . . .) can greatly improve your comfort and health.

A nontoxic bedroom makes heavy breathing a much safer activity.

🐝 NONTOXIC BEDROOM SUMMARY

DUST REDUCTION

1. Replace synthetic-filled pillows and comforters with feather- or down-filled pillows and comforters.
2. Protect pillows, comforters, and blankets with tightly woven washable cotton covers.
3. Please refer to chapter six for more information on dusting and general cleaning techniques.

FUME REDUCTION

1. The finishing resins in many permanent-press or easy care fabrics emit formaldehyde fumes. Avoid buying permanent-press or easy care cotton/polyester sheets. Cotton flannel and knit cotton T-shirt sheets are not treated with resins.
2. American-made mattresses are frequently treated with flame retardants, miticides, and stain repellents, all of which may be harmful. Mattresses that are filled with cotton, wool, or pure latex foam are nontoxic, though expensive. A cotton-filled futon is an inexpensive alternative.
3. See chapter six, "General Cleaning," page 229, for information on choosing nontoxic bedroom furniture, flooring, carpeting, draperies, wall coverings, and other furnishings.

CHAPTER 5

Laundry

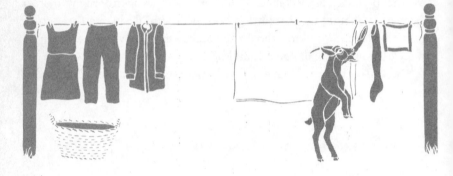

Great-Grandma's Washday

Before the invention of the electric washing machine in 1908, washing clothes was a strenuous and almost solely feminine endeavor. Washing and rinsing a single load of clothes required approximately fifty gallons of water (four hundred pounds), which generally had to be carried in buckets from the pump or well to the wash boiler. Over the course of several hours, the clothes were boiled clean over a hot fire. Stirring the wet, heavy clothes, wringing them out, then hanging them up to dry was hot, heavy, exhausting work. Doing the wash took up an entire day.

The day after washday, the clothes were ironed with heavy clothes irons that were heated on the stove. In those days, ironing was a necessity, not a luxury: After being boiled and wrung out, the cotton or linen clothes were so severely wrinkled and malformed that they were impossible to wear unless they were ironed and stretched back into shape.

The Beauty of the Lowered Standard

The drudgery of washday is something that we contemporary Americans cannot truly comprehend. We are no longer in danger of dying of laundry-induced exhaustion, but that is not a good enough reason to wantonly increase our wash loads. Instead of taking the extra free time and running with it, we have increased the amount of laundry we are doing. Rather than spending a single week day doing laundry, we have spread laundry chores across the entire week. According to Harvard economist Juliet Schor, the amount of time the average householder spent doing laundry increased after the advent of the modern washing machine and dryer.

Sometimes, because we are not paying attention to a chore that no longer requires enormous outputs of time and energy, we make extra work for ourselves. For instance, clean, damp laundry, if allowed to sit in the washing machine long enough, will become dirty, mildewed laundry that needs to be rewashed. Clean, dry, unfolded laundry, if allowed to sit in the dryer or clean clothes basket long enough, will acquire wrinkles. And last but not least, clean laundry that is sitting in a basket in a child's room may be thrown back into the dirty laundry hamper by a child who is too lazy to put his clothes away.

Great-grandma's laundry aids were homemade soap, boiling water, sunshine, and elbow grease. She made the soap herself by boiling down animal fat with lye extracted from wood ashes. By the end of washday, great-grandma was exhausted, and the harsh, homemade lye soap had made her hands rough, red, and sometimes even bloody. Our washdays are no longer physically exhausting, thanks to indoor plumbing, automatic washing machines, and store-bought detergents, but the synthetic ingredients in detergents can damage us as well as our environment. Armed with just a little knowledge, we can have the best of all possible washdays—and save time, money, and resources by utilizing machinery and techniques simple enough that a ten-year-old can run a family's laundry.

Modern automatic washers and dryers are very effective; when used correctly with the proper settings, the laundry that emerges from them is clean and germ-free and has sustained remarkably little damage, though it is perhaps not as blindingly white as the laundry that our great-grandmothers boiled for a day with harsh lye soap. It is high time we started creatively lowering our standards so we can take full advantage of our push-button washing capabilities. If we can cease our fretting over whether our laundry is white enough to dazzle our rivals—either with envy or by blinding them—we may be able to carve large chunks of time out of our laundry chores.

Choosing the Equipment

Top-loading washing machines use agitators to swish clothes back and forth through the wash water; a large top-loading machine may use up to forty-four gallons of water per load. Front-loading washing machines (also known as horizontal-axis or tumble-action) spin clothes horizontally through the wash water. The most efficient front-loading machines (made by ASKO, a Swedish company) use as little as 5.7 gallons of water per load. (American manufacturers make efficient front-loading machines, but none are quite as efficient as those made by ASKO and most are more expensive.) An average household that is using a front-loading washing machine can save up to 16,000 gallons of water per year as well as greatly reduce its energy costs.

The spinning action of front-loading washing machines is easier on clothes, and the very fast spin cycles of front-loading washing machines extract water from laundry quite efficiently, greatly reducing dryer times. According to a fascinating article entitled "Facts about Laundry" published by *Laundry & Cleaning Today*, a typical top-loading machine can leave a load of towels damp enough to need forty minutes in a tumble dryer, while a high-speed front-loading machine can extract enough water to cut that drying time in half.

We have had the pleasure of owning an ASKO washing machine for more than five years, and I have discovered that if I send the wash through an extra spin cycle, it emerges from the washing machine barely damp, needing very little time in the dryer. That extra twirl through the spin cycle is quite efficient; a front-loading washing machine uses far less energy than does a clothes dryer.

Compared to washing machines, clothes dryers are fairly simple. The best clothes dryers have moisture sensors that automatically stop the machine when the clothes are dry; this feature protects clothes from heat damage, saves energy, and helps prevent dryer fires. When buying a new dryer, choose an efficient one that fits your needs and has been given an Energy Star recommendation. (For more information on the Energy Star program, see page 84.)

A Few Words About Lint

Most lint is composed of tiny bits of fuzz that have worn off fabrics in the washer and dryer. The rougher the action of the machine and the more the fabrics are damaged, the greater the volume of lint that will be produced. The use of chlorine bleach can also greatly increase the amount of lint created, as chlorine weakens and damages fabrics.

Lint can be more than simply annoying. If it is allowed to build up in the dryer vent, it becomes a fire hazard. According to the National Fire Protection Association (NFPA), in the mid-1990s clothes dryers caused an average of 14,800 home fires annually, and these dryer fires caused an average of 16 deaths, 309 injuries, and $75.8 million in property damage.

Many of these fires were caused by excessive lint build-up in exhaust vent pipes. The vent pipe removes excess heat and moisture from the dryer and dumps it outside the house. If the vent pipe becomes clogged with lint, the dryer starts working harder and hotter as it strains to remove the trapped moisture. Unfortunately, it doesn't take long for a pile of hot lint to become flaming lint.

Dryer Fire Prevention

1. Clean the lint filter and wipe lint off the inside of the dryer drum each time the dryer is used. Never start a dryer without checking to make sure that the filter is clean.
2. Never run the dryer without its lint filter.
3. Store combustible items, such as piles of dirty clothes, cardboard boxes, stacks of newspaper, and cans of paint and solvent, well away from the dryer.
4. Periodically check to make sure the outdoor vent flap opens easily. (It is also an excellent idea to install a rodent-proof screen

over the whole outdoor assembly. When the chipmunk hits the fan, the results are spectacularly grisly.)

5. Exhaust pipes should be as short and as straight as possible so they don't catch excessive amounts of lint. Because they are smooth and nonflammable, sheet metal vent pipes are the safest. If you can't use sheet metal pipes, choose flexible metal exhaust pipes. Plastic or vinyl exhaust pipes are not considered safe.

6. At least once a year, clean out the exhaust pipe and the exhaust outlet of the dryer. The ribbed surface of a flexible metal pipe will catch far more lint than the smooth surface of a sheet metal pipe, so if you have flexible pipe, it may need to be cleaned more often.

    How to clean out a dryer exhaust pipe:

    a. Unclamp the pipe from the back of the dryer.

    b. Put a dusting brush on the end of your most flexible vacuum cleaner hose.

    c. Turn on the vacuum and snake the vacuum cleaner brush up the disconnected exhaust pipe.

    d. If the exhaust pipe is badly clogged, you might want to replace it with new pipe, which is quite inexpensive.

Washing Machine Lint

Though a washing machine is unlikely to ignite, the lint that washes out with the rinse water can clog waste pipes and septic systems. Putting a mesh trap on the end of the outlet hose will avert both of these potential problems. Hardware stores sell both metal and plastic lint traps.

Plastic mesh orange or onion bags also make excellent lint traps: Just slide one over the end of the washer outlet hose and clamp the bag on with a thick rubber band or a plastic fastener from a garbage bag.

Water and Energy Use

A warm water wash followed by a cold water rinse uses a third less energy than a hot wash followed by a warm rinse. Washing a full load of laundry is more energy efficient than washing a partial load.

Ironing is not a particularly energy efficient way to dry clothes, but if you iron clothes that have just been spun nearly dry by a high RPM front-loading washing machine, you will achieve maximum ironing efficiency. (I wouldn't dare let my damp clothes sit in a plastic bag until I got around to ironing them. While they waited they would probably be completely consumed by mildew, or, if they begin to decompose, could catch fire when the bag was opened. For more information, see "Red Hot Laundry" on page 331. The only thing I iron regularly is the waxy bottoms of cross-country skis.)

Sorting

Though diversity is generally a virtue, laundry should be segregated before it is washed.

By Color, Three Degrees of Separation

Most fabric dyes will bleed color into the wash water for at least the first few washings. Some dark and brightly colored fabrics (especially reds) will bleed dye until the day they die. The only way to avoid accidentally dying your clothing pink, mauve, or lavender is to wash similar colors together. I like to separate my clothes into three color-coded piles: light (white, yellow, and pastels), black-and-blue, and red-and-pink.

The cooler the wash water, the less the dye will bleed. White fabrics and heavily soiled fabrics can be washed in hot water, but brightly colored or dark fabrics should be washed in warm or cool water.

By Sturdiness, Two Degrees of Separation

Protect delicate items such as lingerie, loosely knit sweaters, and clothing with delicate trim or lace by separating them from the tough, heavy, sturdy fabrics such as denim, heavy corduroy, and cotton duck. Wash these dainty items in cool water, and choose the delicate or hand wash cycle.

It is perfectly safe to wash clothing in cooler water, using gentler washing machine settings than the manufacturer recommends, but one should try to avoid subjecting clothing to hotter temperatures and rougher handling than recommended. When in doubt, read the label.

By Dirtiness, Four Degrees of Separation

Due to the nature of our vocations and avocations, our family has been washing at least one full load of filthy, grimy, and often reeking laundry every week for the last twenty years. We have learned to separate the nearly clean wash loads from the gritty, the dirty, the greasy, and the rank.

Heavily soiled clothing needs to be washed vigorously in hot water, while lightly soiled clothing may be clean after being lightly swished through lukewarm, soapy water. There is no point in throwing a barely worn white T-shirt in the washing machine with a mud-caked pair of sweat socks; the ultimate result may be a cleaner pair of socks and a dirtier T-shirt.

Here are the categories for degree of dirtiness. The following should be washed only with their own kind. Categories one through three need to be washed in hot water:

1. Heavily soiled work clothes and play clothes that are caked or impregnated with mud, dirt, sand, limestone, fertilizer, manure, compost, paint, etc.

COLOR SEPARATION

1. White and Light Pastels
2. Black, Blue, and Green
3. Red, Pink, Orange, and Purple

TOUGH SEPARATION

1. Wash Delicates Together
2. Wash Tough Fabrics Together

DO SEPARATE LOADS FOR THE FOLLOWING

1. Lightly soiled items
2. Filthy items
3. Dirty work clothes
4. Kitchen laundry
5. Cleaning rags
6. Diapers
7. Large heavy items (A single quilt or a single sleeping bag makes a full load.)
8. Fuzzy items such as chenille, corduroy, flannel, and new terrycloth (Never wash synthetic clothing with fuzzy items. Synthetic fabrics such as polyester fleece are lint magnets.)

2. Diapers, soiled baby clothes, soiled bed linens.
3. Kitchen towels, napkins, tablecloths, placemats, dishcloths, cleaning rags.
4. Everything else.

Hampering Rips, Tears, Stains, and Broken Zippers

A lot of damage can be prevented if you batten down the hatches before throwing clothing in the washing machine:

1. Close fasteners. Open zippers can inflict and sustain a lot of damage in the washing machine and dryer; not only can they snag and tear fabric, they may also be damaged beyond repair by the force of the washing machine and dryer. Fasten hooks, snaps, and Velcro fasteners to prevent tangling and snagging. Remove pins and belts.
2. Empty pockets. Foreign objects left in pockets can cause problems in the wash cycle or dryer: A single tissue left in a pocket can create enough paper lint to cover an entire load of laundry; washed pens, chocolates, and lipsticks can cause impressive stains; nails, screws, and staples can rip holes in clothing and damage the interior of the washer or dryer; pocket watches and penknives may cease to function after being washed. Try to remember to empty the pockets before you throw items in the hamper.
3. Shake out dirt. Before you throw those clothes in the hamper, try to remember to unroll cuffs and socks and shake the dirt and sand out of them. Scrape off mud or caked-on dirt. Impressively filthy clothing should be presoaked and wrung out before it is put in the washing machine.
4. Mend first, wash later. The tumbling and agitation of washing machines and dryers will enlarge holes and tears and induce fraying; if you want to reduce your mending chores, repair your clothes before you launder them, rather than after.

Inside Out

The stress induced by a washing machine or dryer can make some garments old before their time. The following items will last longer if they are turned inside out before they are laundered:

1. Articles of clothing with attached belts, ties, or strings that may get tangled.
2. Clothing that is embellished with delicate trims, lace, hooks, or fancy buttons that are easily damaged; further protect these items by laundering them inside a zippered mesh lingerie bag or tied-shut pillowcase. Wash delicates in cold water and set the machine to the gentle or hand wash setting.
3. Anything made out of napped or fuzzy fabrics, such as corduroy, chenille, velveteen, or polyester fleece; turning these items inside out will protect the nap from excessive wear.
4. Black jeans; inverted washing will help prevent them from turning prematurely gray.
5. Brightly colored clothing and printed T-shirts.

Washing Frequency

In the days before vacuum cleaners, most homes sheltered populations of unpleasant insect life such as fleas and bedbugs. These insects were controlled through frequent washing and changing of bed linens and thorough spring cleaning, which included restuffing mattresses and painting entire beds (frames, head- and footboards, and each individual bedspring) with kerosene to kill the bedbugs.

Most modern homes are free of these tiny, bloodsucking vermin, so unless one of your family members has a nasty communicable skin disease, it is highly unlikely that anyone will fall ill if the towels and sheets are not changed every day, every other day, every week, or even once a month. And bed linens certainly stay cleaner when they are slept in by pajama-wearing office workers who bathe daily, than they did in the old days when everyone did farm work and bathed only on Sundays.

If everyone in your household is mature enough to wash all the dirt off before they dry themselves, changing your towels once a week is more than adequate. But if the weather is so humid that the hand towels never dry on the rack, you may want to change them every day.

A safety manual entitled *Guidelines for Laundry in Health Care Facilities*, released by the Centers for Disease Control and Prevention (CDC), states "Although soiled linen has been identified as a source of large numbers of pathogenic microorganisms, the risk of actual disease transmission appears negligible."

Unnecessary cleaning wears out people as well as their belongings. Change your linens often enough to keep yourself comfortable, but if it ain't dirty, don't clean it.

Caveat: If you have family members with dust allergies, please disregard my linen-changing opinions. Follow the advice of your allergist about how often to change your linens.

Soap vs. Detergent

Laundry soap is made of animal fat, vegetable oil, and lye; pure soap is environmentally benign, but it tends to leave a residue when used with hard water. Though this residue acts as a fabric softener, it can interfere with the flame-proofing of children's clothing. The only true laundry soap still on the market is Fels Naptha, which is sold in bars or in grated flakes. It is a harsh, animal-fat-based soap, which also contains cleaners, soil and stain removers, chelating agents, colorants, and perfume. All other commercial laundry soaps are actually detergents.

Detergents are designed to rinse completely out of fabrics without leaving a residue behind. Laundry detergents are so effective that they have essentially squeezed laundry soaps right off the market (that old standby, Ivory Flakes, disappeared from market shelves in 1978).

Detergents can contain the following components: surfactants, which help dissolve oil or grease; builders, which soften water and increase the efficiency of detergents; bleaches, which fade stains; optical brighteners, which make clothing glow in the dark (and appear blindingly bright in the daylight); enzymes, which digest organic stains; and solvents, which help dissolve dirt.

The Environmental Protection Agency has analyzed these components and has made recommendations about which detergent ingredients to avoid and which are harmless.

Harmful Detergent Additives

Here are the most common of the additives that are considered dangerous:

Alkyphenol ethoxylates are surfactants. They are persistent in the environment and may damage aquatic ecosystems. Alkyphenols are endocrine disrupters and are considered persistent organic pollutants (POPs), a category composed solely of chemicals that are extremely toxic, that travel far from their origins, and are quite resistant to decomposition. Other POPs, such as PCBs, dioxins, and DDT, have already been banned through international treaties.

Phosphates are builders. They overfertilize the algae in lakes and ponds. Then when the overabundant algae dies and begins to decompose, it uses up all the oxygen in the water, killing the fish and other aquatic animals.

Sodium hypochlorite is also known as chlorine bleach. It can react with other chemicals to release poisonous gas, and it can combine with organic materials to form dangerous chlorinated organic compounds.

Fragrances or *perfumes* may exacerbate allergies and asthma.

Harmless Detergent Additives

Alcohol ethoxylates or betaine esters (surfactants)
Zeolites (builders)
Hydrogen peroxide or ozone (bleach)
Propylene glycol ethers (solvent)
Enzymes (stain removers)

Natural Detergents

Natural or environmentally friendly detergents are designed to prevent environmental and health problems. They should not contain petroleum products, should be phosphate free (phosphate is a water-pollutant), and should contain no chlorine, fabric brighteners, fragrances, or dyes.

Powdered natural detergents, which usually contain washing soda (sodium carbonate), sodium percarbonate, borax (sodium borate), and often some coconut-oil based surfactants, can be found at natural food stores and whole foods co-ops.

Liquid natural detergents are usually plant based. Many of them contain citrus-based cleaners or fragrance.

I once spent several miserable and unsightly months because my husband had bought a citrus-scented natural detergent rather than our usual unscented natural detergent. Eventually I finished the book I was working on, went down to the laundry room, and realized that my innocent husband and children had been inadvertently irritating me every time they did the laundry. If you have sensitive skin, I recommend unscented, mineral-based detergents. Most allergic reactions are triggered by reactions to organic substances, not to minerals.

But, you may ask, what about reactions to chemicals? An allergy is an overreaction to an otherwise harmless substance. For instance, I can comfortably pet a cat, but my friend Ed cannot. When people are sickened by exposure to toxic substances, they are not having allergic reactions, they are being poisoned. It is incorrect to say of a man whose wife was lacing his hot cocoa with arsenic: "Mr. Jones died of an arsenic allergy." This would be the correct statement: "Mr. Jones died of arsenic poisoning." Similarly, it is incorrect to say that your aunt is allergic to the formaldehyde in perfume, since formaldehyde is poisonous. We are all damaged by these chemical toxins; it's just that some of us can tell when we are being poisoned, while others cannot.

A Tribute to Canaries

In the olden days, miners carried caged canaries down into the mines with them so the birds could serve as an early warning system: If the birds were healthy, the air was clean; if the birds died, the miners knew that toxic gases were building up, so they headed for the surface as quickly as possible.

The majority of laundry products are very heavily scented. It is all too easy for those of us who appear immune to the unpleasant symptoms of chemical sensitivity to ridicule those who are affected by the fumes wafting from dryer vents. But people differ greatly in their response to chemicals. Those who are genetically resistant to one chemical may be extraordinarily susceptible to damage induced by another. It is possible that the "human canaries" who tear up, sneeze, and wheeze when they are exposed to domestic chemicals are the lucky ones; they tend to avoid the long-term exposure that may induce chronic health problems such as liver and kidney damage, infertility, or cancer.

Maybe I'm just old-fashioned, but no matter how pretty it smells or how soft it feels, I don't consider anything clean if it can cause permanent health problems.

Recommended Natural Detergents

Full disclosure: My skin is very reactive and I am unwilling to test different brands of detergent at the risk of getting hives. Any fragrance, no matter how naturally derived, makes me itch.

Dianna von Rabenau, the proprietress of The Green Mercantile, a charming little natural department store, was my source for these recommendations. If you cannot buy these products locally, they can be ordered through www.greenmercantile.com.

Liquid

Restore Laundry Detergent is Dianna's favorite. It is concentrated, plant-based, perfume-free, biodegradable, and effective.

Shaklee's Liquid-L Laundry Concentrate is plant-based and contains enzymes (can also be used as an enzyme pretreatment).

Powder

Earth Friendly ECOS powder laundry detergent is mineral based.

Natural Choices Oxy-Prime powdered laundry detergent is mineral-based and contains oxygen bleach.

Country Save detergent is the brand I use. It is mineral-based, completely free of perfume, and keeps me comfortable.

These detergents are available at many natural food stores; they can also be ordered online.

User Precautions

Avoid breathing dust from powdered detergents; no matter how natural they are, they are still very strong chemicals. If you spill some on your skin, rinse, rinse, rinse!

Always use the smallest amount of detergent that will get your laundry clean. Excess detergent can be difficult to rinse out, and may make your laundry gray and dingy.

Front-loading machines require the use of low-sudsing detergents (also known as High Efficiency, or HE detergents) in very small amounts. Standard or high-sudsing detergents in a front-loading washing machine can wreak frothy havoc worthy of *I Love Lucy*.

Anything but White . . .

Keeping white laundry white can be a difficult, destructive business: Most commercial laundry bleach contains chlorine, which is one of the most dangerous and reactive elements on the planet. Not only is it a human and environmental health hazard, it also damages fabrics and makes them wear out far more quickly.

Many natural fabrics yellow as they age: Polyester fabric tends to turn gray. Attempting to keep white fabrics white can be a frustrating as well as a time- and resource-consuming endeavor. Why not splurge a little and buy a brand new shirt or blouse to wear on those rare occasions for which you must be kitted out in snowy white? After the shirt has served its purpose, let it follow the natural trajectory for a white garment as it degenerates from a snow-white dress shirt, to a functionally white office shirt, to an off-white work shirt with a few minor spots, to a gardening shirt with grass and dirt stains, to a paint shirt, to a rag, then to its final resting place in the compost pile or the trash.

Why not choose off-white or colored clothing, towels, and bedding, and make your life simpler and easier? After I mentioned this idea to a friend of

‌ PRODUCT SAFETY

Almost all of the heavily advertised detergents and laundry aids contain at least one harmful detergent additive. Many contain more than one. If you want to check up on your brand of detergent, go online to a search engine and type in the name followed by the letters MSDS, like so: Country Save Detergent MSDS. Many listings will pop up.

MSDS stands for Material Safety Data Sheet. Federal law requires that safety information be made available for all chemical products. The MSDS should list the potential hazards contained in your brand of detergent. *Never* use any product that has an incomplete or uninformative MSDS. The following pathetic MSDS specimen contains the information divulged by the manufacturer of an extremely well-known fabric softener. The product name is being withheld in order to protect the disingenuous:

Chronic Health Effects: MSDS: No chronic effects are given.

Carcinogenicity: Carcinogenicity cannot be predicted from information in the manufacturer's Material Safety Data Sheet (MSDS) because no actual chemical ingredients are listed . . .

Health Rating: N (No information provided by manufacturer)

Flammability Rating: N (No information provided by manufacturer)

Reactivity Rating: N (No information provided by manufacturer)

Ingredients from MSDS/Label

Chemical CAS No / Unique ID Percent

Fragrance(s)/perfume(s) 000000-00-1

Surfactant(s) (unspecified) 000000-00-4

Colorant/Pigment/Dye(s) 999999-49-3

Quality control agent(s) 999999-49-8

The Material Safety Data Sheet is the information that emergency workers, poison control centers, physicians, and veterinarians use when they are dealing with chemically induced emergencies. I imagine that these professionals find it rather difficult to treat victims who have been exposed to this product.

If the package doesn't tell you in very precise chemical detail what it contains, do not, under any circumstances, buy the product!

mine, she decided that she was tired of bleaching the henna stains out of her white pillowcases, so she went to a department store and bought bed linens to match her hair. Her new henna-colored linens are beautiful and will remain that way for a long time.

Laundry Balls and Discs, the Handy Little Devices that Clean Out Your Wallet and Leave Your Laundry Dirty

Laundry balls and discs are plastic devices that are designed to be thrown in the washing machine along with the dirty laundry. The advertising campaigns for these devices are targeted at consumers who want to reduce their impact on the environment. The manufacturers claim that their products change the molecular structure of water and increase cleaning efficiency,

---

In 1997 the State of Oregon prosecuted a case against a company that was making fraudulent claims about its laundry ball. In sworn testimony, Andrew W. Blackwood, the state's expert witness, stated that his company analyzed samples from water that had been exposed to the type of laundry ball in question and read the company's claims that its SuperGlobe laundry detergent replacement produced a new substance or phenomenon called "IE crystals," which ionized the water in a washing machine. Blackwood testified: ". . . there is no theoretical basis for believing that the structures described as 'IE' do or could exist, let alone be stable, at room temperatures or anything approaching room temperatures."

The expert witness testified that he had analyzed the ball and found that it was essentially a polyethylene container filled with water and a little blue dye. He further stated that some of the company's promotional claims about the transmission of electricity through the polyethylene ball conflicted ". . . with basic scientific principles, including the laws of thermodynamics and the conventional understanding of electricity."

As to the actual identity of the "IE" structures as shown in the company's promotional material, Blackwood stated that he and other professionals in the field ". . . customarily refer to such structures as 'bacteria,' though they may be another form of microorganism." The case was ultimately settled out of court, and a fine was paid, although the company denied all wrongdoing.

Moral: Wash your laundry with a little bit of detergent and warm water. If your clothes look dingy afterward, try using less detergent.

thus making laundry detergent unnecessary; this claim is very attractive to many consumers who are concerned about water pollution.

According to Jodie Bernstein, director of the Federal Trade Commission's Bureau of Consumer Protection, "Tests show that these gadgets do little more than clean out your wallet." Plain water cleans clothes every bit as effectively as these expensive doodads.

The first few washings with just laundry balls and water may very well get clothes cleaner than usual because most of us use far too much detergent when we wash our clothes, and the alkaline residue left behind tends to attract dirt. Once the clothes have gone through a few cycles without detergent, the laundry balls will suddenly stop being effective.

General Whitening

Keeping white clothing white need not be a toxic and dangerous endeavor, as long as one avoids using chlorine bleach.

Chlorine Bleach

This type of bleach works by oxidizing stains, but if used full-strength, it will remove both the stain and the cloth. (The technical term for rapid oxidation is "burning.")

Though chlorine bleach makes pure cotton fabric white, it can cause permanent, irreversible yellowing in linen, nylon, spandex, and resin-treated permanent-press fabrics, and it can react with iron-rich water, leaving rust stains behind. Chlorine bleach will ruin silk, wool, leather, mohair, feathers, and other protein-based materials.

Never mix chlorine bleach with other laundry products! Chlorine is extremely reactive and can combine with acids or alkalis to produce deadly gas.

Oxygen Bleach

Like chlorine bleach, this type of bleach works by oxidizing and breaking up stains. But oxygen bleaches, which are also known as all-fabric bleaches, are gentler and far less toxic than chlorine bleach. Though any bleach product is likely to fade colored fabrics, oxygen bleaches are advertised as all-fabric bleaches because they cause minimal fading and very little fabric damage. Follow the directions on the bleach package, and never use any type of bleach on fabrics that are labeled Do Not Bleach.

Look for a Natural Laundry Bleach that is chlorine- and fragrance-free. Powdered oxygen bleaches can contain any of the following compounds, which when dissolved in water release hydrogen peroxide: sodium percarbonate (a solid combination of hydrogen peroxide and soda ash), sodium perborate (borax), and potassium monopersulfate. Most solid oxygen bleaches also contain sodium carbonate (washing soda). Liquid oxygen bleaches contain hydrogen peroxide.

Oxygen bleaches work best in hot water and require time to work. Presoaking or extending the washing period helps improve the effectiveness of oxygen bleach. Follow the directions on the package for optimal results.

When used regularly, oxygen bleach is wonderful for keeping fabrics white and bright, but clothing that has acquired a well-aged brown, yellow, or gray patina is very difficult to restore to pristine whiteness through the use of oxygen bleach.

If your white laundry has achieved a permanent state of dingy yellowness or grayness, it is time for a change of tactics, such as a switch to . . .

Color Removers (Reduction Bleaches)

Color removers, which contain sodium hydrosulfite, are reducing agents that are commonly used to remove fabric dyes before cloth is redyed. Unlike oxidizing bleaches, which destroy stains by adding oxygen to them, reductive bleaches destroy stains by stealing oxygen from them. These products are found in the laundry sections of hardware stores, drugstores, supermarkets, and in the dyeing sections of craft and fabric stores. The most common are Rit Color Remover and Rit White-Wash.

Sodium hydrosulfite is used in the paper industry as an environmentally friendly alternative to chlorine bleach; our friend Al at the sewage treatment plant deals with tons of the stuff every day, and he has no objections to it. If it's good enough for Al, it's good enough for me.

Color reducers can even be used on nonbleachable fabrics, but are recommended for use only on white fabrics. Clothes can be treated in the washing machine or in a pot of hot water on the stove. The stovetop method is recommended for difficult stains.

Color removers are not suitable for use on white clothing with colored trim and should never be used on blue denim. Follow the directions on the package.

Yellowing or Graying

Nonbleachable fabrics that have been yellowed by chlorine bleach are not salvageable, since the yellowing is caused by fabric damage. Most other yellowing or graying, including stains caused by mineral-rich water, can be lightened by color reducers. Follow the instructions on the package.

If your white laundry tends to acquire a romantic brown patina due to the richness of your water, try adding a pinch of color remover to the detergent each time you wash a white load. *Caution:* Color remover is *incompatible* with chlorine bleach and other chlorine-based cleaners and laundry aids! Combining these products may produce toxic gases.

Color Bleeding

If a red lipstick has deposited pink grease stains all over your light blue dress shirt, a shred of red crepe paper has disintegrated and "tie-dyed" the entire load, or you have simply gotten tired of wearing mauve undies, try using a packet of color remover, carefully following the directions on the label, to banish the misplaced color. Many dyed fabrics are colorfast enough to withstand color remover, so if the alternative is discarding a stained garment, try using a color remover first.

Cooking Grease

When the kitchen towels and dish cloths get so saturated with cooking grease that even the hottest water will not eradicate the greasy smell, try adding color remover to the load along with your regular detergent. The reducing bleach will remove all the grease and smell.

Mother Nature's Bleach

The most nontoxic way to whiten natural, untreated fabrics is to expose them to the bleaching power of sunlight. (Resin-treated permanent-press fabrics tend to yellow in sunlight.) Sun-dried clothing ends up fresh-smelling and bright. You can augment the bleaching power of sunlight with the bleaching power of oxygen by laying damp clothing on the grass or over bushes to dry; sunlight and the oxygen being emitted by the green plants make a powerful combination. Be sure to shake your clean, dry, sun-bleached laundry vigorously before you bring it inside in order to dislodge any invertebrates that may have taken up residence.

Recommended Laundry Aids

Hard water contains large amounts of dissolved minerals that can impede the cleaning abilities of soaps and detergents. Whole-house water softening systems add large amounts of salt to the water in order to counteract the effects of the dissolved minerals. Sending large amounts of salt down the drain is not an environmentally friendly action; it is certainly preferable to treat just the laundering water. The following laundry aids are all commonly available at drugstores, supermarkets, and discount department stores. Try one of the following:

Borax

A naturally occurring mineral salt, borax is composed of boron, sodium, oxygen, and water. It acts as a water softener, a fabric softener, a deodorizer, and a mild bleach. 20 Mule Team Borax has been around since 1891.

When using borax, measure out the recommended amount of detergent or soap for your machine, then add an equal amount of borax. Avoid breathing the dust or getting it on your skin or in your eyes; it is an irritant. Do not ingest.

Washing Soda

Another mineral salt (sodium carbonate) that is used to soften water and boost the action of detergents and soaps, washing soda can be used in the same way as borax. Arm & Hammer Washing Soda is the standard. Avoid using washing soda on silks and woolens; it will damage them.

Caution: Avoid contact with eyes and skin. Mixing washing soda with acids (vinegar, for instance) will release carbon dioxide gas, which may accumulate in enclosed spaces and pose a suffocation hazard.

Distilled Vinegar

A cup of distilled white vinegar added to the rinse water kills bacteria and helps prevent a buildup of detergent and mineral residue. You can utilize your machine's fabric softener compartment to dispense vinegar at the proper time.

Bluing

This nontoxic dye is added to wash water to make white fabrics look brighter and whiter. Mrs. Stewart's Liquid Bluing has been on the market since 1883.

Fabric Softeners

Fabric softeners are meant to keep fabrics from stiffening after they are washed and dried and reduce the static charge that can build up in the dryer. Fabric softeners should never be used on children's sleepwear or other flame-resistant clothing because it increases the fluffiness and thus the flammability of fabrics. Fabric softener will also "waterproof" items such as towels and diapers, thus preventing them from doing their job.

If you feel the need to use a fabric softener, there is one fabric softener that was highly recommended by Ms. von Rabenau of The Green Mercantile: Natural Choices Fabric Softener. It is vegetable based, biodegradable, fragrance free, and contains no volatile organic compounds or solvents. This natural fabric softener may be found at your local natural food store or ordered online at www.oxyboost.com.

I Smell Pretty, but I Feel Awful

Most fabric softeners are heavily perfumed. The exact formulas of fragrances are considered proprietary information, so we will never know exactly what chemicals are wafting out of our dryer vents and off of our static-free clothes.

Rosalind Anderson, Ph.D., and Julius Anderson, MD, Ph.D., of Anderson Laboratories, Inc. published a study entitled "Respiratory Toxicity of Fabric Softener Emissions" in the May 2000 issue of *The Journal of Toxicology and Environmental Health*. When the doctors exposed laboratory mice to air that was contaminated with the fumes from fabric softener sheets, the rodents developed irritation of the eyes, nose, throat, and lungs, and some had severe asthma attacks. The mice also had adverse reactions to a T-shirt that had been "softened" in the dryer.

The researchers then did a chemical analysis of the fumes. A partial list of the chemical emissions from just one brand includes the following:

- *Isopropylbenzene*. A narcotic and a central nervous system depressant. Chronic exposure may damage the lungs, liver, and kidneys.
- *Styrene*. A toxic carcinogen that also causes genetic damage. Chronic exposure may affect the central nervous system.
- *Trimethylbenzene*. Inhalation may cause circulatory collapse, severe respiratory damage, coughing, wheezing, choking, nausea, and vomiting. It may also cause fainting, convulsions, and coma.
- *Phenol*. Inhalation may cause severe irritation to the respiratory tract, breathing difficulty, burns, and possible coma. Inhalation of high concentrations may be fatal. Chronic inhalation may cause liver and kidney damage, reproductive damage, and birth defects, and it may affect the central nervous system.
- *Thymol*. Affects the central nervous system, is a respiratory irritant, and may cause kidney and liver damage.

The Andersons were able to analyze the ingredients in consumer products using a gas chromatograph and mass spectroscope. Most of the rest of us must depend upon the completeness and accuracy of labels.

Naturally Soft but Not Clingy

Static electricity builds up in the dryer as fabrics brush past one another, rubbing off electrons, and only occurs when fabrics are quite dry. Fabric softeners leave a waxy coating on fabrics that reduces the friction and prevents the electrons from escaping. Cotton doesn't conduct electricity, so it doesn't

~ It is all too easy to assume that people who cannot tolerate being around heavily scented products and complain of acute symptoms such as shortness of breath, burning eyes, or dizziness, are simply imagining things. It is interesting to note that mice, who are presumably immune to psychosomatic disorders, develop all of these symptoms when they are involuntarily exposed to fabric softeners.

Whether you are a mouse or a human being, chemical irritation of the trigeminal nerve in the face causes stinging and burning sensations in the eyes and nose; chemical irritation of the vagus nerve in the lungs causes shortness of breath. Dizziness and nausea can also be symptoms of chemically induced central nervous system depression. These are all short-term symptoms caused by short-term exposure to chemicals.

Immediately after I read that some of the chemicals found in fabric softeners can irritate the trigeminal nerve, I called a friend of mine who has been battling trigeminal nerve pain on and off for more than twenty years, ever since she had a tumor unwrapped from the nerve, leaving it sheathless and uninsulated. The pain, which occurs when the nerve goes into spasms, had been so constant and unrelenting for the past year and a half that her doctor had put her on epilepsy medication.

I told her about the Andersons' research and e-mailed the article to her. She immediately stopped using fabric softeners. The pain disappeared three days later, and as of this writing it hasn't returned.

build up a static charge; synthetic fibers build up huge amounts of static, especially if they are over dried.

To prevent static cling, add 1 cup vinegar to the final rinse cycle and remove the laundry from the dryer while it is still slightly damp—before it has a chance to build up a charge. This works because acidic water conducts electricity well and steals the extra electrons that might otherwise build up on the tumbling fabric. Unlike commercial fabric softeners, vinegar leaves no smell behind.

Stain Removal

Wet stains are much easier to remove if they are treated immediately after they occur. Gently blot up excess liquid with a clean white rag or paper towel, working toward the center of the spot. Do not rub, lest you damage the fabric and spread the stain. (Never try to remove a stain by rubbing with a colored rag or sponge. The dye may migrate and create another stain.)

Protein-Based Stains

While they are still wet, food, milk, mud, vomit, and blood stains should be scrubbed out under cold running water, then allowed to soak in cold water before the stained clothing is laundered. Do not use soap on protein stains; use detergent.

Crusty protein stains that have already dried should be scraped or brushed off the fabric, then soaked in cold water with liquid laundry detergent or dish liquid before laundering.

Read the presoak directions on the detergent container for specific instructions.

You can also soak blood spots in hydrogen peroxide and cold water until the stain fades, then rinse the fabric with cold water. Repeat if necessary.

Hot water, heat drying, or ironing can set a stain by cooking the protein into the cloth. A heat-treated stain can be very difficult to remove.

Sweat Stains

Underarm stains on clothing can be caused by sweat or by deodorants or antiperspirants. The bad news is that sometimes the chemicals in these products can react with fabrics and dyes to cause permanent color changes that are not reversible; since sweat is not chemically reactive, old-fashioned sweat stains are relatively easy to remove.

Sweat Stain Preventive Methods
The best offense is a good defense.

- A thick layer of deodorant or antiperspirant will tend to rub off on your clothes; apply a thin layer, then let your underarms dry completely before you get dressed.
- Disposable paper underarm shields that can be stuck to the underarm seam are the surest way to protect clothing from sweat and

deodorant stains; if you are wearing expensive formal clothing, underarm shields are indispensable. The shields are comfortable and can be trimmed to fit invisibly under your clothing.

Sweat Stain Removal

It is much easier to pretreat sweaty clothes in order to prevent stains from setting than to attempt to remove stains from laundered clothing. Try one of these methods:

- Shortly after you remove your washable shirt or blouse, spray the armpits with white vinegar to help prevent the sweat from setting. The garment can then be laundered as usual whenever you get around to it. Or fill a bucket with warm water, pour in 1 cup white vinegar, and soak the sweaty garment in the vinegar water for a few hours. Then launder the garment as usual.
- Apply liquid detergent or dish liquid to the sweaty bits of the garment, then soak the item in warm water for half an hour before throwing it in a hot water wash.
- Sweat stains can also be removed with a paste made of meat tenderizer and water. Rub the paste into the stains, then launder the shirt as usual. Meat tenderizer breaks down the proteins in the sweat, making them easier to wash out.
- Pour ammonia over the stained area, then rub.

If the formerly stinky garment has already been laundered, consumer-grade (3 percent solution) hydrogen peroxide can be used to bleach out sweat stains. Peroxide will not harm most fabrics, but may cause color changes in colored fabrics; test the colorfastness by dabbing a little peroxide on a hidden part of the garment, such as the inside of the hem, and checking for color changes. If the color is unaffected, it is safe to soak the garment in hydrogen peroxide for half an hour before laundering it.

Wool can be damaged by hydrogen peroxide, so wait only a couple of minutes before washing hydrogen peroxide out of woolen clothing. Other fibers of animal origin, such as silk, cashmere, and angora, are quite delicate and should not be exposed to hydrogen peroxide. They will need to be professionally cleaned. (See "Dry Cleaning," page 206, for information on choosing an environmentally friendly establishment.)

Oil-Based Stains

- Pretreat cooking oil and food grease, hair-oil stained collars, and machine oil stains by applying liquid detergent or a paste of powdered detergent and water to the spot, and scrubbing. Rinse the area well with hot water, then wash the stained clothing in hot water with a mineral-based powdered detergent. Do not mix oil-stained clothing in with other laundry.
- Dab a paste of salt and water on the spot, then remove the salt with a clean paper towel before laundering.
- Rub "ring-around-the-collar" with oily-hair shampoo, which is formulated to remove hair oils.
- Rub cooking oil stains with liquid dish soap, which is formulated to cut cooking grease.
- If the garment cannot be washed right away, sprinkle some cornstarch or baking soda on the stain, then put a rag on top of your ironing board and lay the stained part of the garment on the rag, stained side down. Iron over the grease stain. The heat of the iron will melt the grease into the rag. Grease stains are the only stains that can be removed with heat. Heat will set all other types of stains.

Note: Petroleum-based stains make clothing extremely flammable. Never put clothes or rags that have been contaminated with fuel in the dryer! Hang them up to dry outdoors.

A cup of vinegar added to the wash water can help remove the stench of fuel.

Vegetable-Pigment (Tannin) Stains

Red wine, brandy, beer, fruit, coffee, chocolate, cocoa, ketchup, tea, and soft drink stains should be washed in hot water with detergent (which does not contain fats or oils). Soap (made of vegetable oil or animal fat) will set these stains. Natural detergents such as Country Save, which contain washing soda and sodium perborate, are ideal for this. Do not attempt to pretreat tannin stains with castile soaps.

- Remove fresh wine and fruit stains from table linens by stretching the stained item over a bowl or over the kitchen sink, then pouring boiling water over the stain until it washes out.
- If your loved one sloshes red wine or grape juice on your clothing, calmly remove the garment, put waxed paper or a plastic bag under the stain, then pour on enough table salt to soak up the moisture. This will help prevent the spill from soaking farther into the fabric. Brush the wine-soaked salt off before laundering the garment in hot water and detergent.

Dye Stains

Stains from food coloring (Kool-Aid, condiments, candy), felt-tip pen, and ink can be difficult to remove. To pretreat the stain, rub in liquid detergent or dish liquid, then rinse thoroughly before washing in hot water.

- Felt-tip pen may come out if it is rubbed immediately with vodka then flushed with hot water.
- To remove ball point pen ink, put several thicknesses of paper towels under the stain, then use a rag to push liquid detergent down through the stain. When the towels get inky, put a clean section under the stain.

Pencil

Lift the pencil mark off the fabric with a kneadable art gum eraser. Rub in liquid detergent or dish liquid, rinse in warm water, then launder.

Kneadable art gum erasers are lumps of malleable gray rubber that are available at art supply stores. Kneadable erasers are excellent for removing marks from delicate paper, fabrics, or unwashable wall surfaces. To remove marks, knead the eraser until it is warm and pliable, then press it down on the mark you wish to remove. Do not rub, just press. Repeat as necessary. When the surface of the eraser becomes soiled, knead it again to renew it.

Paint

Latex Paint

Soak the spot right away in cold water, then wash the garment in cool water with heavy-duty detergent. If you allow the paint to dry, removal may be impossible.

Oil Paint

Spot treat oil-paint stains dry before they dry. Blot the spots with alcohol (vodka) or turpentine.

Rust

Never use chlorine bleach on rust stains or the stains will become permanent.

If the garment is white, you can sprinkle salt on the rust stain, squeeze lemon juice on it, then put the garment in the sun to dry. But be careful because lemon juice may bleach colored fabrics.

Or rub the stained area with cream of tartar and lemon juice.

🌿 STAIN PREVENTION

If you really want to cut down on your laundry chores, make sure everyone in the family owns work clothes and play clothes, aprons, and art smocks, and knows when to wear them. It is far easier to allow old work clothes to accumulate stains than it is to remove stains from dressy clothes.

Teaching children to wipe their hands on their napkins, rather than on their shirts or pants, goes a long way toward reducing food and grease stains.

Finally, if you avoid buying food or drinks that contain large amounts of food coloring, spills will be much less likely to cause permanent stains.

Dry Cleaning

Dry cleaning strikes me as among the least convenient of the modern conveniences; it is certainly one of the most toxic. Much dry cleaning can be avoided simply by reading the labels when buying clothes and avoiding garments that sport a Dry Clean Only label.

Dry Clean Only indicates that the manufacturer of that garment deems the fabric too delicate to withstand machine laundering. Sometimes the fabric itself is quite delicate and can be damaged by machine washing and drying: Some rayons and handmade lace, for instance, are very weak and cannot withstand agitation. Other dry clean only fabrics shrink: Subjecting wool to overly strenuous machine washing and drying can turn big, comfy wool sweaters into stiff felted doll's jackets.

Occasionally the Dry Clean Only label means that the manufacturer was cutting corners and did not bother to preshrink the fabric or chose dyed fabrics that were not colorfast. The first time one of these cheaply made items is washed, the fabric will shrink or the dye will bleed and/or fade. And sometimes manufacturers put the Dry Clean Only label on their wares because they are too cheap or lazy to test their garments for shrinkage, or they want to avoid liability for shrunken clothing. If you don't have too much invested in a garment and you are willing to take a gamble, gentle hand washing in cool water and Woolite can work quite well for some dry clean only items.

Though fine quality tailored jackets and pants are difficult to clean and press properly at home, other types of garments that are labeled Machine Washable or even Hand Wash Only are certain to be sturdier and more well-made than garments made of the same fibers yet labeled Dry Clean Only.

When you are contemplating purchasing a garment, ask yourself these questions: "How much do I want to spend on this garment, and how much time, effort, and money do I want to spend on keeping it clean?"

When my dad was a boy in the beginning of the twentieth century, his mother took in dry cleaning. The hand-cranked machine was in their back yard; the cleaning solvent was gasoline. Because the family was too poor to afford a bicycle, my dad traveled on roller skates as he delivered the clean, dry, neatly pressed clothing to the customers.

Now and then, in idle moments, I wonder whether my father's and aunt's short-term memory problems were caused by exposure to gasoline fumes. Though the danger of chronic exposure to petroleum products was unknown when my father and aunt were growing up, we know now that occupational exposure to solvents can damage brain cells.

The first solvents used in the modern dry-cleaning process were all petroleum based: camphene, benzene, kerosene, and gasoline. These highly flammable solvents made dry cleaning a very hazardous business until the invention of nonflammable dry-cleaning solvents. Perchloroethylene (also known as "perc," perchlor, tetrachloroethylene, 1,1,2,2-tetrachloroethylene, tetrachloroethene, ethylene tetrachloride, or carbon dichloride), one of the first of these nonflammable solvents, was introduced in the 1930s and is still the most commonly used dry-cleaning solvent.

Though freshly dry-cleaned clothing is not likely to burst into flames, it poses another kind of hazard: Chronic exposure to perc fumes can damage the nervous system, liver, and kidneys. It is sad, but certainly not surprising, that one out of every hundred dry cleaning workers develops cancer, most commonly cancer of the kidney, bladder, or intestines.

Just living near a dry-cleaning establishment can be hazardous. A study conducted by the Environmental Protection Agency showed that residents who live in the same building as a dry-cleaning business have an increased incidence of cancer that ranges from 1 in 100 to 1 in 1 million, depending on the type of dry-cleaning equipment that is being used. The Environmental Protection Agency considers a 1 in 1 million chance of cancer worth worrying about.

There is some risk involved in wearing recently dry-cleaned clothing. In 1996, researchers from the Consumers Union measured the amount of perc fumes wafting from freshly dry-cleaned garments. Based on their data, the researchers estimated that wearing a freshly dry-cleaned blazer and blouse just once a week for forty years would give the wearer a 1 in 6,700 risk of developing cancer caused by perc exposure.

Several studies have shown that the fumes emitted by dry-cleaned clothing can build up to toxic levels in small enclosed spaces, such as closets. The Consumers Union recommends that conventional dry cleaning should be used only as a last resort, and that newly dry-cleaned clothes be aired out before they are worn: Hang the garments either outdoors or in an open garage or outbuilding.

Dry Cleaning Comparisons

Luckily, there are excellent alternatives to toxic dry-cleaning chemicals. Researchers from the Consumers Union compared the results of dry cleaning using four different solvents: perchloroethylene, the highly toxic industry standard; and three more environmentally friendly solvents: liquid carbon dioxide (CO_2); a silicone-based solvent; and "wet cleaning," which uses very small amounts of water.

Much to the researchers' surprise, they found that the liquid CO_2 dry cleaning was the most effective as well as the most gentle: none of the lamb's wool jackets, silk blouses, or pleated rayon/linen skirts shrank, changed texture, stretched, changed color, bled dyes, pilled, or came unstitched during repeated cleanings. The liquid CO_2 cleaning method was done at Hangers Cleaners franchises. Website: www.hangersdrycleaners.com.

The researchers considered the silcone-based solvent cleaning process to be nearly as good as the liquid CO_2 cleaning, though the silicone-based cleaning caused a slight bit of shrinkage and some pilling. The silicone-based cleaning was done at GreenEarth cleaning franchises. Website: www.greenearthcleaning.com.

The standard, perc-based dry cleaning caused severe pilling in the wool jackets, shrank the skirts almost a full size, and faded the silk blouse.

The wet cleaning caused pilling and considerable shrinkage.

Since standard dry cleaning is both dangerous and ineffective, perhaps the best solution for those who do not live near an alternative dry cleaner is to make arrangements to ship your dirty delicate clothing to the nearest Hangers or GreenEarth facility.

Fabric Care

If you like your clothing to last for more than a few washings, it is important to buy well-constructed garments made of good materials and follow the manufacturer's laundering instructions. But before you buy the clothing, it is helpful to know a little about the properties of different types of fabrics.

Synthetic Fibers

Synthetic fibers, such as nylon, polyester, acrylic, polypropylene, and spandex, are made from petroleum, a nonrenewable resource. Though synthetic fabrics possess many positive attributes (some are even made from recycled pop bottles), most melt when exposed to high heat and are thus too dangerous to wear while cooking or around campfires. Petroleum-based fabrics also have an affinity for oil stains—the darkened splotches are quite difficult to remove from synthetic fabrics.

Cleaning Synthetic Fabrics
- Read and follow the label instructions for cleaning.
- Synthetic fabrics tend to soak up the oil that is released from natural fabrics during a wash cycle. Try to avoid washing synthetic clothing in a load with anything oily, such as kitchen towels.

  Oil stains on synthetic fabrics should be washed out immediately after they occur. If that is not possible, pretreat the spots by scrubbing them with a little dish liquid (which is designed to cut grease) and rinse thoroughly with cool water before you throw the clothing in the washing machine. Hot water will set in the stains, as will the heat from a clothes dryer or an iron.
- Synthetic fibers melt and shrink at high temperatures; a hot-water wash can cause permanent wrinkles, and a hot dryer can induce permanent clothing deformities.

  Wash synthetic fibers in warm or cool water, then hang them up to dry. (Synthetics dry rapidly and are spun nearly dry by the fast spin cycle of front-loading washing machines.)
- Ironing synthetic fabrics can be rather tricky, since the heat of the iron is enough to melt holes in the material. If you hang synthetic clothing up to dry, the wrinkles should smooth out on their own unless they have been melted into the fabric (see above).

  If your synthetic clothing has been afflicted with melted-in wrinkles, it is probably worth attempting to salvage the garment with a little strategic iron work. Work carefully, use the synthetic setting (warm), and use a pressing cloth under and over the clothing in case it melts.

Plant Fibers

Cloth made of plant fibers—which include cotton, linen, ramie, rayon, and acetate—is usually absorbent, breathable, and relatively durable. Plant-based fibers are flammable, but do not emit toxic smoke and don't melt onto the skin as synthetics do.

Cotton

Most cotton fabrics shrink substantially only once: the first time they are washed and dried. If the fabric is prewashed before the garment is cut from the cloth, shrinkage should not be a problem.

Read the label and follow the manufacturer's laundering recommendations. In my opinion, everyday clothing should be machine washable, dryer safe, and any color but white. (The chemicals that are used to make cotton fabric wrinkle resistant tend to yellow when they are exposed to sunlight. This yellowing is not reversible, and bleaching will eat holes through the cloth before it removes the yellow coloration.)

Remember that a Dry Clean Only or Cold Water Wash Only label on a cotton garment may be a sign that the manufacturer was trying to maximize profits by squeezing extra garments out of unshrunken, unwashed cotton cloth.

Cloth Diapers

Cloth diapers are made of cotton for exactly the same reasons that cotton is the most common fiber used to make clothing: It is soft, durable, absorbent, allows the skin to breathe, and is easily washed.

Health Effects of Disposable Diapers

A study entitled "Acute Respiratory Effects of Diaper Emissions" by the intrepid doctors Rosalind C. Anderson and Julius H. Anderson was published in 1999 by the National Institutes of Health (NIH). (No, not that kind of emissions. The diapers they studied were new and unoccupied, and the emissions were nonorganic.) The authors wrote, "The airborne emissions of some disposable diapers can produce acute respiratory toxicity—including asthma-like reactions—in normal laboratory mice. . . . Several of the chemicals identified in the emissions (of the diapers) . . . cause respiratory toxicity."

The emissions included chemicals such as toluene, xylene, ethylbenzene, and isopropylbenzene. Their respective Material Safety Data Sheets state that all of these substances are dangerous if inhaled, eaten, or absorbed through the skin, and that exposure can cause the following problems: serious skin irritation, severe irritation of the respiratory tract, birth defects, impaired fertility, liver and kidney damage, and central nervous system disorders.

Our babies' tender little bottoms deserve better treatment than this.

The researchers concluded, "New cloth diapers produced very little respiratory effect and appeared to be the least toxic choice for a consumer. Cloth diapers, however, could acquire toxic properties from detergents, fabric softeners . . . or fragrance products . . . associated with laundering."

The Bottom Line

In 1992, the State of Michigan Office of Waste Reduction Services compared the time, energy, financial, and material costs of using cloth diapers or disposable diapers in a day care setting and came to the less-than-surprising conclusion that using cloth diapers was better for the pocketbook as well as for the environment.

It requires a staggering amount of energy, water, and renewable and non-renewable resources to paper a baby's hindquarters from birth until the child is toilet trained. The eighteen billion diapers that are discarded each year make up about 4 percent of the nation's total household solid waste stream.

Growing enough cotton to produce the few dozen diapers necessary to sop up after a baby for a couple of years is a light task compared to growing enough pulp and manufacturing enough plastic to produce the more than five thousand disposable diapers that will be used for an average of seven changes per day in those same two years.

Washing Diapers

But what about the energy and water used to wash and dry cloth diapers? Studies that compare the environmental impact of cloth diapers and disposable diapers vary; it is certainly not surprising that research sponsored by disposable diaper companies tends to show that cloth diapers use as much water and energy as do the paper variety. Other studies show savings of between 25 and 50 percent for parents who home launder their babies' diapers.

Diaper services are even more energy-and-water efficient than home laundering, and they are less expensive than using disposable diapers. The State of Michigan's study showed that day care centers that switched from disposable diapers to using a diaper service saved 13.4 percent per year in diaper costs.

Getting Off to a Nappy Start

If you decide to forgo a diaper service, make sure you buy enough diapers to last a couple of days so your baby won't have to go naked while you do the wash. We started with about six dozen and never ran out, even when we had two offspring in diapers. Two decades later, those diapers are still serving as useful cleaning rags.

Managing the Messy End of the Diaper Cycle

1. Half fill the diaper pail with warm water and add ½ cup borax. The borax will help reduce odors and staining.

   Or if your baby is having trouble with diaper rash, soak the diapers in water with a couple cups white vinegar instead of the borax-and-water. The vinegar will help kill the bacteria that can cause diaper rash.

   Note: Make sure the diaper pail lid cannot be opened by tots. Very young children can drown in an inch of water.

2. Rinse out the urine and scrape the solid waste into the toilet before putting diapers in the diaper pail. (You can keep a plastic spatula in the bathroom for this purpose; store it as you would a toilet brush.) Soak the baby's waterproof pants in the diaper pail as well.

3. When the diaper pail is full, drain as much of the water as possible into the toilet, and lug the pail to the laundry room.

4. Put the diapers in the washing machine, and set the dial to the heaviest wash cycle and the hottest water setting. (If your machine has a separate setting for the spin cycle, you may want to use it to spin the excess liquid out of the diapers before starting the wash cycle.)

5. Soap can leave a residue that may irritate a baby's skin. Use a gentle unscented detergent: For the sake of the baby's future, try to choose a detergent that is biodegradable and phosphate free. For the sake of the baby's skin, try to choose a detergent that is free of fragrances, dyes, bleaches, and brighteners; your baby's tender little bottom will be sitting in these diapers all day long, every day, and these chemicals can cause irritation and allergic reactions. (See detergent recommendations on page 188.)

6. Add 1 cup vinegar to the final rinse cycle.

7. Dry the diapers using the cotton setting of the dryer. Do not dry the nylon or plastic pants in the dryer lest they melt. Hang the pants up to dry, preferably in the sun.

8. If your baby is having problems with diaper rash, try drying the diapers outdoors in the sun. Sunlight is a very strong disinfectant.

Baby Clothes

Most flame-retardant baby clothes are made of synthetic materials that have been treated with fire retardants. These types of clothes must be washed with detergent because soap will ruin the flame retardant.

The only naturally flame-retardant fabric is wool. If you are concerned about exposing your child to the dangers of flame-retardant chemicals, dress him or her and the crib in washable wool. To order washable woolens for babies, go online and search for "baby washable wool." There are many companies that sell washable wool baby blankets, mattress pads, and clothing. Follow the manufacturer's instructions for washing these items.

Baby laundry should be washed with the same type of gentle detergent that is used for washing diapers (see above). Never wash the baby's clothes in the same load as the diapers; no matter how filthy the clothes may be, they generally are not as soiled as the diapers. Baby clothes that are heavily soiled should be treated as if they were dirty diapers and washed separately from the family's general laundry.

Baby Stains

Presoak stained baby clothes in cold water with detergent or borax. Rubbing milk stains with a paste made of baking soda and water will help remove them from baby clothes.

Linen

Linen is made from the stems of the flax plant. High-quality linen is a tough, durable fabric. In fact, the oldest extant pieces of linen fabric are the several-thousand-year-old wrappings of Egyptian mummies.

Undyed linen—which ranges in color from cream and pale yellow to tan and dark brown—is really tough; nonetheless, the dyes in many modern linen fabrics are not colorfast and the weave is so loose that many of these materials cannot be machine washed.

Though you should always follow the washing instructions on the labels of linen clothing, here are some do's and don'ts for washable linens:

- Washable linen should be laundered with pure soap or a very gentle detergent that doesn't contain additives (chlorine bleach and/or optical brighteners can cause blotching and color changes).
- The time-honored method of bleaching is to spread damp linen articles over bushes to dry in the sun. If you have no obliging bushes, lay out a groundcloth or sheet before spreading your linens out on the ground.
- Chlorine bleach will turn linen fabrics yellow. If you must use a bleach, use a nonchlorine bleach or hydrogen peroxide. (See page 192 for information about bleach.)
- Throwing linen in a tumble dryer verges on fabric abuse: Linen dries very quickly and is so brittle that it may be damaged by the tumbling action of the machine. Even if the fabric escapes the dryer undamaged, it will emerge horrendously wrinkled and will be annoyingly difficult to iron.

- Washable linens look best if they are ironed dry immediately after they are washed.
- Never let any damp clothing sit in a pile for more than a few hours, lest it grow mildew. If you are not going to iron your washable linen clothing right away, hang it up to dry as soon as you remove it from the washing machine. Shake the garment sharply before you hang it up, and smooth out the pockets, sleeves, and collar in order to minimize the amount of ironing that will eventually be required.

Rayon

Rayon is a man-made fiber manufactured from cellulose that is extracted from wood fibers and reconstituted into fibers with varying strengths and properties. Rayon fibers are used to manufacture products ranging from silky women's blouses to disposable diapers to the cords that reinforce automobile tires.

Some rayon fabrics may not be colorfast, so beware using water to wash any rayon fabric that is labeled Dry Clean Only.

The most common rayon is also known as viscose rayon. It is quite weak when wet, and it must be washed carefully to prevent shrinkage or stretching.

To clean viscose rayon that is labeled Hand Washable:

1. Use lukewarm water and very gentle soap, such as Dr. Bronner's Pure-Castile Soap.
2. Gently squeeze the soapy water through the cloth.
3. Rinse the garment with lukewarm water.
4. Do not wring or twist the garment. Roll it up in a clean, dry bath towel, and press firmly to squeeze out as much water as possible.
5. Unroll the damp garment and hang it on a rustproof hanger.
6. Rayon sweaters or other knit rayon garments must be smoothed out and dried on a flat surface. A wooden clothes rack or mesh clothes-drying platform is ideal; if you don't own either, spread the garment out to dry on a clean towel on a waterproof surface. A garment drying on a solid surface will need to be turned occasionally.
7. If a rayon garment needs ironing, use a moderate setting with a clean cotton press cloth between the garment and the iron.

The other types of rayon are more durable. If you want to buy rayon clothing that is easier to take care of, read the label and look for the following varieties:

High wet modulus (HWM), also known as polynosic rayon or Modaltm, is designed to be strong when wet and stands up well to machine washing and drying.

Tencel or lyocell is relatively strong, colorfast, and machine washable and dryable; but as always, heed the manufacturer's instructions.

Because rayon is such a variable fiber, one should not make assumptions about the way to wash it. Reading and following the manufacturer's fiber care instructions is essential.

Ramie

The plant ramie is related to nettles; its strong fibers are used to make fabrics that can resemble either silk or linen. Ramie does not tend to shrink when washed; in fact, a study conducted by Louisiana State University showed that ramie sweaters tend to increase in size if dried flat. The researchers found that gentle hand laundering does not agree with ramie and ramie blends; they stay softer and don't stretch out of shape when they are machine washed and dried.

As usual, you should read the label and follow the manufacturer's washing instructions, but if your newly washed ramie sweater stretches out of shape, try throwing it in the washer and then in the dryer.

Animal Fibers

Animal fibers are made of protein and include silk—which is extruded from the back ends of silkworm caterpillars—and hair, which includes wool, cashmere, angora, mohair, camel, alpaca, and qiviut (the soft undercoat of the fierce musk ox). Strong chlorine bleach will dissolve fabrics made of animal fibers; weak solutions of chlorine bleach will permanently yellow and stiffen them. These protein-based fibers should be washed with a gentle soap, such as Woolite or Dr. Bronner's Pure-Castile Soap.

Silk

Silk has a very high tensile strength, which means it would make a very strong rope, but it is not abrasion resistant, which means that the rope would fray badly if it was pulled over a rock or the rough bark of a tree. Exposure to chemicals, oil, and strong sunlight will also damage silk. All of these characteristics affect the way silk can be cleaned.

Hand Washing Silk

Read the label and follow the manufacturer's instructions.

Silk garments that are labeled Washable can be hand washed in very mild soap in exactly the same way as wool (see below), but silk should be hung up to dry indoors, out of the sunlight, on a smooth, waterproof, rust-proof hanger.

Wool

Though it may be a bit more expensive than synthetic clothing, heavy-duty woolen clothing is so durable that it can last a lifetime with a minimum of care. I have a woolen work jacket that I have been abusing mercilessly for more than three decades. It needs a little repair around the buttonholes and the cuffs are a bit frayed, but otherwise it is in excellent shape.

Wool resists both dirt and moisture; really high-quality wool seldom needs to be cleaned if it is aired out frequently and allowed to dry thoroughly between wearings. Unlike synthetics, wool does not accumulate body odors. Wool is also heat- and fire-resistant.

Unless wool is marked with the Superwash label, it is not safe for regular machine washing and drying. Extreme changes in temperature and rough handling while wet will shrink most wool. Both hot water and very cold water will shrink wool, as will the agitating action of a top-loading washing machine. Never throw woolens in the dryer: The tumbling action will shrink the woolen fabric into metamorphic felt. Drying your woolens in front of a fireplace or heater will not cause felting, but the wool will probably shrink.

Felted wool is wool that has been shrunken and matted together through heat and agitation. For instance, when knitters make felted berets, they loosely knit an item that is large enough to serve as a lace tablecloth, but after it has been machine washed in hot water and run through the dryer, the "tablecloth" shrinks down to the size of a beret.

Hand Washing Wool

1. Fill a basin with tepid water and squeeze in a few drops of either a gentle castile soap or Woolite. These will gently clean the wool without removing its protective lanolin (the natural oil in the wool).
2. Swish the woolen fabric gently through the water. Do not twist or wring.
3. Drain the wash water, gently squeeze the excess water out of the garment, and fill the basin with tepid rinse water.
4. Gently swish the garment through the rinse water. If the water gets very sudsy or dirty, empty the basin, squeeze the garment out again, and fill the basin with clean tepid rinse water.
5. Roll the garment in a dry towel and pat it to remove some of the excess water.
6. Lay the garment on a flat surface, then stretch and pat it back into shape.

    If you are washing a very precious garment, you may want to trace its outline on a large piece of paper before washing it. Then, after you wash it and remove the excess moisture, you can lay the garment out on its own outline and pat it back into its previous shape.
7. Wet or damp wool is delicate; it shrinks when exposed to heat, and turns yellow when exposed to sunlight. Allow the garment to dry away from all sources of heat.

Machine Washing Wool

Front-loading washing machines are not as hard on wool as are top-loading machines. Many front-loading washing machines have Hand Wash/Wool cycles, which are gentle enough for sturdy woolens. The wash water and rinse water should be the same temperature: tepid. Use Woolite or a gentle plant-based liquid natural detergent, such as Restore Laundry Detergent.

My work sweaters emerge clean and unscathed from the hand wash cycle of my front-loading washing machine. (They remain unscathed unless someone throws them in the dryer or carefully lays them out in front of the furnace to dry.)

Shrunken Wool

If someone who shall remain nameless has transgressed against your favorite sweater, and it is merely shrunken, not felted, you can try resurrecting it by boiling it in vinegar and water. The vinegar will help relax the wool and should make it possible to stretch the sweater back into shape.

(When wool has become felted rather than merely shrunken, its fibers have inextricably twisted and matted into each other so that all traces of the separate stitches have disappeared. Felting is irreversible.)

Salvaging Shrunken Wool

1. Make a solution of 1 part vinegar to 2 parts water.
2. Put your sweater in a large stock pot and drown it with the vinegar water.
3. Boil the sweater for half an hour.
4. Turn off the heat, and carefully use a strong wooden spoon or two to remove the hot sweater and lay it out on a thick terrycloth towel.
5. Roll the sweater up in the towel to remove some of the water.
6. Unroll the sweater and lay it out on another thick towel, and try to stretch it back into shape.
7. Let it dry.
8. Remove any pills from the sweater by brushing them off with a dry sponge.

Hopelessly felted sweaters can be cut up to make wonderfully warm woolen insoles for winter boots.

Rain Washing

Wind alone cannot clean a truly dirty item such as a muddy work jacket. If, like me, you are averse to dry-cleaning chemicals and live several states away from the nearest dry-cleaning establishment that utilizes liquid carbon dioxide, you can engage Mother Nature to clean your delicate or very large woolen items. These techniques work for items ranging in size from baby sweaters to large carpets. Rain washing is the gentlest possible washing technique, since it requires no agitation of any kind. (See page 250 for information on rain washing carpets.)

Letting the Rain Blow through Your Clothes

1. If a rainstorm is in the forecast, choose a shady spot and hang your more heavily soiled woolens outdoors over a sheet on a clothesline, or lay them out on a clean flat surface in the shade. Let the rain wash through them. (A rustproof metal-mesh table would be an ideal surface for this operation.) I have rain-washed sweaters, blankets, sleeping bags, and rugs with great success.

2. If your wool blanket is in need of cleaning and a big rainstorm is in the forecast, hang the blanket over a set of paired clotheslines, fill a spray bottle with water, add a couple drops of Woolite or a protein shampoo, and spray the blanket with the shampoo water. The pouring rain will rinse the shampoo and the dirt right out of the blanket.

3. Whenever you hang woolens outside in mild weather, you should shake them vigorously before bringing them inside in order to dislodge and kill any insect eggs that may have been laid on the wool. Alternatively, the tumbling action of a dryer will kill insect eggs. It is perfectly safe to put dry woolens in the dryer and tumble them without heat in order to exterminate insect eggs.

Snow Cleaning

Snow was one of the first dry-cleaning solvents. Snow cleaning is still one of the most efficient and effective dry-cleaning methods, and it is recommended by many dealers of fine handmade woolen rugs.

Dry or "sugar snow," rather than very wet snow, is best for this, so do your snow cleaning during very cold weather. Your belongings will get clean without getting wet. (See page 251 for information on snow-cleaning wool and silk carpets.)

To Snow-Clean Woolen Garments

1. Hang clothing outdoors during a snow storm (not during a blizzard, however; you don't want your clothing to blow into the next county). Hang the clothing so it is as open as possible.
2. Let the falling snow brush the dirt off.
3. Shake the snow off the garments and bring them indoors.

Storing Woolens

Wool should be cleaned before it is stored: Clothes moths are attracted to clothing that is soiled with bits of food, body oils, and flakes of skin. Fend off moths by storing your woolens in closets, drawers, or chests that are scented with incense cedar or intensely fragrant herbs such as lavender, rosemary, or bay leaves.

There is no such thing as a good reason to use moth balls. They may repel moths, but they poison humans. (See page 380 for details.)

Bedding

Down Maintenance

Comforter covers or duvets help protect down comforters from dirt and grime. Though a well-covered down comforter or pillow may need to be cleaned only every two or three years, it should be fluffed up and aired out regularly. (I like to hang things out to air on breezy days, to take advantage of the wind's power.)

If you are a city dweller who cannot air your downy and feathery bedding outdoors, try hanging them up in front of a sunny window.

Comforters

Down comforters can be machine washed, though not in the average home machine. When your down comforter needs to be cleaned, take it to a commercial laundry, put it in a large capacity front-loading washing machine (the spinning action is gentler than an agitator), and wash it in warm water with a small amount of Woolite, which won't strip the protective natural oils out of the down. (Hand washing a down comforter in a bathtub is a job that is just as wet and almost as awkward as washing a reluctant Saint Bernard, though not nearly as much fun. And the Saint Bernard, unlike the down comforter, will dry rather quickly after the operation.)

The spin cycle of modern front-loading washers removes excess water so efficiently that, if at all possible, you might want to send the comforter through the spin cycle twice: Machine drying down-filled items can be a very slow process. If the comforter emerges nearly dry, you might want to take it home while it is still damp and hang it up.

If you want to machine dry your comforter, put it by itself in a large commercial dryer, and set the heat on low.

Note: There is conflicting information about drying down-filled items. Some sources suggest that putting clean tennis balls or canvas tennis shoes in the dryer helps fluff up the down; others say that the pounding of the tennis balls or tennies damages the down and reduces its useful life. I prefer to err on the side of caution and keep the tennis equipment out of the dryer.

Feather Pillows

I have had such awful luck with feather pillows exploding in the washing machine that I usually either hand wash or rain-wash my pillows, then line dry them. But if you're feeling lucky, there is no reason that you can't wash your pillows in a large commercial machine. If they survive the washing machine, maybe they'll also survive the dryer.

Drying Techniques

Preferred Equipment

- *Nylon cord* with a plastic sheathing is the most common type of clothesline. The plastic coating keeps the clothesline clean and dry so your drying clothes will stay cleaner.
- *Spring clothespins* are more versatile and hold more securely than the old-fashioned, one-piece variety.

  A handy clothespin holder can be made by cutting a hand-size access hole in the side of a one gallon jug, and slicing through the handle near the bottom. The jug can then be hung by its handle from the clothesline. Store wooden clothespins indoors when they are not in use; they will stay cleaner and will be less likely to stain your clothes.
- A *sturdy laundry basket* with comfortable handles is a necessity for hauling heavy, wet laundry. Wicker is pretty, but plastic is waterproof and easier to keep clean.
- *Thick, heavy-duty plastic hangers* and some attachable plastic clips are handy for hanging up pants and skirts as well as smaller items such as socks, bras, and hats.
- *Adjustable pants-stretchers* are indispensable for ironing avoidance.
- A *clothes rack, retractable clothesline*, or *wire shelf* for hanging wet garments indoors.

THE SOLAR CLOTHES DRYER

A while back the brilliant scam artist, Steve Comisar, cleverly exploited the efficiency of line drying laundry by advertising a "Solar Powered Clothes Dryer" for only $49.95. When the suckers, er, customers, opened the eagerly awaited packages, they discovered that the "Scientifically proven, space age clothes dryer" was a piece of clothesline. I'm sure quite a few of them were amused.

The equipment necessary for line drying clothes is usually inexpensive, unless you mail-order it.

Outdoor Line Drying

Drying clothes outdoors on a clothesline is the most energy-efficient drying method of all. The aroma of line-dried laundry is hard to beat; so is the fact that the wind tends to blow the wrinkles out of the drying clothing.

Very still, humid days are virtually useless for line drying; conversely, a high wind can damage or relocate your laundry. The best line-drying days are moderately warm, dry, and slightly breezy.

If you are lucky enough to live in a neighborhood where line drying is allowed (residents of planned neighborhoods should not try this at home!), string up your clothesline where there is plenty of room for your linens to blow freely without contacting trees, buildings, fences, or other obstructions. It is a good idea to have at least part of your clothesline in the shade: Brightly colored garments tend to fade rather quickly in the sun. To increase the odds that your laundry will stay clean while it dries, avoid the "drop zone" under your local birds' favorite perching tree, and before you hang out the wash, wipe the clothesline with a clean, damp rag and check to make sure your clothespins are clean.

Front-loading washing machines have such fast spin cycles that the laundry is spun almost dry. This is a real advantage when laundering clothes that you should not dry in a machine.

Crack-the-Whip

Snap your damp clothes and linens as if you were cracking a whip before you hang them up; this helps straighten out wrinkles and fluffs towels. (The wetter the towels when they are hung on a line, the more likely they are to be stiff when they dry. Towels that are washed and then spun in high RPM front-loading machines are quite close to dry when they come out of the washing machine, so they tend to stay flexible after they are line dried.)

Clothing that is not dryer-safe should be hung up immediately after it is removed from the washing machine.

Plastic or rustproof metal hangers are necessary for hanging up wet or damp clothes; steel or wooden hangers may stain wet clothing. Carefully flatten and smooth the hung-up clothing, button the buttons, straighten the collars and cuffs, then let them dry. Hang your trousers and skirts on hangers that are equipped with rustproof clips. Pants are rather top heavy, so if you hang them upside down, their own weight will straighten out most of the wrinkles.

When you are line drying your shirts and dresses, use two plastic hangers for each item. The hangers' hooks should be facing in opposite directions so the wind can't blow the garment off the line.

Fold linens and towels in half over the line so their hems are even (if the linens were people, their waists would be flopped over the clothesline, and their fingers and toes would be touching). When your linens are folded this way and each edge is pinned to the line, it takes quite a gale to blow them off.

Indoor Line Drying

If your winters are dry enough that you must run a humidifier, you may safely dry your clothes on an indoor clothesline in the winter without causing moisture problems such as dripping windows or damp walls. Laundry will not dry satisfactorily indoors during humid weather unless a dehumidifier is running. (If your domicile is that damp, mildewed walls and books are inevitable. Turn on that humidifier!)

I find that putting damp garments on plastic hangers then hanging them from wire mesh shelving is most convenient. Smaller items can be suspended from plastic clips.

The bathroom tends to be rather humid and is not a good place to hang clothing to dry. Try hanging clothes from a curtain rod in front of a warm window or over a radiator or hot air register.

Delicate Drying

Garments whose labels state that they should be kept out of the sun can be hung to dry indoors. Delicate items such as silks or loosely knit sweaters that may stretch out of shape should be dried flat, not on a clothesline.

Stretched Trousers

Old-fashioned pants stretchers are one of those inventions that simply can't be improved. They are designed to be used on trousers that are still wet from washing. The pants are stretched tightly over the thin adjustable metal frame of the stretcher, and as the pants dry, they shrink and lose all inclination to wrinkle.

The stretchers come in pairs, one for each pant leg, and are quite simple to use: Put a stretcher inside each damp, newly washed pant leg, line it up along the crease line, and adjust it to fit. Hang the stretched trousers upside-down and they will dry wrinkle-free and with perfect knife-edge creases.

If your clothesline is strung up very tightly, you can dry your dress pants with pants stretchers in them. If the line is a bit loose, you may need to dry your stretched pants indoors so they don't drag on the ground.

Pants stretchers are nearly a necessity for the ironing averse. I was lucky enough to be given several pairs of pant stretchers, but they are available through the following outlets:

Cumberland General Store: www.cumberlandgeneral.com
Lehman's: www.lehmans.com
Vermont Country Store: www.vermontcountrystore.com

Oh, if only someone would invent a blouse-, shirt-, and dress-stretcher!

Ironing

If, despite your best efforts, you just cannot avoid ironing, it is my duty as a lifelong shirker to remind you that scorching is forever, unless the fabric is thick enough and tough enough that you can actually remove the scorched surface of the material by brushing it with a stiff brush, rubbing it off under cold water with another piece of cloth, or sanding it with very fine sandpaper.

Safe Ironing

- Put a clean cover on your ironing board. A stained or rusty ironing board can produce permanent stains.
- In order to avoid damaging your clothing, read the care label and follow the manufacturer's ironing instructions.

- Never set the iron for a temperature that is higher than recommended; you may burn or melt your clothing.
- Always use a clean cotton pressing cloth between the iron and the garment when ironing delicate fabrics.
- Use distilled water in your steam iron. The dissolved minerals in undistilled water can build up and clog the holes. (The water that your dehumidifier has pulled out of the air is free of minerals and is perfectly safe to use in a steam iron.)
- Keep your steam iron clean by emptying the water reservoir after each ironing session.
- An iron is hot enough to start a fire. Never leave a hot iron unattended. If you must answer the door, unplug the iron first.

Do Not Iron, Do Not Starch

Try to refrain from ironing items that are meant to be soft and absorbent: towels, napkins, and underwear, for instance. Though stiffly starched, ironed, and origamied napkins look lovely on a formal dining table, they are fairly useless for wiping and sopping-up duties.

Starches, which are derived from plants, make fabrics much more attractive to destructive insects such as silverfish and firebrats. One should only store linens in an unstarched state.

If you want your freshly ironed textiles to smell wonderful, try mixing a couple drops of lavender oil with distilled water in a spray bottle. Use the lavender water to dampen your wrinkled items before ironing. Unlike starch, the lavender spray will repel insects.

A Message from the Department of Redundancy Department

There is almost nothing less efficient than having to do a job over again. Whether you do your laundry daily, every other day, or weekly, paying a little more attention can save you a lot of time and effort. Gratuitous laundry chores can be easily avoided.

- Prevent mildew by emptying the washer promptly and dealing appropriately with its contents.
- Remove laundry from the dryer while it is still warm, then immediately fold it or hang it up to minimize wrinkling. If you remove your laundry before it is completely dry, it will form fewer wrinkles, and it will not have a chance to build up static electricity.
- Prevent the premature cycling of clean clothing by teaching your kids to do their own laundry; though they may be quite willing to make extra work for you, they won't make extra work for themselves. Even young children are capable of carrying a small basket of their clothes to the laundry room, putting them in the machine, adding detergent, and pushing the appropriate buttons.

Roughing It

The standards for the camp laundry are of necessity much lower than the standards for home laundering. There are only a couple of objectives for cleaning clothes while camping: Avoid polluting the water, keep the clothing flexible, and prevent blisters, rashes, and chafing. A small bottle of Dr. Bronner's Pure-Castile Soap is adequate for the average camper's laundering, dishwashing, bathing, and hair washing. Exceptionally stoic campers may also use Dr. Bronner's to clean their teeth.

Grime Prevention for Sleeping Bags

A sleeping bag liner is a washable cloth bag that fits inside a sleeping bag and functions as a sheet. If you use a liner every time you sleep in your sleeping bag, you may never need to wash your sleeping bag at all (you don't wash your mattress, do you?).

Many types of ready-made sleeping bag liners are available. Or you can fabricate a simple liner by folding a sheet in half lengthwise, pinning, then sewing one long seam and one short seam, leaving the other short edge open.

❧ LAUNDRY ROOM SUPPLIES

WASHING

• Natural fragrance-free detergent: A mineral-based powdered detergent is preferable for allergic individuals.
• Hand washing: Woolite or Dr. Bronner's Pure-Castile Soap
• Pretreatment: An enzyme stain remover, such as Nature's Miracle Stain & Odor Remover or Restore EnzAway
• Water-softening, residue removal, and disinfecting: 20 Mule Team Borax or white distilled vinegar
• Whitening and brightening: Hydrogen peroxide; Oxy-Boost; Rit Color Remover, Rit White Wash, or Mrs. Stewart's Liquid Bluing
• Damage prevention: Nylon mesh lingerie bag

OUTDOOR DRYING

• Plastic-coated nylon clothesline
• Spring-closing clothespins
• Sturdy plastic hangers

INDOOR DRYING

• Clothes rack, retractable line, wire mesh shelving, or a convenient pipe for hanging wet clothing indoors
• Sturdy plastic hangers, plastic hangers with attached plastic clips for hanging skirts and trousers, or plastic hooks with clips for hanging socks, bras, hats, and other small items
• Pants stretchers

MISCELLANEOUS

• Large, sturdy clothes baskets
• Hamper for storing dirty laundry
• Wastebasket

It All Comes Out in the Wash . . .

Great-grandma's washday may have been long and exhausting, but at least there was only one washday per week. Life was much simpler then: Great-grandma had only one brand of soap (her own) and far fewer types of fabrics to choose from. All the clothes were boiled, then wrung out and dried in the sun. The next day, all the clothes were ironed back into wearable shape.

Great-grandma divided her clothes into categories before she washed them for the very same reasons that we do: to protect delicate and less soiled items and to reduce the amount of work we have to do. Here are Great-grandma's washday imperatives:

- Mend, then wash.
- Wash the cleanest and most delicate items separately.
- Wash dark-colored items separately.
- If it ain't dirty, *don't wash it!* (And here's a modern-day addendum: Clean it, don't chemically contaminate it!)

There is a big difference between the health effects caused by exposure to clothes that have been soiled with natural substances and exposure to clothing that has been "chemically enhanced." Though gardening clothes may be caked with dirt, streaked with grass stains, and reek of sweat, it is highly unlikely that any healthy person would become seriously ill from wearing them in that state for a week or two; unfortunately, many of us have adverse reactions to clean clothes that have been prettied up with scented detergents or fabric softeners.

Which is cleaner, a pair of mud-caked jeans or a spotless blouse that reeks of fabric softener? I'd much rather take my chances with the muddy jeans!

CHAPTER 6

General Cleaning

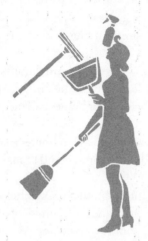

The Well-Tempered House

Up until the eighteenth century, most music in the Western world was performed in only a few keys. Keyboards were tuned to a single perfect scale, and all the other scales were more or less out of tune: Keys with a single sharp or flat were tolerable; those with two or three sharps or flats sounded decidedly strange; and scales that contained more than three accidentals were unbearable. It is no wonder that composers never ventured beyond the tried and true keys.

This entrenched conservatism ended with J. S. Bach, who demanded a different method of tuning that would make it possible for him to compose in all keys. The solution to the problem was to tune a single key (usually middle C) perfectly, and make subtle compromises in tuning the rest of the keyboard. These compromises meant that all the scales were equally imperfect and minutely out of tune: None were perfect, but all were usable. Bach composed a series of preludes and fugues in all the keys to celebrate the invention of this new tuning method, and called the series of compositions the "Well-Tempered Clavier." Tuning has never been the same since, and neither has music composition.

Living a well-tempered life is like playing a well-tempered instrument: Neither is possible without compromise. If the keyboard is perfectly tuned to one scale, the rest of the scales suffer; and a house that is perfectly adjusted to the needs and desires of a single occupant is unlikely to make the other occupants sing.

By adjusting the tension between its inhabitants, it may be possible to turn a house into a harmonious home. The choices we make when we furnish, decorate, clean, and organize our homes can increase or decrease household harmony.

Most people are happiest and at ease in homes that are moderately clean and neat. Both extremes of housekeeping tend to make people unhappy and uncomfortable.

This chapter contains information that will help you clean your home with nontoxic cleaning products and a minimum of effort, so you can spend more quality time with your family or pursuing your hobbies. (Quality time does not include time spent yelling about spills and tracked-in dirt.) It also contains information about how to choose low-maintenance, healthy furnishings that will enhance your quality of life, as well as how to cope with less than ideal furnishings.

Healthy Decor

The United States Environmental Protection Agency (EPA) has ranked indoor air pollution as one of the top five environmental risks to Americans' health. A large percentage of indoor pollution emanates from our furnishings. Upholstery fabric, carpeting, carpet padding and carpet glue, draperies, paint, wallpaper, paneling, plywood, particleboard, and fiberboard can emit a variety of pollutants, including benzene, chloroform, trichloroethylene, carbon tetrachloride, and phthalates. Petroleum-based and scented cleaning products are also big contributors to the problem. The term "Sick Building Syndrome" (SBS) refers to buildings with indoor air pollution problems and the symptoms they cause, which include dry or burning sensations in the nose, eyes, and throat, stuffy or runny nose, sneezing, fatigue or lethargy, headache, dizziness or nausea, irritability, and forgetfulness. The more tightly sealed and energy efficient the building, and the newer its furnishings, the more likely it is to cause Sick Building Syndrome.

We can no longer act as if interior decoration is frivolous and irrelevant, since Sick Building Syndrome is largely caused by our household furnishings and the cleaning products that we use to maintain them. The only cure for SBS is to choose low-emissions furniture, carpeting, paints and varnishes, cleaning products, and personal care products.

Plank, Board, and Parquet Flooring

If you prefer an easily cleaned and resilient natural flooring material, traditional wooden floors are hard to beat. They will outwear all their synthetic competition.

Hardwood floors are so durable that sometimes they outlast their original home. Deconstruction businesses are springing up in many urban areas; these companies carefully take buildings apart and salvage valuable materials. Disassembling condemned houses rather than demolishing them saves materials, energy, money, and landfill space. Older materials are often of higher quality than their newer counterparts, and salvaged materials can be considerably less expensive than buying new materials.

Though wood is a renewable resource, you can reduce your impact on the environment by buying recycled wood flooring. You can also save trees by buying flooring made of bamboo, one of the most renewable resources on the planet (bamboo grows so fast that you can actually hear it crackle as it grows); or buy flooring made of natural cork (cork is the bark of the cork oak, *Quercus suber*, a Mediterranean native whose bark is harvested approximately every ten years). In the future, more varieties of natural flooring will become available.

Sheet Flooring

Perhaps if the performance of vinyl flooring were truly an improvement over linoleum, its predecessor, choosing between the two might be troublesome. I tend to have great difficulty deciding between products that have different but equal virtues; choosing an ice cream flavor can, if you will pardon the pun, stop me cold. But the differences between linoleum and vinyl are stark.

Vinyl flooring could be uncharitably described as decorated sheets of solidified petroleum. It melts easily and, like other chlorinated plastics, it produces horribly toxic smoke when it burns, so it is certainly not the floor of choice for anyone who is worried about fire safety.

Vinyl not only melts and burns; it is also easily cut, gouged, ripped, and abraded. We once wore out a brand-new vinyl floor in less than a year. Vinyl flooring is not biodegradable, so unless it is sent to an incinerator (where vinyl doesn't belong), discarded vinyl flooring will take up space at a landfill forever.

When our son was about eleven years old, he was cooking with his class at school. He picked up a hot saucepan and the handle started to bend so he quickly put the pot down on the vinyl floor, which ignited, producing enough smoke to set off the fire alarm, which caused the evacuation of the entire school.

A Real Environmental Bargain

Most people are understandably reluctant to buy environmentally friendly products whose performance is inferior. This is only right and proper. Buying durable items reduces the need for landfills and helps conserve energy. Luckily for those of us who are worried about indoor air quality and fire safety, yet covet resilient sheet flooring, linoleum is superior to vinyl flooring in absolutely every way.

Vinyl flooring is manufactured from polyvinyl chloride, a toxic, carcinogenic chemical that can cause problems at virtually every stage of its life: If not properly ventilated, the vinyl manufacturing process may poison workers as well as area inhabitants; newly laid vinyl flooring offgasses toxic fumes; and used vinyl flooring is difficult to dispose of and impossible to recycle.

Real linoleum is manufactured from linseed oil (pressed from the seeds of annual flax), sawdust and natural cork, pine rosins, limestone dust, and pigments. These ingredients are mixed together then baked onto a backing made of natural jute fiber. This combination of materials makes linoleum remarkably resistant to fire—unlike vinyl, linoleum cannot melt.

Under normal conditions, linoleum is very durable and has an expected life span of thirty to forty years; it is not easily gouged or ripped, a dropped cigarette will not melt it, and since the colors go all the way through the sheet, linoleum can be buffed and refinished. After it has outlived its usefulness, discarded linoleum can be composted.

Marble, Stone, Ceramic, Concrete, Tile, and Rubber Flooring

Marble, slate, granite, brick, ceramic tile, concrete, and natural rubber floors are all tough and long lasting. Marble and stone can be damaged by contact with acidic liquids. Rubber is resilient, easy on the feet, and recyclable. These are all preferable to synthetic flooring.

Carpeting and Rugs

Natural carpets made of coir, sisal, seagrass, jute, hemp, and cotton are nontoxic and fairly inexpensive, but they are not very durable, and they are flammable. The best carpets and rugs are made of wool. Wool is nontoxic, durable, naturally fire retardant, repels stains and liquid, and absorbs and digests odors. If you buy wool carpeting, make sure you buy a color you can live with because by all accounts, wool carpeting lasts a lifetime!

Wool carpeting may seem expensive, but if you compare its price to the cost of replacing synthetic carpeting every few years, the wool carpet will begin to look like a bargain. If you really can't afford wool carpeting, the next best choice is carpeting made of recycled and recyclable materials.

> Rugmark is a nonprofit organization that rescues children from rug-weaving factories in India, Nepal, and Pakistan, then educates them. The organization is working to stop rug manufacturers from illegally exploiting child weavers.
>
> When you are shopping for a handmade wool rug, look for a Rugmark label, which indicates that the rug was made by adults rather than by exploited, overworked children. E-mail: info@RUGMARK.org

Synthetics

New synthetic carpeting, rugs, carpet padding, and carpet backing can emit chemical fumes for several years. In many sick buildings, synthetic carpet is the source of the majority of the airborne toxins that make people ill. If you are buying synthetic carpeting, either choose a low-emissions carpet that meets the Carpet and Rug Institute's Green Label criteria for indoor air quality, or buy recycled or reconditioned carpeting, which has finished out-gassing. Look for the green and white Green Label logo on carpet samples in the showroom.

Some of the worst chemicals associated with carpeting are the stain and liquid repellents and the fire retardants that are used to coat synthetic fibers in an attempt to make them perform more like wool.

Perfluorinated chemicals (PFOS) are a slippery class of chemicals that are used in the manufacture of coatings that repel oil, grease, and water. These chemicals are apparently imperishable. They have never been known to biodegrade. The levels of these toxins have been steadily rising in the environment and bioaccumulating in mammals (including humans) since 1938, when the first perfluorinated chemical was concocted. Studies have shown that exposure to PFOS can cause birth defects, liver damage, and cancer.

Studies conducted in 2002 by 3M Corporation found that children are more heavily contaminated with these chemicals than are adults. One former researcher speculated that the levels were highest in children who played on stain-repellent carpeting. 3M ceased manufacturing perfluorinated products in 2000, including its original formulation of Scotchguard, which has since been reformulated without the hazardous compound.

Dirtiness and cleanliness can be defined in many different ways. Is a spotless, stain- repellent white rug really cleaner than a stained wool rug?

Dusty Carpets

Even older carpets that are chemically stable may contribute to indoor air pollution. Studies have shown that the air and dust in most American homes is contaminated with worrisome levels of a wide variety of dangerous chemicals. Every spritz of hairspray, spot remover, or deodorant, every dab of nail polish, makes our household dust a tiny bit more poisonous.

The list of contaminants found in household dust during the ongoing Cape Cod Breast Cancer and Environment Study, which began in 1994, includes the following banned chemicals: PCBs, dieldrin, chlordane, heptachlor, pentachlorophenol, methoxychlor, chlorpyrifos, and DDT. Though

DDT has been off the market for more than thirty years, it was detected in the air and dust of 65 percent of the homes that were tested.

Where are these banned chemicals hiding? According to John Spengler of the Harvard School of Public Health, "Carpets are very effective at re-suspending materials." Every time someone walks across a carpet, dust is wafted into the air. Vacuuming also re-suspends particles.

Carpet Choices

Textures

Some carpet textures are easier to live with than others. Dirt is more easily trapped in loosely woven carpets, sculpted carpets, and textured carpets than in carpets with level surfaces and tightly packed fibers.

The most durable carpets have tightly twisted yarn and short, densely packed fibers; longer and looser fibers are more easily frayed, dented, and compacted.

Padding

The padding beneath a carpet protects the carpet as well as the floor beneath. Choose carpet padding with a moisture barrier that will protect the floor from liquids seeping down through the carpeting.

Carpet padding made of 100 percent recycled materials will not release fumes into your home. There are two different types: The most common is multicolored synthetic padding, made of chopped and shredded bits of foam called bonded polyurethane foam or rebond; the other type is made of felted recycled (nonvirgin) wool.

GreenFloors manufactures both types of padding. Website: www.greenfloors.com.

Self-Cleaning Carpeting

Odor-Eaters carpets and carpet pads are impregnated with natural bacterial enzymes that are activated by moisture. These enzymes are similar to those that transform milk into yogurt and cheese, and water, malt, barley, and hops into beer. These self-cleaning carpets will consume the aftermath of any organically based accident. This means that neither the odor nor the stain from spilled milk, broken eggs, greasy burgers, dropped beer, sick dogs, or drunken debauches will become permanent. This is almost as good as growing a low-maintenance groundcover in the living room.

If your accidents are inorganic, you may be out of luck. Try to avoid spilling ink, paint, tar, or nail polish on your carpet.

Odor-Eaters carpet cushions come in six-foot-wide rolls and can be used under wall-to-wall carpeting or area rugs. They are available at retail carpet stores.

Location, Location, Location

If you have a choice, avoid bathroom and kitchen carpeting. Kitchen carpeting tends to absorb airborne cooking grease, and as discussed the only kind of rug that belongs in a bathroom is the kind that can be thrown in the washing machine once a week (especially if young boys live in the house).

End of Carpet-Life Issues

When natural-fiber carpeting reaches the end of its useful life, it can be easily composted. Unfortunately, most modern carpeting is made of synthetic, petroleum-based fibers that cannot be composted.

The Minnesota Office of Environmental Assistance sponsored a waste-sorting study that determined that 5 percent of the material interred in Minnesota's landfills is carpeting. The amount of petroleum-based products thrown in American landfills annually is staggering. (In fact, the amounts are so vast that they have apparently made statisticians woozy: Estimated amounts vary from 1.8 to 2.5 million tons per year.) Efforts are underway to recover as much of this fuzzy petroleum as possible and either recondition it and send it back out to cover floors, or melt it down and use it as a raw material for making products ranging from new carpeting to flooring to car parts.

Reclaimed Carpeting

If your wallet cannot stand the strain of acquiring wool carpeting, the next best alternative is to buy refurbished carpet that has been reconditioned by the manufacturer. After the carpet has been superheated, cleaned, retextured, and redyed, it is actually better than new: Refurbished carpeting comes with a warranty, costs 40 to 45 percent less than "virgin" carpeting, and does not emit fumes.

Most refurbished carpeting comes in the form of carpet tiles, which are also known as modular tiles or modular carpeting. Carpet tiles, which are usually about seventeen inches square, are easy to transport, install, and replace. Once installed, modular carpeting looks seamless.

Carpet tiles make sound financial and environmental sense: When a path is worn in a broadloom (wall-to-wall) carpet, the whole thing must be replaced; when a path is worn in a modular carpet, the worn tiles can be removed and replaced, leaving the rest of the carpet intact. Image and bottom-line conscious businesses and institutions have been using carpet tiles for years.

RECOMMENDED RECYCLED-CARPET MANUFACTURERS

Refurbished Carpet Tiles
Milliken Floorcovering, *Earth Squares:* www.millikencarpet.com

Recycled Carpets and Carpet Recycling Programs:
C & A Floorcoverings: www.cafloorcoverings.com
GreenFloors: www.greenfloors.com
J&J Industries: www.jjindustries.com
Lees Carpets: www.leescarpets.com
Mannington Mills: www.mannington.com

Carpet Recycling Program
The DuPont Corporation accepts used carpeting for recycling. The carpeting is melted down and used to make flooring, soundproofing material, and padding. The company accepts used carpeting from other manufacturers, too.

Carpet Formerly Known as Pop Bottles
It takes about two cases of recycled pop bottles to make one square yard of carpet. These companies make carpeting from recycled PET bottles:
Beaulieau of America: www.beaulieu-usa.com
talismanmills: www.talismanmills.com

The Carpeting Solution

It is probably impossible to clean all the chemical contamination out of wall-to-wall carpeting. The most effective way to reduce chemical contamination in an old home is to rip out and dispose of this carpeting.

Wood, cork, bamboo, stone, or ceramic tile flooring and area rugs made of natural fibers such as wool, cotton, jute, or sisal are all nontoxic, and they are far easier to maintain than are wall-to-wall carpets.

Hardwood floors are the most care free floors of all; they are the easiest to keep clean and last far longer than carpeting. When your hardwood floor eventually needs refinishing, there are nontoxic, water-based floor finishes that are far more durable than the less-expensive, solvent-based finishes.

If you must have wall-to-wall carpeting, wool carpeting is the best choice; it is the most durable, as well as nontoxic and naturally fire-resistant. Wool carpeting is usually free of chemical treatments.

Window Coverings

Glass conducts heat readily, making windows the weakest link in a house's thermal shell. Though insulated, reflective, sealed window units help reduce heat loss in the winter and heat gain in the summer, it is a rare window that cannot use help from well-chosen insulated or heat-reflecting window coverings.

A wide variety of styles of custom or ready-made insulated window coverings are available. Many fabric stores and do-it-yourself centers also sell materials and instructions for constructing window treatments in styles ranging from sophisticated insulated Roman Shades that glide on vertical tracks to tightly woven conventional draperies made of insulating material to the unsophisticated but impressively energy efficient sections of Reflectix (a thin layer of bubble wrap sandwiched between two layers of reflective plastic sheeting) that many of us in frigid northern climates put in our windows during frigid winter nights in order to reduce our heating bills.

Window Blinds

If someone in your household has asthma or a dust allergy, window blinds or shutters, which are easily vacuumed and dusted, are better choices than even the most tightly woven draperies.

Choose metal or wooden slatted window blinds and cloth roller blinds; they are durable and nontoxic. PVC blinds, the cheap alternative, are not durable and may not be safe: In the 1990s, researchers at the U.S. Consumer Product Safety Commission (CPSC) discovered that many imported vinyl (PVC) mini-blinds contain high levels of lead. Vinyl breaks down quickly in sunlight, and lead is one of the additives that can be used to make it more stable. Even with stabilizers, PVC still gradually breaks down and becomes toxic dust. The CPSC found that the lead-laced dust produced by some mini-blinds was so toxic that a child who ingested the dust from one square inch of one of these blinds every day for two weeks could sustain brain damage. (This is unfortunately easy to do: Touch blind. Suck finger.)

Though the problem with vinyl mini-blinds has been well publicized, imported products are not always tested for toxicity, and unless you test them yourself, you cannot be sure that they are safe. (Just this year, high levels of lead have been found in imported costume jewelry, children's jewelry, and gumball-machine toys. Millions of these items have been recalled.)

Building Materials and Furniture

Most of the glues that are used to manufacture press-board, particle board, and plywood generally contain formaldehyde. Formaldehyde fumes are emitted from these materials for several years after they are manufactured.

Solution: If you are in the market for new furniture, either try to buy solid wood furniture or look for used furniture that is old enough so it no longer outgasses formaldehyde. (Ten-year-old furniture should be somewhat stabilized.)

If you are building a new home or are remodeling an old one, look for building materials that are labeled Formaldehyde Free. These less toxic materials usually cost more, but if you are sensitive to chemicals, you may have no choice. In the long run, nontoxic materials may cost less because they help prevent large medical bills.

Choosing Upholstery and Drapery Fabrics

Remember that loosely woven materials are more delicate than tightly woven materials; in addition, loose and knobby weaves are magnets for dust and pet hair, and are difficult to clean.

Petroleum-based synthetic fabrics are quite flammable and are frequently treated with toxic flame-inhibitors. Choose natural materials when you can and avoid fabrics that have been treated for stain and water repellence.

Natural Fibers

The following are plant- or animal-based fabrics: Cotton, linen (linen thread is spun from the stalk fibers of the flax plant), ramie (fiber from a plant in the nettle family), hemp, bark cloth, wool (sheep hair), cashmere (hair from goats that are native to Kashmir), camel hair, alpaca, qiviut (the undercoat of musk oxen; qiviut is the softest natural fiber in the world), horsehair, angora (the hair of angora goats or rabbits), silk (fiber spun by silk worms, which are the larvae of silk moths).

The following stuffing materials are plant- or animal-based: down (the soft under-feathers of geese), eider down (down from the breasts of eider ducks), horsehair, kapok (silky fibers from the seed of the ceiba tree), feathers, latex rubber (processed from the sap of the rubber tree), wool, cotton, cattail fuzz, milkweed silk.

A Separate but Natural Category

Leather, made of dehaired, softened animal skins, is very durable and fire resistant. It is an excellent choice for sofa upholstery that will resist the depredations of small children, pets, and smokers.

Petroleum-Based Materials

The following fabrics are synthesized from fossil fuel, so they melt easily and produce toxic smoke when they burn: nylon, polyester, polypropylene, polyethylene, Capilene, Polartec, Thinsulate, acrylic, modacrylic, olefin, vinyon, Saran, and spandex.

Vinyl (PVC) cannot really be called a fabric, but it is one of the most potentially toxic petroleum-based materials.

Wood Pulp-Based Fibers

The following fibers are spun from natural cellulose derived from wood pulp. When they burn, the smoke they produce is similar to that of other plant-based materials: rayon, viscose rayon, high wet modulus (HWM) rayon, Modaltm, polynosic rayon, acetate, triacetate, lyocell, Tencel.

Rayon is a versatile fiber that is used to make clothing, home furnishings, surgical products, feminine hygiene products, and tire cord.

A note about microfibers: Microfiber refers to the diameter of the synthesized fibers that make up the fabric. These very thin, fine fibers can be made of either polyester or rayon, so check the label.

Corn-Based Fibers

Since the 1980s, researchers have been working on biodegradable, plant-based replacements for petroleum-based fibers and materials. One promising material is Polylactic acid (PLA), which can be synthesized from corn sugars and used to manufacture fibers, fabrics, foam, and plastics. A few PLA products, such as PLA foam pillows and PLA fiberfill comforters, are already on the market. The automobile industry is researching the use of PLA carpeting, foam, acoustic fibers, and PLA plastic panels in order to facilitate the recycling of scrapped cars.

It will be a happy day for all of us when petroleum-based mattress and upholstery foam is replaced by safer, biodegradable foam!

Harmonizing

The furnishings and decor of your home should help make you comfortable and bring you joy; the other people you live with should also be able to experience this joy. Small children, inattentive adults, and pets are often made unhappy by delicate, easily damaged furnishings. Try to choose your furnishings based on your actual, rather than your ideal, lifestyle.

Annoying Building Syndrome

Annoying Building Syndrome (ABS) is caused by unfortunate decorating choices. ABS can waste large amounts of time and may cause familial discord. Knowledge is the only protection against ABS. Unfortunately, most people learn about ABS the hard way: by purchasing high-maintenance furniture or rugs that make their lives miserable.

I have interviewed many householders about their experiences with ABS, then compiled their hard-won knowledge. Here are some suggestions for designing a low-maintenance household.

Color Choices

- White and light colored rugs are generally not improved by association with children, pets, or messy adults. Many a first-time homeowner has indulged in a light, sophisticated decorating theme, only to regret it when the children began arriving: "I loved my white carpeting and couch until we had kids!"

    Solution: If you are neat, tidy, and happily single or your native soil is white, by all means, buy that ecru carpet and the sofa to match. Otherwise, stick to medium-dark fabrics and carpeting.

- Very dark carpets and upholstery show every bit of dust, lint, and pet hair that sticks to them.

    Solution: Choose medium-

 A friend once told me about a woman who lived in Oklahoma, who had just begun housecleaning when a passing tornado destroyed her house. She was convinced that the tornado had been attracted by her housekeeping activities, and she vowed never to clean again. While the workmen were rebuilding her house, she set white carpet samples outside every door. After several weeks, the workmen had completely saturated the carpet pieces with good red Oklahoma clay; the good lady brought a sample to the carpet store and told them to match the color. She is thrilled with her spot-free carpeting.

dark fabrics and carpeting. Better yet, match your upholstery and carpeting to your pets. A friend of mine owns a little tan cairn terrier that perfectly matches her wall-to-wall carpeting; she also has a large black Newfoundland that doesn't. You never see a single cairn terrier hair on her carpet. You never see a single Newfoundland hair on her carpet either: It's all in clumps. Next time she should get a large tan dog and a small black one.

- Dark-colored bathroom fixtures highlight every molecule of soap scum, and black or brown toilets actually look dirty more quickly than do lighter-colored toilets.
  Solution: Choose white or light-colored bathroom fixtures.

Finishes and Fabrics
- Many synthetic upholstery fabrics build up a static charge that attracts and tenaciously holds dust, dirt, and pet hair.
  Solution: Choose natural fabrics.

- Hair tends to twine through the large openings in coarsely woven fabric; these intertwined hairs are nearly impossible to vacuum out. Sometimes the only way to remove the hair is to pull each strand out of the fabric by hand.
  Solution: Choose tightly woven fabrics.

- Mirrored or polished metal, stainless-steel, and shiny black surfaces highlight dust, dirt, water spots, and grease, and preserve a record of every hand, finger, and dog nose that touches them between cleanings. Kitchen appliances with textured surfaces are hard to wipe clean of the grease that settles into their surface crevices.
  Solution: Choose kitchen appliances with smooth, shiny, light-colored finishes, rather than shiny black or stainless steel. Plumbing fixtures with a white, satin, or gun metal finish will hide water spots.

- Matte paints and other rough wall coverings such as textured, flocked, or woven wallpaper cannot be scrubbed or otherwise washed.

Solution: Unless you really enjoy painting, choose smooth, washable wall coverings for high traffic areas, kitchens, bathrooms, halls, and children's rooms.

- Large knickknack collections take hours to dust.

   Solution: Put your knickknacks and other small decorative items in glass-fronted cabinets. It takes far less time to dust the top of one cabinet than to pick up and dust 148 separate ceramic ducks.

Cleaning Methods

Not long after you acquire a home and furnishings, they will accrue a coat of dust, dirt, or grime. Here's how to clean it off.

Equipment
Broom with soft nylon bristles
Dutch Rubber Broom (see page 67 for full description)
Clean rags
Sturdy wash buckets
Scrub brush with stiff nylon bristles
Long-handled scrub brush with stiff nylon bristles
Spray bottles
A vacuum cleaner with a high-efficiency filter system (HEPA)
Synthetic "Cousin It" duster that attracts dust through static
    electricity (these come in short- and long-handled versions;
    the long-handled dusters are handy for dusting ceiling fans
    and pulling down cobwebs from ceiling corners and can be
    purchased at hardware stores, discount stores, and cleaning
    supply stores) *or* handkerchief-size squares of synthetic fleece
    fabric

Recommended Cleaning Products
White distilled vinegar made from grain
Baking soda
Liquid Castile Soap (Dr. Bronner's)

Murphy's Oil Soap
Pet Stain Remover that is enzyme-based
Olive oil
Beeswax
Glycerin-based liquid saddle soap
Hydrogen peroxide
Citrus solvent (There are two different types of citrus solvent:
    One is extracted from citrus peels and the other is synthesized
    from petroleum. Before buying, read the labels, then choose
    citrus-derived solvent.)

Hardwood, Resilient, and Tile Floors

Most modern floors have a tough, long-lasting factory finish. If the floor is kept free of grit, this finish will last for many years. Most of these finishes do not require waxing, but read and follow the manufacturer's care instructions. When the finish begins to wear off, the floor will need to be stripped and given a new coat of urethane. Urethane finishes are preferable to slippery, high-maintenance waxed finishes.

Note: Refinishing a floor used to be a grueling, sickeningly toxic job. The job is still grueling, but modern water-based urethane floor finishes are nontoxic and fume-free; they are also tougher and longer lasting than the older, solvent-based finishes. If you don't have strong muscles, high tolerance for noise, dust, and boredom, and at least a week to devote to the job, you should probably hire a professional floor-refinisher.

Protective Measures

It is much easier to prevent grit from entering your home than to remove it.

- Put large rubber-backed, commercial floor mats inside and outside all entrance doors. These mats will remove a lot of the grit, sand, road salt, water, and dirt that would otherwise end up on your floors.
- It is standard procedure in some areas (Japan and northern Minnesota, for instance) for residents and guests to remove their shoes

when they enter a home. This practice helps keep the homes much cleaner.
- Wipe your pets' feet when they come inside.
- Put felt-bottomed furniture glides under furniture feet.

Dry Mopping, Damp Mopping, Sweeping, Vacuuming
All floors should be swept, vacuumed, or dry mopped frequently to remove dirt and grit that can scratch and damage the finish.

When you clean a floor, start at the farthest corner and move out the door. Avoid traipsing through your dust piles, and try not to walk over cleaned areas. Sweep gently to avoid sending dust aloft.

Cleaning Organic Flooring
Cork, linoleum, hardwood, laminate, and bamboo flooring are all environmentally friendly materials that are made of renewable resources.

Standing water can cause these organically based floors to warp, swell, or buckle. Wipe up spills immediately, and clean the floor with a barely damp cloth, then towel dry.

Sweep, dry mop, or vacuum the loose dust and debris off the floor before attempting to wet or damp mop or you will make mud.

Avoid using cleaning products, waxes, or polishes that contain natural or synthetic waxes or oils on floors that have shiny surface finishes. Wax and oil can make these floors dangerously slippery and may void the manufacturer's warranty.

Cork Flooring
- Sweep or vacuum frequently to remove finish-damaging grit.
- Wipe the floor clean with an almost-moist cloth, then wipe dry.
  (Try washing your hands, shaking off the excess water, then drying your hands on a clean, dry cleaning rag. The amount of water on the rag is the amount you can use for cleaning your cork floor.)

- Never wet mop. Wipe up spills promptly.
- Follow the manufacturer's recommendations about rewaxing and buffing.
- Do not use acrylic wax.
- When the floor finish begins to show signs of wear, have it professionally refinished.

Hardwood, Bamboo, Wood Parquet, Linoleum, and Laminate Floors

- Sweep or vacuum frequently to remove finish-damaging grit.
- Wipe clean with a lightly dampened cloth, then wipe dry. (The easiest way to accomplish this is to give the clean cloth one quick spritz from your spray bottle of cleaning vinegar, drop the cloth on the floor, and push it around with a Dutch Rubber Broom.)
- Never wet mop. Wipe up spills promptly.
- Do not use an acrylic floor wax on a floor with a urethane finish.

Marble, Stone, Ceramic Tile, Rubber, and Vinyl Floor Care

- Sweep, vacuum, or dry mop the floor frequently to remove abrasive grit, dirt, or sand.
- Wipe up spills immediately. Most beverages are mildly acidic and can etch stone surfaces.
- Wet mop the floor weekly with warm water and a clear, nonabrasive, nonacidic soap such as Dr. Bronner's or Murphy's Oil Soap.

How to Wet Mop

- Fill a cleaning bucket with warm water. Add a squirt of liquid soap.
- Drop a clean dry rag into the bucket of soapy water, then wring it out slightly.
- Put the rag on the floor, place the head of your Dutch Rubber Broom on the rag, and scrub the floor.
- Replace the used rag with a clean one each time you need more water.

This is an efficient, effective, puddle-free way to wash a floor. The wash water stays clean, and the floor gets cleaner because you never put a dirty rag in the bucket.

Caveat: If your floor is very smooth and tends to be slippery, *do not use oil soap!* Use Dr. Bronner's instead. Oil soap can make a smooth floor dangerously slippery.

Floor Wax

Manufacturers of some types of flooring do not recommend waxing their floors. Follow the manufacturer's recommendations.

Most modern floor waxes do not contain natural wax, which is softer and more slippery than the more common synthetic polyethylene or polypropylene waxes. The synthetic finishes are not only tougher, longer lasting, and clearer than the old-fashioned natural wax finishes, most also contain fewer volatile solvents than did their waxy predecessors.

Many floor finishes contain large concentrations of volatile organic compounds (VOCs) that contribute to indoor and outdoor air pollution, as well as other chemicals that can damage human and planetary health. Look for floor finishes that are labeled Low Emissions or have been awarded the Green Seal.

Product Testing

Green Seal is an independent, nonprofit, nonpolitical organization that tests chemical products in order to determine how safe and environmentally benign they are. The best products are awarded the Green Seal.

Green Seal Recommended Floor Finishes

Enviro Solutions High Gloss Finish #80
Enviro Solutions High Traffic Floor Finish #96
Hillyard Industries Super Hil-Brite
JohnsonDiversey, Inc. Butcher's Neon Floor Finish
Johnson Wax Professional ZF1500+ UHS Floor Finish
M.D. Stetson Transcend Floor Finish
Pioneer Eclipse Corporation EnviroStar Green Floor Coating

Rochester Midland Corporation EC Resilient Tile Coating
Spartan Chemical Company Green Solutions Floor
Seal & Finish

Green Seal Recommended Floor Strippers
Enviro Solutions ES-85 Scrub Free Floor Stripper
Fuller Brush T.E.T. Power Stripper
M.D. Stetson EPS (Environmentally Preferable Stripper)
Orison Marketing, LLC Eco Natural Floor Stripper
Pioneer Eclipse Corporation Envirostar Green Floor Stripper
Rochester Midland Corporation EC Floor Finish Remover

CONTACT INFORMATION

www.enviro-solution.com
www.fuller.com
www.hillyard.com
www.johnsondiversey.com
www.mdstetson.com
www.orisonllc.com
www.pioneer-eclipse.com
www.rochestermidland.com
www.green-solution.com

How to Apply Floor Wax
1. Clean all dirt, grime, and grease off the floor using the appropriate technique for the flooring type.
2. Choose a floor finish that is recommended for your type of floor.
3. Follow the instructions on the product container.
4. Each time you wax, apply the finish to the heavy traffic areas of the floor. Areas that are rarely or never walked on—such as corners, close to the walls, and under the furniture—may never need to be waxed at all. If you do wax these seldom trod-upon areas, apply the finish lightly and quite infrequently (once every couple of years is probably plenty).

Rug and Carpet Care,
with a Little Upholstery Thrown In

Nontoxic Dry Cleaning
- To sweeten a rug and make it smell better, sprinkle it with baking soda, use a stiff-bristled broom or scrub brush to work the baking soda into the rug, then vacuum up the baking soda.
- Salting a rug will loosen dirt and kill flea and moth eggs. Sprinkle the carpet with salt, work it into the nap with a stiff broom, then vacuum up the salt.

Cleaning Area Rugs
Many hand-knotted wool rugs are not dry-cleanable and are too fragile for carpet-cleaning machines. Rain-washing is an excellent method for cleaning these delicate carpets and can even be used to renovate musty old wool carpets that you might otherwise be tempted to throw out.

How to Rain-Wash a Carpet
Carpets should never be hung up for rain washing, lest their own weight damage their backing. They should be laid out on sheets or towels on a flat, clean surface such as a lawn, a patio, or a picnic table (the wire-mesh type of picnic table is absolutely ideal for rain washing). If your rug is made of wool, choose a washing venue that is in the shade, since wet wool may yellow when exposed to sunlight.

This technique may be unsuitable for large, room-size carpets, which become prohibitively heavy when wet.

1. Listen to the weather forecast, and wait until a heavy rain followed by several days of fair weather is expected.
2. Roll the carpet up and carry it outside.
3. Lay it face down on the sheet- or towel-covered flat surface.
4. Let the rain wash through the carpet.
5. Let the carpet dry in the shade. If the forecast was wrong and the rain lasts for days, you may need to roll the rug up and carry it into an outbuilding or garage where you can lay it out for further drying.

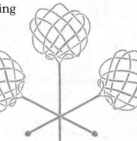

If the rug is drying very slowly, try hanging it over several taut clotheslines to dry.

6. Before bringing the dried carpet indoors, shake it briskly or beat it vigorously with a broom in order to dislodge and kill any insect eggs it may have acquired.

Snow Cleaning

Snow cleaning is recommended by many dealers of fine handmade woolen and silk rugs. Any carpet that can be rolled up and carried outside can be safely snow cleaned.

Snow cleaning works best during very cold weather when the snow is too dry to make decent snowballs or snowmen.

How to Snow Clean a Carpet

1. Roll up the carpet.
2. Stand the carpet on end and let it cool down for a couple of hours so its residual heat doesn't melt the snow beneath it. (The cooling down can be done in an unheated porch, garage, or outbuilding.)
3. When the carpet has cooled down, unroll it pile side down on a clean patch of sugar snow.

Our local bed & breakfast had an oriental rug in the entryway that was nearly ruined by the foot traffic during the Holiday Tea Open House, which was held during a heavy ice and snow storm. Road grit, salt, and dirt tracked in by revelers turned the rug's tassels completely black, and the entire rug was filthy. The owner had just learned about snow washing, so she decided to try it. After the holidays the rug was rolled up and hauled into the snowy backyard, where it was unrolled onto some pristine snow and stomped on. To the owner's astonishment, the rug was restored to its original glowing colors, which hadn't been seen for years, and its tassels actually turned white again.

The owner has begun snow washing her entire carpet collection.

4. Beat the back of the carpet with a broom or stomp on it, until the snow beneath gets dirty.
5. Move the carpet to a clean patch of snow. Repeat steps 4 and 5 until the snow beneath stays mostly clean.
6. Sweep the snow off the rug.
7. Roll the carpet up and bring it inside.

Maintenance Cleaning

Wall-to-wall carpeting can be tricky to maintain because it must be cleaned without ruining the underlying floor. But whether your floor covering is a room-size Persian rug or wall-to-wall carpeting, its preventive maintenance requirements are the same:

- Abrasive particles can damage carpet fibers. Vacuum frequently to remove dirt, sand, and grit before it gets ground deeply into the carpet fibers. Vacuum diagonally across small area rugs to avoid sucking the edges into the vacuum cleaner.
- Fluff up the dents caused by furniture legs by spraying steam from a steam iron or steam cleaner into the depressions. Spray the steam from a couple inches above the carpet; do not allow the iron to touch the carpet. Apply enough steam to heat up the carpet, then gently fluff the nap up with your fingers.

  Furniture coasters under the legs of furniture will help spread out the weight of the furniture and reduce or prevent dents in carpeting.

Cleaning specialists maintain carpeting by cleaning it lightly and frequently, rather than deeply and seldom. The light cleaning method they use is called bonnetting, and it involves a specialized machine with a fitted cloth pad (the bonnet) that is dampened in a cleaning solution.

Here is a simple, low-tech approximation of bonnetting: This method uses a very small amount of full-strength white vinegar to clean the surface of the carpet. Unlike other cleaning solutions, vinegar does not need to be rinsed out, and it doesn't leave a sticky, dirt-attracting residue. Wiping a carpet down with vinegar will brighten its colors and remove dirt.

1. Vacuum the rug or carpet thoroughly, using a carpet head with a powered beater-bar, if you have one.
2. Use a heavy-duty rubber band (the kind that is used to bundle produce works well) to clamp a large, clean rag or towel over the working end of a Dutch Rubber Broom, stiff-bristled corn broom, or sponge mop.
3. Set a spray bottle of white vinegar on fine mist. Working from a standing position, pull the trigger once per one-foot-square section of carpet. Dampen about four square feet of carpet at a time. The carpet should feel barely damp, as if a mouse had sneezed on it.
4. Use a gentle pulling motion to wipe the vinegar-misted carpet with the rag-swathed mop or broom. Do not scrub, lest you damage the carpet's pile. Wiping the vinegar off the top of the carpet should take only a couple of strokes.
5. When the rag gets dirty or too wet to soak up vinegar, replace it with a clean, dry one.
6. After you finish the first four-foot section, bend down and feel the carpet; it should feel completely dry to the touch within minutes.
7. Repeat steps 1 to 6 for the next four-foot section of carpet.

Note: This is one cleaning job that works best when done very lightly. If you work hard enough to wear yourself out, you are also wearing out your carpet.

The same vinegar-mist method can also be used to clean the surface of upholstered furniture. Spray the furniture very lightly with vinegar, then polish the surface with a clean, dry rag.

Steam Cleaning

The best way to deep-clean wall-to-wall carpeting or upholstered furniture is with an extractive steam-cleaning machine. These machines use steam to loosen the dirt, then vacuum up the dirty water. The best carpet shampoo in the world cannot compete with water, the Universal Solvent, when it is in the form of steam. Newly shampooed carpeting looks nice, but the shine may wear off rather rapidly as the shampoo residues attract and hold dirt; a steam-cleaned carpet is free of residue and will not attract dirt.

Consumer-grade steam cleaning machines are quite effective, but if you need more power, larger, commercial-grade steam cleaners are readily available at rental centers. Follow the manufacturer's instructions, but use plain water only.

All-Purpose Carpet and Upholstery Cleaning Foam

Check the label on your upholstery before attempting any wet-cleaning methods.

Mud spots and many other garden variety stains may succumb to this all-purpose foam: Pour a half cup distilled white vinegar into a small mixing bowl. Add a tablespoon of dish liquid. Use an egg beater or electric mixer to whip the mixture to a stiff froth.

1. Apply the foam to the carpet with a stiff brush.
2. Avoid making scrubbing motions, which can ruin the texture of the carpet. Instead, push the foamy bristles deep down into the carpet. While keeping the brush tips stationary, jiggle the brush handle to work the foam into the carpet pile.
3. Blot up the suds with a clean, dry rag.
4. Rinse by blotting the area with a clean, damp rag, then blot dry.
5. Go over the area with a wet vac or steam cleaner, if possible.

Stains

It is much easier to prevent spills and stains than to clean them out of carpeting and upholstery. Try to limit your eating and drinking to uncarpeted rooms, and supervise young children's art projects.

But into even the most well-regulated life, rogue liquids will fall, and when they land on the carpet, deal with them efficiently, like so:

- Clean quickly. The more quickly you attend to a spill, the less likely it is to stain. Use a clean, dry rag and blot the spot from the outside in; try to prevent the stain from spreading outward.
- Blot gently by pressing straight down on the wet spot. Rubbing may damage the carpet fibers, and a fuzzy spot may be just as unsightly as the stain it is replacing.
- As soon as the rag gets wet, replace it with a clean one. Continue blotting gently until a clean rag stays dry when pressed against the spot, or use a wet/dry vac to suck up the excess liquid.
- Use a minimum of liquid for cleaning, and blot up spills as quickly as possible.
- Any soap or detergent that is left in the carpet will attract dirt like a magnet. So after you have finished cleaning up the spot, use a wet/dry vac to suck up the excess cleaning solution and speed the drying. Or go over the area with a steam-extraction cleaner.
- If the carpet pad or upholstery stuffing gets wet and stays wet, it may mildew, stink, and stain.
- After the excess liquid has been removed but before the spot has dried, you can take stock of the situation and act accordingly, based on the nature of the "accident."

Here are some tried and true spot cleaning methods:

Animal-Based Protein Stains

1. Remove all solids. Blot up as much liquid as possible. If you have a wet dry vac, use it.

   If you are cleaning up vomit, pour at least half an inch of baking soda onto the wet spot. The baking soda will wick up and neutralize the liquid. Digestive juices are extremely acidic and may bleach your carpet if they are not rapidly neutralized. Pick up the clumps of baking soda.

2. If your carpet is synthetic or plant-based (cotton, jute, coir, hemp,

seagrass, etc.), you can use an enzymatic pet urine remover product (these are available at pet shops and at hardware and building supply stores), which will digest all traces of animal protein, including milk, eggs, urine, feces, vomit, and blood. (Unfortunately, enzyme cleaners cannot be used on protein-based materials such as wool, silk, feathers, fur, or leather: These enzymes will happily digest the spilled milk as well as the wool carpet.)

Remove as much of the liquid and solid material as possible before applying the enzyme product. You must carefully follow the directions on the label: Usually the spot must be covered and kept damp for a few days to give the enzymes a chance to work. Covering the area with aluminum foil will prevent the pet from rebaptising the rug while the enzymes are working.

3. If the offended surface is made of wool, silk, leather, fur, feathers, or any other protein-based material, proceed as in step 1, then sprinkle the spot with another quarter inch of baking soda and spray on enough vinegar to soak the soda. A lot of bubbling and fizzing will ensue. Let the spot dry, then vacuum up the powder. (This technique is used by cleaning specialists who take care of the mess that inconsiderate corpses leave behind on carpeting.)

4. After you have finished the initial steps, cleaning the area with an extractor-type steam cleaner can help restore the texture of the rug.

Spot Training

It is easier and more pleasant to prevent accidents than to clean them up. Dogs desperately want to please us and to be good. Do your newly acquired puppy a favor and begin housebreaking him immediately. We have found the kenneling method to be simple and effective. Here's how to do it:

- Dogs are very reluctant to soil their dens. When you are not watching or playing with your puppy, put him in a portable crate or kennel that is big enough for him to comfortably lounge in. Put some clean folded towels in the bottom of the kennel to pad the floor. This kennel will become your puppy's den, his place of refuge.

- When you are ready to feed, play with, or keep careful watch over your puppy, open the kennel door and carry him outside to relieve himself. When he accomplishes his task, praise him effusively, then bring him indoors and play with him.
- While the puppy is out of the kennel, watch him carefully for signs that he needs to relieve himself (squatting, wandering aimlessly, etc.) and try to take him outside before he has a chance to wet or soil your floors. If he starts to mess indoors, grab him and run outside with him. *Do not hit or yell!* Remember, a puppy is only a baby; be encouraging when he does his duty outdoors.
- When you leave the house or need to get something done, put the puppy back in the kennel. Do not leave the puppy incarcerated for extended periods of time, and make sure to keep the kennel clean.
- For more detailed, expert dog training advice, consult your veterinarian, a professional dog trainer, or your local kennel club.

Kitty's Accidents

Though methods for cleaning up cat accidents are exactly the same as for canine accidents, the strategies for preventing feline accidents are different.

Using a litter box is normal feline behavior. A cat that regularly goes outside the box is usually either sick, angry, or a territorial male that should have been neutered before he matured.

REDUCING ACCIDENTS

1. Cats dislike dirty litter boxes. Clean the solids out of the litter box daily and replace the litter when it gets damp.
2. Experts recommend that each household should have one litter box per cat, plus a spare, like so: One cat should have two litter boxes; two cats should have three litter boxes; three cats should have four litter boxes, etc.
3. Cats dislike change. Do not suddenly switch brands of kitty litter. If your cat doesn't like the new litter, there will be accidents.

If you want to switch brands, try putting the new brand in only one of the litter boxes to give your cat(s) a chance to get used to it.

4. If a formerly sedate cat suddenly starts relieving himself outside of the litter box and there is no obvious external reason, the cat may be ill. Take him to the vet.

Grease

Soap is made from fats or oils that have been heated and combined with a strong alkali, such as lye; this process is called "saponification." When we use alkaline substances such as soap, baking soda, washing soda, or borax to break up grease, we are taking advantage of the reaction between grease and alkalis.

- The best way to deal with greasy spills or stains is to immediately smother them with enough baking soda to soak up all the liquid, then use a shop-vac to remove the greasy baking soda.
- If a greasy spot remains, complete the cleaning by patting the soiled area gently with a clean rag dampened with a mild dish detergent or Woolite and water.
- Steam cleaning can also work wonders on grease stains.

Ink

1. Cover fresh, wet ink with table salt, then vacuum up the stained salt. Repeat until the spot is dry.
2. Apply cheap full-strength vodka to the salty, inky spot with a clean rag. Blot and repeat until the spot disappears.
3. Wet vac or steam clean the area if possible.

Indelible or permanent ink may not be removable. Now is the time to gloat if your wall-to-wall carpeting is made up of carpet tiles.

Soot Marks

If the chimney sweep has walked across your ecru carpeting, vacuum up the loose soot then use an art gum eraser to erase the residual marks. (Art gum erasers are small blocks of pure natural rubber that are available at art supply stores.)

Chewing Gum

Chewing gum gets brittle when it is cold. This fact will help get it out of your carpet.

- Cool the blob with ice cubes. When the gum hardens, hit it with a hammer to break it off the rug. Pick and scrape the pieces out of the rug. After you have removed as much of the cold, brittle gum as possible, pour a small amount of very warm vinegar on the gummy spot, then gently agitate the area with a clean, stiff brush. The warm vinegar will dissolve the gum residue so it can be blotted up.
- If you happen to have a container of dry ice lying around, freeze the gum with dry ice, then proceed as above. (Never touch dry ice with your bare hands; it is cold enough to blister your skin.)
- Cold weather sometimes comes in handy. If the weather is very cold and the gum is on a portable rug, take the rug outside. Leave it there until the rug is very cold, then hit the gum with a hammer.

Red Wine and Other Alcoholic Beverages, Tea, Coffee, and Other Plant-Based Stains

1. Pour a thick layer of salt on the wet spot, let it absorb the liquid, then use a wet dry vac to suck up the damp salt.
2. Dip a clean rag in a solution of warm water and a little borax or dish liquid, and gently blot the stain until it disappears.
3. Blot the spot dry with a clean dry towel.
4. Rinse with a clean rag dipped in warm water.
5. Blot dry with a clean rag.
6. Wet vac or steam clean the area if possible.

Have you ever noticed that no one ever seems to spill white wine or mineral water? When the elbow hits the glass, the glass usually contains red wine, milk, or grape juice.

Candle and Crayon Wax

Cover the waxy spot with ice cubes to make it brittle, then hit the wax with a hammer. Pick out and scrape off as much of the wax as possible. Then put a clean, damp, white rag over the spot and iron it with a warm iron. The steam will melt the wax, and the hot, damp cloth will suck it out of the carpet. (Do not use a hot iron, lest you melt or ignite a synthetic carpet or shrink a wool one.)

Citrus solvent will remove residual stains from crayons and candle wax.

Tar

Scrape off as much of the tar as you can, working from the outside of the blob to the inside to avoid spreading the stain. Pour citrus solvent on a clean rag and apply it to the stain. Blot gently, then apply more citrus solvent with a clean section of the rag. Repeat until the stain disappears.

Soak up the excess citrus solvent with baking soda, and vacuum it up. Spray the area with full strength white vinegar, and blot up as much of the moisture as possible. Use a wet vac or steam cleaner to remove residual moisture.

Walls and Ceilings

Unfortunate wall- and ceiling-covering choices can be physically and/or psychologically unpleasant: Paints and wall coverings that emit volatile organic chemicals (VOCs) pollute indoor air and cause health problems, while walls and ceilings that are difficult to keep clean can be a source of great frustration. Wall and ceiling finishes should be both nontoxic and easy to clean.

Toxic Wall Coverings

The following wall coverings are not recommended:

- Vinyl wall coverings, like other vinyl products, may emit toxic pollutants for many years after they are installed. Unfortunately, vinyl wallcoverings don't just give off pollutants, they actually produce new ones: Experts in the building trades, as well as in the vinyl industry, have stated that vinyl wall coverings, because they are impermeable and trap moisture in the walls, are the primary cause of indoor mold and mildew infestations, some of which are toxic.

A vinyl-clad wall may look clean and easy to care for, but what is the point of being able to easily clean the nontoxic crayon marks off vinyl wallpaper that is exhaling endocrine-disrupting phthalates while protecting and concealing a crop of toxic mold?

- Water- and stain-repellent wall coverings are coated with less-than-salubrious chemicals. Choose untreated wall coverings. Better yet, stick with painted or stenciled designs and faux finishes, which are safer as well as much more durable than wallpaper. Most paint stores and hardware stores sell ready-made faux finish paints, along with the necessary gadgets and instructions.

  You can also find many fine books on the subject of faux finishes and stenciling at your local library or bookstore.

- Fiberboard- and plywood-backed paneling may emit formaldehyde for many years after they are installed. If you want the look of wood-panelled walls, use real wood, preferably salvaged or recycled wood.

Paint

There are good reasons why paint is the most common wall finish: It is the least expensive, easiest to apply, and easiest to replace—and if you make a mistake, you can simply paint over it.

The days of dangerously toxic interior paints are waning: Lead paint was outlawed in the United States in 1978 (the nontoxic white pigment, titanium dioxide, is now used instead of white lead), and mercury, which was used as a fungicide, was banned as a paint additive in 1991.

Children who live in buildings that have old lead paint are still at risk of lead poisoning. If you suspect that your home contains lead paint, contact your local health department and ask for advice.

Homeowners should never attempt to scrape, sand, strip, heat, or burn off lead paint.

Generally, the lead paint must be covered with another building material, such as wallboard, to sequester the lead-contaminated dust and paint chips. Removing lead paint is a job for lead abatement experts.

Nontoxic Paint

There are two main types of interior paints: water-based (latex) and oil-based (alkyd). Water-based paints dry more quickly, emit fewer fumes while they are drying, and can be cleaned up with soap and water. Oil paints take longer to dry and continue to emit toxic fumes—which may include acetone, toluene, turpentine, and xylene—until they are completely dry. (If you can smell it, it's emitting fumes.) Oil paint cleanup requires paint thinner or other volatile solvents. People who are chemically sensitive may react to new oil paint for months.

The least toxic latex paints are labeled Low VOC. These are paints that have been formulated to emit the lowest possible amount of fumes, both before and after they dry.

Specialty Finishes

Milk paint is made of milk protein, lime, clay, and earth pigments. Milk paint is one of the oldest known surface finishes: Wooden items in King Tutankhamen's tomb were painted with milk paint. Milk paint forms a durable, nontoxic, matte finish, which nowadays is most commonly used on furniture, toys, and woodwork. You can find milk paint at these websites: The Old Fashioned Milk Paint Company (www.milkpaint.com) and The Real Milk Paint Company (www.realmilkpaint.com).

Shellac is a hard, clear finish that is made of the resin secreted by a scale insect cultivated in India. Shellac is a natural, nontoxic alternative to petroleum-based wood finishes. It can be used on furniture and wood paneling, but it is not recommended as a floor finish because it is not water resistant. Look up Zinsser Co. Inc. (www.zinsser.com).

Choosing Finishes

Matte or flat finishes, whether paint, cloth, or wallpaper, are not washable. Those who prefer to wash a wall rather than repaint or repaper should choose paints that have a bit of shine, such as satin, semigloss, and gloss paints. Heavily used areas look cleaner when painted with glossy paint. Bathrooms, kitchens, and other rooms that tend to be damp should only be painted with high-gloss paint, which is more water resistant than matte paints.

Insulating Paint, the Wave of the Future

Paint can do far more than simply provide pretty colors and textures. Insulating paint can increase the comfort level of a home, reduce utility bills, and help prevent the growth of mildew caused by condensation on cold outside walls.

Most insulating paint utilizes the ceramic technology used to make the insulating heat shields on space vehicles. This material is used to make microscopic, hollow ceramic balls that turn ordinary paint into reflective insulating paint.

Reflective insulating paint is more expensive than plain paint, but it is also thicker and far more durable, fills in small cracks and irregularities in walls, muffles sound, and is fire-resistant. When painted on interior walls, it acts as a radiant barrier that helps prevent heat loss and keeps the walls warmer, thus making your home more comfortable in the winter. Reflective insulating paint applied to roofs and the outside of a house reflects solar energy and will help keep the building cooler in the summer. Painting interior wooden shutters with insulating paint would transform them into paragons of energy efficiency. Insulating paint can also be applied to hot water pipes to help prevent heat loss.

When we moved into our country home, we painted the bathrooms and some of our exterior walls with insulating paint. In the winter, these surfaces are noticeably warmer than the exterior walls without insulating paint. In fact, I am occasionally fooled into thinking that a careless family member has forgotten to turn off the baseboard heater in the bathroom; only after I pass my hand over the heater do I realize that the heat I am feeling is my own body heat reflecting back at me.

INSULATING PAINT DISTRIBUTORS:

Hy-Tech Inc. (www.hytechsales.com)
Kwik Company (www.heatshield-r20.com)
Pawnee Specialties (www.koolcoat.com)

Choosing Wallpaper

Nontoxic wallcoverings are generally made of paper, cloth, or coarsely woven plant materials such as grasscloth, burlap, or sisal. These porous materials need to be vacuumed frequently and do not take kindly to liquids. Compared to glossy paint, these are extremely high-maintenance wall finishes.

Good old-fashioned wallpaper paste is made of plant starch or cellulose; wallpaper adhesive is an acrylic. Neither type of wallpaper stickum exhales toxic fumes.

Ceiling Textures

It's difficult to clean dull, flaky, nonwashable, absorbent surfaces that you can reach. Unless you are running a recording studio, why choose a surface like that for a ceiling?

Acoustic tiles, which are used to make sound-muffling drop ceilings, are not washable and they lose their sound-muffling qualities if they are painted. If an acoustic tile gets too dirty to be vacuumed or wiped clean with a rubber dry-sponge (available at most hardware stores), you should probably just replace it.

Cottage cheese textured ceilings are well-nigh impossible to clean. If you can't make a cottage cheese ceiling look presentable by vacuuming it with a dusting-brush attachment, you will probably need to paint it.

Gloss or semigloss paint and a minimum of texture are my ceiling preferences: I like to be able to clean without getting glitter and grit in my eyes from a disturbed cottage cheese ceiling.

Cleaning Walls and Ceilings

The coal furnaces, wood burning stoves, and open fireplaces of our great-grandparents' era produced large quantities of soot. By winter's end, house interiors were quite filthy, necessitating energetic spring cleaning.

Modern heating and cooking equipment doesn't leave sooty deposits on all the walls, ceilings, and furniture in a home. Though kitchen and bathroom walls do need washing now and then, other walls that are vacuumed regularly—before the dust hardens into grime—may never need a floor-to-ceiling washing.

Note: If a ceiling or wall has water stains, peeling or flaking paint, or if chunks are falling off, you don't have a cleaning problem, you have a moisture problem that needs to be fixed before the surface problems can be solved.

Cleaning Dull Surfaces

Matte surfaces are not considered washable because washing or scrubbing will permanently change their texture and appearance. Dry-cleaning methods such as vacuuming or rubbing with chalk, corn meal, baking soda, a dry cloth, or a rubber eraser are the only useful cleaning methods for matte paint and wallpaper, cottage cheese ceilings, and textured or flocked wallpaper.

How to Wash a Smooth Painted Wall

Relatively smooth walls and ceilings that are painted with washable gloss or semigloss paint are easy to clean. A spray of undiluted white distilled vinegar, wiped off with a clean, soft rag is usually sufficient to remove most marks from walls. Vinegar leaves no residue so no rinsing is necessary.

1. Vacuum the entire wall, or dust it with a dust mop or brush.
2. Remove loose deposits of dirt with a dry-sponge.
3. Place a layer of newspapers, towels, or a painting tarp at the base of the wall.
4. Fill a bucket with warm water and 1 cup white distilled vinegar. If the wall is greasy, add 1 teaspoon dish liquid.
5. Drop a clean rag into the bucket, then wring out the excess water.
6. Turn the Dutch Rubber Broom upside down, drape the wet rag over the head, and use a thick, sturdy rubber band to secure it around the handle.
7. Raise the rag-bedecked Dutch Rubber Broom over your head and begin washing the wall a section at a time by starting at the top and working down.
8. When the rag gets dirty or too dry, remove the spent rag from the broom and drop it in the kitchen laundry basket.
9. Wet a clean rag in the cleaning solution, then attach it to the broom head.

10. Continue until the entire section of wall has been washed. Then replace the wet rag with a clean, dry one, and use it to dry the newly washed section of wall.
11. Repeat until the entire wall has been washed.

A friend used the following rubber broom and wet rag technique while doing the spring cleaning at the bed & breakfast she manages:

1. Throw a full load of cleaning rags in the washing machine. After the wash cycle finishes, remove the damp rags from the washing machine and put them in a clean bucket. Put a spray bottle of white distilled vinegar on top of the rags.
2. Use these clean, damp rags to wipe down walls, ceilings, stairs, window blinds, and other dusty or grimy household surfaces. Each time a rag gets dirty, replace it with a new one. With your rubber broom in one hand and your bucket of clean, damp rags in the other, you can clean your way quickly and efficiently through your home, wiping down walls, ceilings, stairs, window blinds, and other dusty or grimy surfaces as you go.
3. Spray the rag with vinegar before cleaning particularly dirty surfaces.
4. Blotting and rinsing are unnecessary.

Varnished or Shellacked Wood Paneling
- Wipe down wood surfaces with a clean rag moistened with water and a few drops of vinegar. Wipe dry with a clean cloth.
- Remove paper that is stuck to a finished wood surface by dampening the paper with a few drops of olive oil. Let it sit for a few minutes, then rub the paper off with your fingers. Wipe the oil off with a clean dry cloth.

Removing Grease
Cooking Grease
That greasy residue can be wiped off washable kitchen walls with a clean rag dipped in either of these solutions:

- 1 quart very warm water and 1 teaspoon dish liquid
- 1 quart very warm water and 1 tablespoon borax

Rinse off the cleaning solution by wiping the walls down with a rag dampened in plain hot water.

Body Grease

Any surface that is touched frequently by animals—whether two or four legged, feathered or furred—will eventually be soiled by body oils. This grease tends to form a dark but thin layer that is easily removed from smooth, washable walls by spraying the begrimed area with full-strength white distilled vinegar, then wiping it down with a clean rag.

- Greasy finger marks can be erased from finished woodwork with an art gum eraser. This technique may also work on wallpaper and matte paint.
- Grease tends to soak in to matte finishes. Matte paint that is stained with grease usually needs to be scrubbed and repainted. If the wall is very greasy, it may need to be painted with a sealing primer before it can be coated with regular paint.

Removing Marks

Marks caused by a wide variety of materials—including crayon, washable marker, rubber, and pencil—can be erased from walls with an art gum eraser, a dry-cleaning pad such as Mr. Clean Magic Eraser, or by scrubbing with a paste made of baking soda and water.

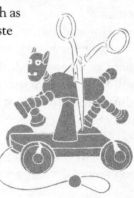

Many of these same marks can be prevented by supervising young children as they work on art projects. There is no good reason why a two- or three-year-old should be allowed unlimited access to crayons, markers, paints, pencils, scissors, clay, tape, or glue.

If you want children's art work to be executed on paper or canvas rather than on the walls, floor, furniture, toys, books, clothing, windows, or drapes, supply the paper, cardboard, or canvas, dole out the art materials, and either do some artwork of your own or work on a project in the same room.

I guarantee that everyone in your family will be happier if an adult controls access to art materials until the child reaches the age of reason.

Removing Soot Marks

Burning food, wood burning stoves and fireplaces, and badly maintained gas appliances can all produce soot.

Soot should be dry cleaned if possible. Wetting soot marks should be done only as a last resort.

- Vacuum soot off walls, ceilings, woodwork, and masonry rather than washing them.
- Use an art gum eraser or a rubber dry-sponge to remove soot marks from woodwork, walls, stone, and brick.
- If the above dry-cleaning methods fail, clean smoke and grease stains off woodwork and painted brick by painting the smudged areas with a solution of laundry starch and water, letting it dry, then rubbing the area with a soft clean cloth.

Cleaning Wallpaper

Washable wallpaper is likely to be made of environmentally unfriendly vinyl. Vinyl wallpaper can be cleaned in the same way as washable paint: with a warm water and dish liquid solution or with a vinegar spray.

Nonwashable wallpaper, flocked wallpaper, and fabric-covered walls should be vacuumed regularly, and very gently, with the dust brush attachment of a vacuum cleaner. Removing dust before it hardens into grime will help preserve these fragile wallcoverings. A rubber dry-sponge can also be used to delicately wipe slight amounts of grime off nonwashable surfaces.

If your valuable antique wallpaper or expensive murals are heavily soiled, spotted, or stained, call in a professional who specializes in cleaning and restoring wallpaper and decorative painted surfaces.

Washing Windows

Plain distilled white vinegar does a wonderful job of cleaning windows, unless they have already been washed with commercial glass cleaners. Before you can utilize plain vinegar as the official window cleaner of your environmentally friendly home, you must remove all waxy residues by washing the windows with a solution of 2 cups water, a half cup distilled white vinegar, and a half teaspoon dish liquid. Pour the mixture into a spray bottle, spray the solution on your window, wait half a minute, then polish the glass with a clean rag. The dish liquid will break down the wax so the next time your windows need washing, you can spray them with full-strength distilled white vinegar, then use a rubber squeegee or a clean, soft rag to dry them.

✑ SEEING THE FUTURE CLEARLY

Eventually, homeowners ascending ladders to wash their windows will be as anachronistic as starting a car with a crank, using a slide rule, or wearing a corset. Some major glass manufacturers are already producing self-cleaning glass that breaks down and disintegrates organic dirt such as tree sap and bird droppings. A layer of titanium dioxide (the same nontoxic white pigment that is used in all modern paints) is incorporated into the outer layer of the glass, forming a photo-catalytic layer that reacts with sunlight to break down and disintegrate organic dirt on the surface of the glass. When rain or water from a hose wets the glass, the water runs off in a solid sheet, washing off all the dirt, both organic and inorganic, and leaving the window perfectly clean and spotless. (The indoor face of these self-cleaning windows must still be washed, but maybe the engineers are working on it.)

If you cannot find a local distributor for self-cleaning windows, here is a list of manufacturers. Contact them to find your nearest distributor:

Pilkington Activ: www.activglass.com

PPG Industries: www.ppg.com

AFG Industries, Inc.: www.afgglass.com

Sunlight will dry the windows so quickly that streaks will form on the glass. Wash windows on a cloudy day, or when they are in the shade.

If you are washing the windows indoors and outdoors on the same day, use a horizontal motion on one surface and a vertical motion on the other. That way you can easily discern whether the streak you need to rub off is on the inside or the outside of the window.

Cleaning Window Screens

Window screens can be cleaned in place using the soft dust-brush attachment of a vacuum cleaner. Screens that need a more thorough washing should be brought outside and hosed off. Use a soft-bristled car washing brush to remove caked-on dirt. Let the screens dry completely before putting them back in the windows.

Cleaning Blinds

The easiest way to dust louvered window blinds is to lower them all the way, then twist the bar that completely closes them. Use a clean, damp rag, a dust mop, or the soft dust-brush attachment of your vacuum cleaner to remove the dust from one side, then twist the control rod to flatten the blinds in the other direction and repeat. If you dust your blinds reasonably often, you may never need to wash them at all. Roller blinds should be lowered all the way and then vacuumed. A rubber dry-sponge can be used to wipe dirt from both types of blind.

If your washable blinds have already built up a layer of grime, here's how to clean them:

- Start on a warm summer day because washing window blinds is a splashy outdoor job.
- Remove the blinds and lay them down outside on towels or on the lawn. Pull the cords to lower them all the way, then twist the control rod to turn them completely to one side.
- Spray the blinds with the hose, wipe them down with a soapy rag, then rinse. Twist the control rod to turn the blinds the other way so you can wash the other side.

- If you are certain that no one will step on the blinds, you can let them dry flat on the ground, otherwise hang them from a clothes-line.
- Put them back in the window after they have dried completely.

Dusting

I am a great believer in using a vacuum cleaner for dusting chores, rather than a dust mop or rag, whenever practicable. Unfortunately, some surfaces in our home hold bits of memorabilia that would be missed if I vacuumed them up, so I am obliged to pick them up occasionally and dust around them. I believe that this sort of mindless activity is best done while talking on a cordless phone with a headset.

There are many different types of dust mops and dust cloths on the market. The long-haired dusters that attract dust through static electricity work quite nicely, as do the microfiber cloths. Small pieces of polarfleece, which are quite soft and staticky, also work nicely.

All of these dusters have one minor drawback: They must be cleaned after they are used. I like to use clean, holey socks and underwear as disposable dust rags. When I am in a dusting mood, I take one of these decrepit bits of cloth, dampen it with a little warm water, wring it out well, and wipe up dust with it. When it is completely dusty, I throw it in my compost bucket and get out another rag. Everyone likes a little disposable convenience now and then!

Cleaning Ceiling Fans

If you are tall enough to use the dust brush attachment on the vacuum cleaner wand to dust the tops of your ceiling fan blades, do it. If you cannot reach, you might want to invest in a long-handled synthetic dust mop with a flexible wire handle that can be bent to exactly the right angle to dust the blades. It is also handy for removing cobwebs from high corners and other inaccessible areas. These dust mops are available at janitorial supply stores.

Spread a dust sheet under the ceiling fan before you begin to clean. The dust on ceiling fans can be very thick.

Dusting, Cleaning, Oiling, and
Polishing Wooden Furniture

Furniture must be thoroughly dusted before it can be oiled, waxed, or polished. Dust mixed with oil forms a gummy substance that resembles children's play clay.

Homemade Furniture Oil and Polish

Most commercial furniture polish contains petroleum distillates, which are flammable, toxic, and pollute indoor air. Choose vegetable oil–based furniture polish or oil, or make your own:

Furniture Oil

- Mix one part lemon juice and two parts olive oil, *or* one part white distilled vinegar and three parts olive oil.
- Mix in a blender or shake vigorously in a tightly lidded jar, then apply sparingly. If the mixture begins to separate, shake it up again before applying.
- Let the mixture soak into the wood for a few minutes, then wipe dry with a clean, soft cloth.

Furniture Polish

Making furniture polish is an excellent way to recycle the stubs of beeswax candles.

- Put four parts olive oil and two parts beeswax in a double boiler.
- Heat the oil and wax over medium heat until the wax melts.
- Remove the double boiler from the heat, and beat the oil and wax with a hand mixer until the mixture is thick and creamy.
- Apply the creamy polish with a clean soft rag. Buff with a clean, soft cloth until the furniture is shiny and doesn't feel oily.
- Store the leftover polish in the refrigerator.

Note: This nontoxic furniture polish also makes a dandy lip balm that helps heal chapped lips.

Homemade Dusting Formula

Add a few drops of olive oil to ¼ cup white distilled vinegar. Dampen your dust cloth with the solution.

Cleaning

You can simultaneously clean and oil your wood furniture by dampening a cleaning rag in a solution of ¼ cup Murphy's Oil Soap per gallon of warm water. Wring the rag out well and wipe down the wood surface. When the rag gets dry or dirty, replace it with a clean one; only clean rags should be put in the cleaning solution.

Water Rings on Wood

To remove the white water stains and rings that form under wet drinking glasses, mix 1 tablespoon white vinegar in 1 cup olive oil, then use a clean cloth to apply the oily solution to the white stains. Let it sit for a few minutes, then rub it dry with a clean cloth. Polish the rest of the wood with the oily rag to even out the color.

Cleaning Wicker Furniture

Clean wicker furniture by scrubbing with a moderately stiff scrub brush that has been dipped in warm saltwater. Use as little water as possible; you don't want to soak the furniture. Let the furniture dry in the sun. You can make saltwater by adding salt to warm water until the salt stops dissolving.

Cleaning Leather Furniture

Leather is a durable, water-repellent, and low-maintenance material that should last for decades, unless it is allowed to dry out. If leather is not kept cleaned and oiled, it will begin to crack and will eventually turn to dust.

Petroleum-based solvents will damage leather, and rubbing alcohol will tend to dry it out. Never use solvents or alcohol to clean leather, no matter what has spilled on it. When leather begins to look dry, dirty, or scuffed, it should be cleaned with a high-quality glycerin-based liquid saddle soap.

- Apply the liquid saddle soap to the leather with a clean dry cloth or with a piece of undyed sheepskin. Apply the saddle soap sparingly, using a circular motion.
- Dampen the leather with the saddle soap; do not soak it. Do not add water to the saddle soap.
- When you are cleaning a large piece of furniture, such as a sofa, apply saddle soap to one section at a time, then polish the damp area with a clean dry rag before saddle soaping the next area. The glycerin will condition the leather without leaving a sticky residue.

Liquid saddle soap is available at saddle and tack shops, or it can be purchased online; search the web for "liquid saddle soap."

Computers

Here are three excellent reasons to choose an LCD (Liquid Crystal Display) monitor rather than an old-fashioned CRT (Cathode Ray Tube) screen:

1. LCD monitors consume about 70 percent less energy than CRT screens.
2. LCD monitors do not emit electromagnetic radiation. (There are questions about the long-term effects of exposure to electromagnetic fields; studies are still being conducted.)
3. LCD monitors do not flicker, and are less likely to cause eye strain.

Computer Care

Computers are delicate machines, and the options for cleaning them are extremely limited.

SCREEN CLEANING

1. Turn off the computer and monitor.
2. Dampen a clean, soft, lint-free cloth with plain water.

3. Wipe the screen with the damp cloth. Never spray liquid directly on the screen.
4. Never clean a computer with alcohol, ammonia, or acetone, or with ammonia- or alcohol-based cleaners. These chemicals will damage the plastic.

KEYBOARD CLEANING

1. Turn off your computer.
2. Dampen a clean, soft, lint-free cloth with plain water.
3. Wipe down the keys with the cloth.
4. Moisten a cotton swab with plain water, squeeze out the excess moisture, and swab the spaces between the keys.

CABINET CLEANING

1. Turn off your computer.
2. Use a clean, soft, lint-free cloth dampened with plain water to wipe down the outside of the computer. Avoid getting moisture in the openings.
3. Refrain from using aerosol sprays, solvents, or abrasives on the computer.
4. If the vent holes are furry with dust, you can use the soft, dusting-brush attachment of your vacuum cleaner to clean them.

The best way to clean your computer is to avoid soiling it in the first place:

- According to computer technicians, the most common cause of computer malfunction is scum from cigarette smoke. Refrain from smoking around computers.
- Also refrain from eating, drinking, sneezing, or spitting near your computer.
- Don't touch your computer screen. Don't touch it with your fingers, don't press your nose or your forehead up against it, don't use a pen-

cil, pen, or crayon to point out interesting details. Don't allow other people to touch it. Ever. Period.

Computer Spills

If you spill a liquid or drop crumbs into your keyboard, or if your computer seizes up due to cigarette smoke, don't say I didn't warn you, but try the following:

- If you spill water or plain unsweetened tea into your keyboard, turn the computer off immediately, unplug the keyboard, and turn it upside down. Let the keyboard drain and dry for twenty-four hours at room temperature. If the keyboard still doesn't work after it dries out, bring it to a repair shop.
- Thick or sweetened liquids leave a residue that will gum up the works. If you spill your coffee, milk, juice, or soft drink on the keyboard, unplug it and take it to a repair shop.
- If you make a practice of eating at your computer, you should invest in a can of compressed air (choose one with a nontoxic, nonflammable propellant) or a "computer mini-vac."

To remove crumbs and other debris, unplug the keyboard, turn it upside down, then suck or blow the crumbs out, using the computer mini-vac or the canned air.

Computer mini-vacs and canned air are available at electronics stores and online. (Do not attempt to use a full-size vacuum nozzle to clean a keyboard, lest you lose the keys.)

Creative Tension

There will always be tension between the urge to preserve things as they are and the urge to create anew, the urge to make messes and the urge to clean them up, but a certain amount of flexible tension may be necessary. The tension between opposing sets of muscles keeps us upright and walking. The voice of a stringed instrument resides in the tension of its strings: If the strings are wound too tightly, something will snap; if they are too loose, they are incapable of producing sound. In compromise lies harmony.

The well-tempered house should be just neat and clean enough to make both the neatest person and the sloppiest person in the household just a tiny bit dissatisfied.

CHAPTER 7

Indoor Air Quality

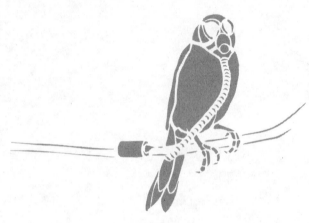

Peeople in industrialized societies spend up to 90 percent of their time indoors. According to the EPA, the air in the average American home is between two and ten times more polluted than the air just outside the threshold. We cannot blame industry, agriculture, or motor vehicles for this excess pollution. As Pogo once said: "We have met the enemy and he is us!"

A certain amount of indoor pollution is inevitable when we burn fuel for cooking or heating. In addition, as we live and breathe, we living beings produce "bioeffluents," such as ethyl alcohol, acetone, methyl alcohol, and ethyl acetate. Mold and mildew can also contribute to an unpleasant, occasionally unhealthy, indoor miasma. And the modern convenience that is not emitting volatile organic compounds (VOCs) is a rare bird indeed. As previously discussed, the particleboard and plywood used to build our homes, our synthetic carpeting and flooring, the glues that hold our furniture together, the wrinkle-free textiles on our beds and our bodies, the toiletries that give us our distinctively nonhuman smell, and the electronics that keep us entertained and employed are constantly releasing a wide variety of VOCs.

The natural byproducts of combustion and respiration and the less natural byproducts of modern synthetic products can foul the air in tightly sealed, energy-efficient buildings. Proper ventilation and an efficient air-cleaning system can help maintain indoor air quality.

Then there is the issue of elective pollutants. Every time we use an aerosol spray can, perfumed toiletries or cleaning products, air deodorizers, or pesticides, and every time we light a cigarette, a scented candle, or a stick of incense, we are voluntarily fouling our own nests with toxins. Eschew elective pollutants! There are perfectly acceptable nontoxic alternatives available.

Domestic Odor Control

Rather than adding chemicals to the air to mask an unpleasant odor, try to hunt down the source of the odor and eliminate it. (This rule should not be applied to family members or pets. They may simply need to be bathed or have their socks or diapers changed.)

Animal Odors

- Cheap cat food is bulked up with large quantities of filler, which increases the quantity and stench of feline waste products. Higher quality cat food will improve your indoor air quality while reducing your feline maintenance chores.
- Buy "natural" unscented cat litter, and change the cat's litter box frequently. Cats do not like using dirty litter boxes and may begin seeking more pleasant venues such as potted plants or secluded closets if the litter box is not cleaned regularly.
- Housebreak the puppy and clean up accidents immediately with an enzyme cleaner (see page 256). A smelly house can be quite confus-

ing to a puppy: If the house smells the same as "his yard" it may be impossible to housebreak the animal. (An odoriferous pile of teenager's clothing on the floor may also confuse a puppy.)

Indoor Air Pollutants

The Environmental Protection Agency (EPA) divides indoor pollutants into three categories: particles, gases, and radon.

Particles (also known as particulate matter) are bits of solid or liquid material that are small enough to float in the air. The smallest particles, which include cigarette smoke, combustion products from unvented gas appliances, viruses, bacteria, and some mold spores, are considered the most dangerous, since they can be drawn deep into the lungs where they may lodge for long periods of time and can eventually cause lung cancer or permanent lung damage. Larger particles, such as mold spores, pollen, animal dander, cockroach dust, and the spoor of dust mites, do not infiltrate the lungs as deeply, but can cause allergic reactions in sensitive individuals.

Gaseous Pollutants

Hundreds of different gaseous pollutants have been detected in indoor air. Cigarette smoke, solvents, cleaning products, personal care products, fragrances, pesticides, and fumes from building materials and furnishings are just a few of the sources of these pollutants. Gases can immediately cause allergic reactions, as well as eye, throat, and lung irritation. Long-term exposure to gaseous pollutants can induce cancer, cause liver damage, and harm the immune, reproductive, nervous, and cardiovascular systems.

Radon is a naturally occurring radioactive gas that emanates from natural sources such as rock, soil, groundwater, natural gas, and mineral building materials, including concrete, stone, and brick. It is suspected of inducing lung cancer in humans, and may be responsible for as many as fifteen thousand lung cancer deaths each year. Experts tell us that the greater the exposure to radon, the greater the cancer risk.

Natural radon levels vary across the country and depend upon the type

✎ PARTICULATE POLLUTION IS PARTICULARLY PROBLEMATIC

Dr. Ronald Wyzga, technical executive for the Electric Power Research Institute, a nonprofit research organization, gave the following testimony in front of the House Science Committee on May 8, 2002: "Among the various pollutants examined, the strongest associations between air pollution and health are for particulate matter." It is estimated that foreign particles in the air cause about one hundred thousand premature deaths per year.

Dusty roads, farming activities, industry, wildfires, and agricultural burning are common sources of the "larger fine particles" (perhaps we should refer to them as oxymoron particles?). These coarse particles are considered relatively nontoxic.

In the 1990s, researchers gradually realized that the most insidious particles are the smallest ones. By analyzing the number of people hospitalized on days with varying types and amounts of air pollution, researchers found a direct correlation between fine particulate matter in the air and hospitalizations: As the amount of fine particulate material in the air increased, more people were stricken by respiratory illnesses and heart disease. Exposure to fine particulate matter (which is defined as particles that are less than 10 microns in size, about one-fifth the diameter of a fine human hair) irritates the respiratory tract and can cause wheezing, asthma attacks, coughing, bronchitis, pneumonia, emphysema, and lung cancer. Very fine particles that are small enough to be inhaled deeply into the lungs are even more dangerous; these particles are defined as those less than 2.5 microns in diameter. Very fine particles can evade the natural cleansing functions of the respiratory system and infiltrate the farthest reaches of the lungs, where they can set up permanent residence. These fine particles also have an unfortunate tendency to attract toxic materials that they carry into the lungs. Once in the lungs, the toxins can be absorbed into the bloodstream.

Some common sources of very fine particles are diesel engines and poorly maintained gasoline engines, wood burning stoves and fireplaces, spray paint, toxic chemical compounds, and cigarette smoke.

of soil and rock found in the area. Granite, phosphate, shale, and pitchblende are natural sources of radon. Radon is not a health hazard outdoors; it is only dangerous when the levels build up in an enclosed space. It seeps up into houses from the dirt floors of basements, through gaps and cracks in foundations or concrete slabs, and through pipes, sumps, and drains.

Indoor Pollution Control

The most effective pollution control strategy is to identify and eliminate the source of the emissions.

Particulate Pollution Prevention

Plastics contain a static electric charge that attracts airborne particles. A black, sooty buildup on plastic items may be an indication that your indoor air quality is unacceptable. Here are some ways to improve that air quality:

- Avoid using unvented natural gas, propane, or kerosene space heaters.
- Keep your gas or propane furnace in good working order.
- Turn on the stove fan when you are cooking to vent out smoke and grease. The kitchen will stay cleaner, and so will your lungs.
- If you burn wood, have the chimney and wood stove or fireplace inspected and cleaned annually.
- Do not let your car idle in an attached garage. When you depart, back the car out as soon as the engine starts; and when you arrive, turn the engine off as soon as you park the car.
- Avoid burning incense indoors. Tests conducted by the EPA showed that burning incense releases fine particulates in larger quantities than any other indoor source. A single stick of burning incense can push the concentration of fine particulate matter well into the danger level.
- Burning candles can give your home a romantic air. Make sure that your air is still safe to breathe by choosing your candles carefully. Natural beeswax candles are the safest as well as the most delightfully fragrant.

Most commercial scented candles contain large amounts of synthetic chemicals that are released into the air as the candle burns. Some candles, especially imported ones, have lead-stiffened wicks which pollute the air with lead as the candle burns. Tests conducted by the EPA showed that

burning a single candle with a lead-stiffened wick can raise indoor lead levels high enough to violate standards set by the Clean Air Act. Luckily, it is
easy to test a metal-stiffened wick for lead: Peel the cotton fiber away from
the metal, then rub the metal core against a piece of white paper. Lead will
leave a gray mark on the paper. If the metal leaves no mark, it is zinc, and
the candle is safe to burn.

- Oil lamps produce large amounts of soot, so they may not be a good
  idea in a very tightly sealed home. If you must use oil lamps, choose
  lamp oil that is free of synthetic perfumes and fragrances.
- Air fresheners that plug into electrical outlets efficiently pollute the
  air with volatile organic compounds.
- And last, but not least, *quit smoking!* (If you can't quit, at least do
  your smoking outdoors.)

  Researchers in northern Italy compared the emissions from cigarettes to the emissions from diesel engines. They ran a diesel
  engine for half an hour in a closed garage while continuously monitoring the concentration of particulate matter. Then they measured
  the emissions produced by three lit cigarettes in the same garage.
  Running the diesel engine produced 88 micrograms of particulate
  per cubic meter of air; the three lit cigarettes produced 830 micrograms of particulate per cubic meter of air. This is perhaps not too
  surprising, since modern engines, even the relatively dirty diesel
  kind, have been engineered to minimize emissions, and cigarettes
  are designed to produce smoke.

Gaseous Pollution Prevention

Preventing Gas Leaks

- A malfunctioning combustion appliance, such as a gas or oil furnace, gas stove, or gas water heater, can emit lethal amounts of carbon monoxide. It is essential to keep gas- or oil-burning appliances
  in good working order by doing regular cleaning and maintenance
  chores. It is a good idea to have gas- or oil-burning appliances
  cleaned and adjusted by an expert at least once a year, especially

before heating appliances are fired up at the beginning of the heating season.

- Plug a carbon monoxide detector into an outlet on each level of your home, and check the detectors periodically to make sure they are functioning. Carbon monoxide is odorless, invisible, and has no taste. Without a detector, you must rely on your own instincts to warn you that you are being poisoned by a gas that impairs mental functioning. (For more information, see page 322.)

I experienced carbon monoxide poisoning one winter day while I was working in a community ceramics studio. I became dizzy and nauseated rather rapidly and went home. The smokers who were using the studio were not sickened by the elevated levels of carbon monoxide in the room. Smokers have built up a tolerance for carbon monoxide, and they may not feel its effects until it is too late; this is a dangerous situation that makes carbon dioxide detectors even more essential.

MISCELLANEOUS FUME REDUCTION

- As much as possible, avoid using volatile fume-emitting products such as solvents, oil-based paints, pesticides, and products that contain synthetic fragrances.
- Choose furnishings that are either made with safe, low-emission materials or are at least five years old, so they have finished offgassing.

Radon Mitigation
New Construction

New homes can be built with radon-resistant techniques that include the following:

1. Pouring the concrete slab over a 4-inch layer of clean gravel. This will allow the radon to move freely under the building so it doesn't get trapped and build up. A vent pipe is run through the gravel bed, then through the house and out the roof. This vent conducts soil gases safely out of the house.

2. Putting a layer of plastic sheeting over the gravel bed before the concrete slab is poured. The plastic sheeting prevents the radon gas from infiltrating the basement. (Radon is not strong enough to fight its way out of a plastic bag.) If the house has a crawlspace, the plastic sheeting is placed on the dirt floor.
3. Sealing or caulking all the openings in the concrete foundation against gas infiltration from the soil.

Old Construction

Lowering the radon levels in existing homes is a little more difficult. The first step toward reducing the danger is to have your radon levels tested. Contact your state radon office or local public health official for information.

Radon testing information is also available online:

Environmental Protection Agency (EPA):
www.epa.gov/radon/pubs/citguide.html

The National Environmental Health Association (NEHA):
www.neha.org

The National Safety Council: www.nsc.org/issues/radon. Inexpensive radon testing kits are also available online through the National Safety Council.

If your home's radon levels are low, you can safely do nothing, but if your home has dangerously high radon levels, radon mitigation work should be done by a licensed contractor who is trained in the appropriate techniques. The NEHA website lists experienced contractors. Some or all of the following work may be involved:

1. Sinking pipes through the concrete slab and connecting a fan to the pipes to suck the gas out of the basement. Sometimes existing drain pipes or sump drains can be used for this purpose.
2. Installing vents or fans to improve the ventilation in crawl spaces.
3. Sealing cracks in the foundation and concrete slab.

4. Opening the windows, doors, and vents on the lower floors to dilute the radon gas with uncontaminated outdoor air. (This method, unfortunately, can prove expensive in all but the most moderate weather.)
5. Investing in an air-to-air heat exchanger (also known as a heat recovery ventilator). This device improves ventilation without increasing your heating or cooling bills because as the fresh air is brought inside, it is heated or cooled by the outgoing air.

Researchers have found that smokers do appear to be unusually suscep-tible to radon-induced lung damage. A study by the National Academy of Sciences showed that the risk of lung cancer caused by radon exposure is ten to fifteen times higher for smokers than for nonsmokers. The study looked at lung cancer rates of deep-mine workers, who are exposed to high levels of radon in the course of their work. If you are truly concerned about the state of your lungs, stop smoking and avoid smoke-filled rooms and deep mines.

Out with the Old Air, In with the New

Ventilation is the next best pollution-reduction strategy after prevention. No matter how polluted the outside air, indoor air is often worse due to the concentration of fumes emitted by modern conveniences.

- If your indoor air is oppressively close, humid, or smelly and the weather is temperate, open your (screened) doors and windows and turn on your bathroom and kitchen exhaust fans.
- Petroleum-based solvents emit large quantities of volatile fumes. Oil-based paints or stains, paint thinner, paint strippers, airplane glue, and other strong-smelling products must be used in well ven-tilated areas only. For most of us, that means keeping all the win-dows and doors open, and running a couple of fans at full-blast to push the polluted air out of the house as quickly as possible. Since uncongenial weather may make the open window policy impracti-cal, try to avoid using all solvent-based products during very hot or

very cold weather. It is expensive to heat or cool the great outdoors via an open window, and even more expensive to replace pipes that have frozen and burst.

Rather than waiting until spring or fall to paint, stain, or glue your next project, purchase water-based products labeled low-emissions and nontoxic, and use them year-round.

Removal or Filtering

The third way to reduce pollution is through air purification. A good air purifier can reduce the amount of dust and mold spores floating in the air. There are three types of appliances that are specifically designed to clean pollutants out of the air: mechanical filters, electronic air cleaners, and negative ion generators.

In addition to particle-removal devices, some air cleaners may contain absorbent materials, such as activated carbon, that can absorb some chemicals, but are ineffective at capturing volatile chemicals and have an unfortunate tendency to gradually reemit the chemicals they have absorbed. Other air purifiers contain chemically treated materials that can capture specific pollutants.

Air conditioners and dehumidifiers can also reduce indoor pollution levels: As they draw excess moisture out of the air, they also draw out pollutants, and the contaminants end up in the drip pan, dissolved in the water.

Air must be allowed to circulate freely around air-cleaning appliances. Do not push an air cleaner up against walls, furniture, or other objects.

Mechanical Filters

A 1992 study by the Consumers' Union found that fan-and-filter air cleaners are the most efficient at removing particulate matter from the air. Mechanical filters can be installed in central heating or air-conditioning ducts; installing a finer filter in your ducts can greatly improve the quality of your air.

There are two types of filters available: flat or panel filters, made of coarse, intertwined fibers that can efficiently collect large particles but let most of the small particles get away; and pleated filters made of finer material, which efficiently capture large and small particles. Pleated filters are the most highly recommended.

Portable air filtering units are also available. Fans can blow dust back into the air, however, so put portable units on a hard, clean surface—not on a carpet.

Electronic Air Cleaners

Electronic air cleaners create an electrical field that attracts particles, zaps them with an electric charge, then attracts and captures the charged particles either on flat collection plates or on an electrically charged filter. These appliances are fairly efficient at capturing airborne particles, but they do have one major drawback: Many of them create ozone (O_3), a toxic gas that is a major component of smog.

Negative Ion Generators

Negative ion generators (also called ion generators) use static electricity to charge the particles in the room. These charged particles are then attracted to, and cling to, all the solid objects in the room, including the walls, ceiling, floor, and objets d'art. Unfortunately, some research has suggested that charged particles are also more likely to lodge in the lungs; this is because charged particles are "stickier" than uncharged particles.

Ion generators, like electronic air cleaners, may produce toxic ozone.

I doubt I'll be using an electronic "air cleaner" of any kind anytime soon.

Removing Particles

Allergy specialists recommend daily vacuuming with a high-efficiency particulate air filter (HEPA) vacuum cleaner and the use of an air purifier to reduce the level of particulates in the air. HEPA filters are supposed to have a minimum particle-collection efficiency rate of 99.7 percent.

Air-cleaning systems can remove the particles emitted by burning cigarettes, but most cannot remove the gases emitted by the cigarettes.

Caveat: If mechanical filters, such as HEPA filters or pleated filters, get damp or moist, bacteria, viruses, and fungi can colonize them. Ever alert,

OZONE BY ANY OTHER NAME IS STILL TOXIC

The oxygen molecule that keeps us alive has two oxygen atoms. Ozone is a form of oxygen composed of three oxygen molecules. Though the two types of oxygen are related, they are not interchangeable. When inhaled, regular oxygen supports respiration and maintains life, while inhaled ozone is a potent toxic gas that can damage lungs, exacerbate asthma, increase susceptibility to respiratory infections, and cause chest pain and eye and throat irritation. Ozone's toxicity is due to its third oxygen atom, which detaches readily from the other two. This lone oxygen atom reacts readily with other molecules, changing their chemical composition; the changes are generally detrimental.

Ozone is a naturally occurring compound, however, and when it is in its proper place, it performs a very important function: High above the earth, in the stratosphere, ozone acts as a protective shield that absorbs lethal ultraviolet radiation that would otherwise kill off most terrestrial life. But here at ground level, excess ozone causes problems. When ozone reacts with sunlight, photochemical smog is formed. Statistics show that more people are hospitalized when ozone levels are high. High ozone levels can also damage crops.

It is rather ironic that many ionic and electronic air cleaners incidentally produce ozone, a toxic air pollutant. It is nearly inexplicable that there are actually "air purifiers" on the market that were purposefully designed to produce and emit ozone. The manufacturers claim that their appliances emit "energized oxygen" or "pure air," which can react with and neutralize almost any chemical. The EPA has labeled these claims misleading. Other ozone aliases are "trivalent" oxygen, "saturated" oxygen, "activated" oxygen, "allotropic" oxygen, "superoxygen," or "mountain-fresh air." Ozone is the gaseous equivalent of snake oil.

Tests have shown that ozone generators are ineffective at removing carbon monoxide and formaldehyde. Other contaminants can react with ozone to create new, more toxic and corrosive chemicals. Running an ozone generator can actually increase the concentration of organic chemicals in the air. Some ozone generators produce dangerously high ozone levels even when they are operated according to the manufacturer's directions.

Some manufacturers of ionic and electronic air cleaners have recently modified their products so that they supposedly convert at least some of the ozone back into oxygen before it's released into the room. I think I'll wait for the EPA or Consumers Union to weigh in on these before I invest in any of them.

many companies now treat their filters with triclosan, and call this treatment "Microban." I fear that it may not be a good idea to expose airborne bacteria to this antimicrobial; we could be hastening the evolution of an easily inhaled, antibiotic-resistant bacteria. Products that are treated with Microban or other antimicrobials will be labeled as such; I avoid them.

Moral: Store your air-cleaning appliances in dry areas, and if a filter gets wet, change it.

Stubborn Gases

The EPA does not consider air-cleaning devices efficient at removing gases. In its document "Residential Air Cleaning Devices: A Summary of Available Information," the EPA concluded that "... none can be expected to adequately remove all of the gaseous pollutants present in the typical indoor air environment."

Watery Air

Water vapor is an essential component of healthy air. Relative humidity is the measure of how much water vapor is in the air. In colder parts of the country, low humidity is a winter phenomenon; arid regions have low humidity most of the year. Parched, cracked lips and fingertips and shockingly lively light switches, carpeting, blankets, and car doors are sure signs of low humidity. Many parts of the country have a "humid season"—a time of year when humidity levels are above 40 percent and mildew becomes a common indoor crop. Controlling indoor humidity is the most important element of fungus prevention and control.

If you are unsure about your household humidity levels, buy a humidity gauge at your local hardware store.

Preventing Fungi, Mold, and Mildew

Home Maintenance

- Mop up indoor puddles or wet spots immediately. Do not allow water to pool outside next to your foundation.

🦋 THE SLIME BEHIND THE WALLS

Recent news stories about homeowners being chased out of their homes by a slimy, black fungus that contaminated their domiciles and made them sick have alarmed the general public.

High humidity levels can encourage the growth of molds, mildew, fungi, and dust mites. These organisms can cause property damage by rotting wood, ruining wallboard, ceiling panels, paint jobs, and wallpaper, and staining books, papers, and stored textiles. Exposure to fungal spores or dust mites can induce allergic reactions or asthma attacks. When exposed to high levels of toxins from certain molds, such as the infamous slimy black fungus *Stachybotrys chartarum,* even the toughest individuals may be afflicted with dizziness, headaches, and damaged immune systems. *S. chartarum* thrives on damp wallboard, gypsum board, and cellulose ceiling panels.

The good news is that mold levels need to be quite high in order to cause health problems. Mike Muilenberg, an instructor in the Department of Environmental Health at the Harvard School of Public Health, said ". . . I think that some of the recent panic is a little bit out of proportion to the risk." He and his colleagues found that it takes extremely high levels of fungal contamination to cause any ill effects. Most buildings do not harbor enough mold to affect anyone's health.

Note: Some people are allergic and have dangerous reactions when exposed to even small quantities of fungi. Allergic reactions are different from reactions caused by exposure to large amounts of fungal toxins. Anyone can be poisoned by exposure to fungal toxins; allergic individuals are endangered by their reactions to all fungi.

- Clean leaves and other debris out of gutters and downspouts regularly to ensure that rainwater is conducted away from the house.
- Slope adjacent soil, pathways, and paving away from the house.
- Fix leaking pipes, water heaters, and roofs.
- Dry out wet building materials, furniture, and carpeting quickly after a flood or a leak. If the materials cannot be dried within a few days, they may need to be replaced.

No matter how long it was damp, if your carpeting or upholstery smells musty, it should be replaced. Musty carpeting releases mold spores into the air every time someone walks across the room; and sitting on musty upholstery puffs mold spores aloft.

- Kitchen exhaust fans should always be vented outside. Use the fan to remove cooking fumes and excess moisture.
- Never leave damp clothing in a pile; mildew will not improve its smell.
- Open a window or run an exhaust fan while you are showering or bathing, and leave the window open or the fan running for at least fifteen minutes after you finish your ablutions.

    If you are installing a new exhaust fan, choose one that can vent twice the air volume of your bathroom per minute. (Calculate the volume of a room by multiplying the length of the room by the width of the room by the height of the room [L x W x H]. The answer, if you have measured in feet, will be the volume of the room in cubic feet.)
- If the bathroom walls are dripping, wipe them dry with a towel. Discourage mildew (surface mold) by spraying the walls with full-strength white distilled vinegar. (See chapter three, "The Low-Maintenance Bathroom," page 130.)

Circulation

The key to mildew prevention is to provide adequate ventilation and prevent moisture from building up. Allow an airspace between furniture, bookshelves, and other large objects and the indoor side of your domicile's exterior walls. Large pieces of furniture can effectively insulate the wall from your central heating and allow the wall to get cold enough to condense moisture out of the air. If the area remains damp, mildew can grow. (If your winters are cold enough, ice may form behind that bookshelf or posterboard.)

Many experts recommend that artworks on paper—such as prints, watercolors, and drawings—be hung on inner walls only. The moisture that can build up behind a framed piece of artwork hung on an outer wall can encourage the growth of mildew that may ruin the art. Inside, you can help protect your valuable framed art from moisture damage by installing small rubber bumpers on the back of the frame at each corner to hold the frame away from the wall and allow air to circulate.

Walls that are the same temperature as the rest of the room are less likely to be damp. The easiest and most effective way to keep your walls warm and dry in the winter is to paint them with insulating paint. These paints contain a tiny amount of insulating ceramic or glass microspheres that form a radiant barrier; they work in the same way as the high-tech ceramic heat shields on spacecraft. The painted-on radiant barrier slows the transfer of heat and helps your house stay warmer in winter and cooler in summer.

Insulating interior paint is a bit more expensive than the cheapest paints, but the cost isn't out of line for higher end paint. (Refer to page 263 for more information on insulating paint.)

Vanquish Evil Dampness with Dehumidifiers or Air Conditioners

Indoor humidity levels should be kept below 40 percent in order to prevent mold, mildew, peeling wallpaper, and drooping wall calendars. Run a dehumidifier during humid weather, or ventilate humid areas with strategically placed fans.

"Dry" air conditioners, which do not have a built-in humidifying feature, are less likely to cause disease than are "wet" air conditioners that increase humidity. Disease organisms can grow in the cooling water of wet air conditioners; the machines then blow the microorganisms into the air. Running a dry air conditioner is an effective way to lower the relative humidity level in a home.

The dehumidifier is one of the very few air-quality appliances that is universally acclaimed by experts. Judicious use of a dehumidifier during damp or humid weather can work wonders. It will prevent the growth of fungi, keep the wallpaper and paint flat on the walls, protect books, papers, walls, wood, and textiles from mildew and rot, prevent condensation on windows, and make everyone in the household more comfortable. Dehumidifiers also improve air quality by sucking in airborne microorganisms and dust and depositing them in the drip pan.

Note: A dehumidifier will not be able to compensate for leaking walls, ceilings, or floors. Fix the structural problems in your domicile, then run a dehumidifier.

Choosing a Dehumidifier

Dehumidifiers work by blowing humid, moisture-laden air over refrigerated metal coils. Moisture condenses on the cold coils, then drips into a container. Warm, dry air is then blown back into the room. Here are some tips from the experts:

- Buy a model that has a larger capacity than necessary to cover the area that needs to be dehumidified. A powerful unit that can do the job, then cycle off, will be more efficient than a struggling, smaller model that needs to run continuously.
- Choose an Energy Star certified model.
- Make sure there is an automatic shutoff feature that will be activated when the water reservoir is full.
- Choose a model that has an adjustable humidistat that will automatically control the relative humidity level.
- Dehumidifiers are warm weather appliances. Some lose efficiency and begin to ice up at temperatures less than 65° Fahrenheit. If your cold, damp basement needs to be dehumidified, look for a model that is Energy Star certified, will run efficiently at temperatures down to 44° Fahrenheit, and has an auto-defrost function that will shut the unit off when the temperature drops below 44° Fahrenheit.
- If your entire house needs to be dehumidified, the Santa Fe Rx Whole House dehumidifier is highly recommended. It can be ordered online through the following companies:

> AllergyBuyersClub.com:
> www.allergybuyersclubshopping.com
>
> National Allergy Supply Incorporated: www.natlallergy.com
>
> Pure n Natural Systems, Inc.: www.purennatural.com

Dehumidifier Maintenance

- Empty the drip container and wipe it dry at least once a day. (During very humid weather, the water may need to be emptied more often.)

- Every couple of weeks, clean the inside of the water bucket to prevent the growth of mold, mildew, and bacteria. Wash it with warm water and a mild detergent, or spray hydrogen peroxide and vinegar in the container, then wipe it off.
- Wipe or vacuum the outside of the unit regularly to keep it clean and dust-free.
- *WARNING! Electrocution hazard! Unplug your appliances before unscrewing service panels!* At the end of the humid season, empty, dry, and clean the appliance. Read the owner's manual and follow the manufacturer's instructions on vacuuming the dust out of the interior refrigerator coils.
- Store your clean dehumidifier in a dry place.

Humidifiers

Low humidity can be uncomfortable and may irritate the sensitive membranes of the nose and throat, but it is generally not a serious health hazard. Unfortunately, a common remedy for low humidity may be hazardous: The U.S. Consumer Product Safety Commission has found that bacteria and fungi can grow in humidifiers, and these organisms can then be dispersed into the air along with the humidifying mist. The contaminated mist can exacerbate asthma or allergies and can cause lung infections, some of which may be fatal.

Legionella pneumophila, the bacteria that causes Legionnaire's disease (a severe and sometimes fatal pneumonia), is one species that thrives in the still waters of humidifier reservoirs. The bacteria was first discovered and named in 1976, after thirty-four people who attended an American Legion Convention died of bacterial pneumonia. Eventually, the outbreak was traced to bacteria that had contaminated the air-conditioning cooling-towers in the hotel where the Legionnaires had stayed. The air-conditioning system had efficiently distributed the *Legionella* bacteria, and the victims had inhaled the airborne bacteria.

Domestic cases of Legionnaire's disease have been traced to shower heads, hot tubs, whirlpools, humidifiers, and air conditioners. Any appliance that may emit mist, steam, or vapor should be cleaned regularly. Viruses and bacteria have traveled on air currents for millennia: Coughs and sneezes propel disease organisms into the air where they can be inhaled by new victims.

Humidifier Choices

There are four different types of humidifiers: Ultrasonic humidifiers use sound waves to break water up into a fine mist; cool mist (impeller) humidifiers use a high-speed rotating disk to break water up into tiny droplets; evaporative humidifiers use a fan to blow air across a wet absorbent wick or filter; and steam vaporizers heat water to form steam (warm mist humidifiers are a variant of the steam vaporizer).

Ultrasonic and cool mist humidifiers are the most efficient microbial and mineral air-transport systems because they break water up into tiny, easily inhaled droplets, and then spray them into the air. Evaporative humidifiers and steam vaporizers are slightly safer because, though they can harbor microorganisms, they do not disperse them efficiently. When water evaporates, it leaves its microorganisms behind.

Prophylactic Measures

If you feel that you must use a humidifier, choose an evaporative humidifier or a steam vaporizer, then keep it clean.

A contaminated humidifier may have film or scum stuck to the sides or bottom of the water reservoir, on the motor parts, or floating on the surface of the water; on the other hand, the contamination may be invisible to the naked eye. If you have not been cleaning your humidifier regularly, you should assume that it is contaminated.

If your sadly neglected humidifier is incubating bacteria and fungi, the unit should be completely dried out, then disinfected with a liberal application of straight hydrogen peroxide. Every surface of the humidifier that has ever been damp must be swabbed down. If your humidifier is heavily contaminated, you will need to wear a dust-filtering mask when you clean out the water reservoir.

In order to prevent a recurrence, you will need to clean, disinfect, and dry your humidifier every day. Fill the reservoir with distilled or demineralized water, or use the demineralization cartridges or filters that are recommended for use with your appliance. Tap water contains minerals that can be dispersed into the air with the mist. These minerals can settle as a fine white dust in the room. Though there is no specific information on the health effects of inhaling this fine mineral dust, there is plenty of information about inhaling fine mineral dusts from sources other than humidifiers, and some of the news isn't good.

Humidifier Maintenance

DAILY

- Unplug the humidifier. This simple action may prolong your future.
- Empty the water reservoir. Dry all the humidifier's surfaces with a clean, dry rag.
- Pour hydrogen peroxide liberally on a clean, dry rag, and wipe the humidifier down, inside and out. Pour hydrogen peroxide through the filter or demineralization cartridge.
- Fill the reservoir with distilled or demineralized water, and reinstall it.
- Plug in the humidifier.
- Repeat the following day.

YEARLY DEACTIVATION

- At the end of the dry season, unplug the appliance, then remove and discard the demineralization cartridge or filter. Drain, clean, dry, then disinfect the humidifier. Store the machine in a dry spot.
- Before you use it again, vacuum or dust off the machine and install a new demineralizing filter or cartridge.

I am not prepared to spend large amounts of time staring at a humidifier's innards every day. This laziness partially explains why I don't own one. A truly lazy organic housekeeper will not put up with babying a humidifier.

Alternative Humidifiers and Air Cleaners

Tightly sealed, insulated homes are energy efficient, but they are likely to have poor indoor air quality. Leaky old homes have good indoor air quality, but are expensive to heat and cool. Air-cleaning devices may remove some pollutants while adding others. If air purifying and air-cleaning appliances aren't quite up to their assigned job, are we fated to either breathe contaminated indoor air, or to greatly reduce the fuel efficiency of our homes?

Not necessarily. Scientists at the National Aeronautics and Space Administration (NASA) spent many years studying the problem of toxic contamination in tightly sealed chambers. The problem had to be solved, or long-distance space travel would be impossible, due to the inevitable build-up of toxic substances in the air inside space vehicles.

In 1980, experiments conducted at NASA's John C. Stennis Space Center in Mississippi showed that houseplants placed in sealed test chambers were capable of removing large concentrations of chemical contaminants from the air. Though all of the oxygen in our atmosphere is produced by green plants during the process of photosynthesis—plant leaves normally take in carbon dioxide (which animals exhale), and give off oxygen and carbon dioxide—scientists were not certain that houseplants could adapt to air that contained large concentrations of toxic contaminants. The experiments showed, however, that not only could the plants clean the air, they gradually became more and more efficient as the experiment progressed.

The scientists found that the plants' leaves absorbed air impurities that were then transported to the roots and to the soil surrounding them. The roots and their associated microorganisms digested these organic pollutants. The following common chemicals were successfully and efficiently removed from the air by NASA's houseplants: benzene, formaldehyde, xylene, toluene, acetone, methyl alcohol, ethyl acetate, ammonia, trichloroethylene, and carbon monoxide.

Many previous studies had shown that soil microbes can destroy a wide variety of environmental pollutants, but the microbes that surround plant roots are particularly efficient at inactivating toxins. Studies have also shown that living plants release phytochemicals that suppress the growth of mold spores and bacterial colonies. NASA experiments showed that houseplants reduced the indoor concentration of molds and bacteria by 50 to 60 percent. The researchers also found some evidence that radon was also absorbed and sequestered in the plants' tissues.

Dr. B. C. Wolverton, who headed NASA's studies, has written an excellent book about the cleansing abilities of houseplants. The book is called *How to Grow Fresh Air: 50 Houseplants that Purify Your Home or Office*, and it contains detailed information that can help you choose houseplants that will thrive in your home and help cleanse your air of toxins.

Dr. Wolverton gave the following houseplants very high ratings: Areca palm (Chrysalidocarpus lutescens), Lady palm (Rhapis excelsa), Bamboo palm (Chamaedorea seifrizii), Rubber plant (Ficus robusta), and Boston Fern (Nephrolepsis exaltata).

The Air Scouts

Houseplants are modest, unassuming, quiet, efficient, and low-maintenance air-improvement devices that beat their plugged-in competition palms down. Plants produce oxygen and water; electrostatic air cleaners produce ozone. Plants absorb dust while electric air cleaners stick it to the wall. Plants absorb and eat toxic gases; electric air cleaners don't. Low-technology wins again.

CHAPTER 8

Hazardous Materials, Fire Safety, Home Maintenance, Automotive Care

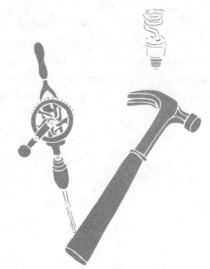

Accidents are the leading cause of death for Americans between the ages of one and twenty-one, and the fifth leading cause of death for adults. Accidents in the home are the second leading cause of accidental death, surpassed only by motor vehicle accidents. This chapter contains information about safety measures and household maintenance chores that can greatly reduce the risk of domestic accidents. We focus on such areas as basements, workshops, garages, and outbuildings, where the more imminently hazardous materials and equipment are usually located.

But as we know, accidents do not always involve a victim running afoul of the laws of physics: Many household accidents are chemical in nature. Because home improvement projects often require large quantities of materials, the choices we make when we purchase supplies for such projects can have a profound effect on our health as well as on the environment. For example, a very picky housekeeper may use a few gallons of cleaning products annually, but painting a house usually requires a couple of dozen gallons of paint. Frequent exposure to small amounts of toxic household products can cause many health problems, as can large but infrequent exposures to paints, solvents, adhesives, and pesticides. The information in this chapter will help you make decisions so your home and automotive maintenance chores will be safer and less toxic.

Hazardous Materials

Hazardous materials are substances that are so dangerous that people may have no time to wonder whether their accidents will ruin their health. The victims are often eligible for Darwin Awards, meaning they have removed themselves from the gene pool.

Some Advice from a Guy Who Picks
Up the Pieces

Captain Marcus Hardin, the hazardous materials coordinator for the Duluth Fire Department, who also oversees the State Emergency Hazardous Materials Team for the northeastern Minnesota region, regularly responds to hazardous material emergencies as well as to fires.

He said, "Household chemicals pose dangers for householders and their families, and for the environment. . . . It's sad, but almost everything you can buy in the store is dangerous. People have a tendency to buy whatever is advertised. From insecticides to fabric softeners, it's all chemicals. If they replaced these synthetic products with more natural products, they'd be a lot safer."

According to the Environmental Protection Agency (EPA), materials can be classified as hazardous if they are easily ignitable or subject to spontaneous combustion, corrosive, reactive, or toxic.

Hazardous Materials Disaster Prevention

Before you buy a chemical product, *read the label.* If you don't feel you can follow the safety instructions exactly, *don't buy the product!*

All products have safety ratings. The federal ratings are based on hazards to the consumer.

DANGER: the highest hazard level, the most dangerous product
WARNING: medium hazard level, a dangerous product
CAUTION: low hazard level, least toxic

If the label has no warning, the product is considered non-hazardous.

Volatile

Volatile organic compounds (VOCs) are substances that catch fire at very low temperatures (140° Fahrenheit or above) and will be labeled as so: DANGER. HARMFUL OR FATAL IF SWALLOWED. SKIN AND EYE IRRITANT. VAPOR HARMFUL. COMBUSTIBLE.

These materials are called volatile because they evaporate readily, even at very low temperatures; this is why gas stations reek of gasoline even when it is 40 degrees below zero. Smoking is forbidden at gas stations because volatile vapors are extremely flammable. A few examples of volatile liquids are petroleum products, paints, solvents, kerosene, gasoline, adhesives, nail polish, nail polish remover, and furniture polish.

Caustic or Corrosive

These strongly acidic or base (alkaline) products will be labeled: DANGER. CORROSIVE! MAY BE ABSORBED THROUGH SKIN. SEVERE RESPIRATORY AND DIGESTIVE TRACT IRRITANT. MAY CAUSE SKIN AND EYE BURNS. These products will eat through any organic material they encounter, including your clothing, skin, hair, and eyeballs. Drain cleaners, oven cleaners, toilet bowl cleaners, rust removers, and battery acid are the most common corrosive products found in house-holds.

Very strong acids and bases, which are particularly dangerous to the eyes and lungs, can cause severe burns similar to those caused by heat. If you must use strongly corrosive products, wear protective clothing—especially safety goggles. (I refuse to use a cleaning product that necessitates the use of safety goggles. I'd rather just clean a little more often and avoid the problem altogether.)

The Nose Knows?

Though inhaling concentrated volatile vapors can cause immediate death, many modern humans have become accustomed to these petroleum-based smells and find them rather pleasant. Some people who strongly object to the odors of natural substances, such as horse manure or dirty socks, don't seem to mind volatile fumes from paint or gasoline.

Just smelling gasoline is actually harmful. Chronic exposure to small amounts of gasoline fumes or other VOCs may eventually damage your nervous system, brain, liver, or kidneys, or cause cancer. The smell of horse manure is perfectly harmless. If you have doubts about your ability to smell the difference between toxic and merely stinky, ask a dog. A dog will revel in the harmless stench of a dead fish, but retreat from the truly dangerous smell of a solvent.

Hazardous Materials Disposal Programs

Hazardous materials should never, ever, be poured down household drains, into storm sewers, put into the regular household trash, or dumped on the ground. They need to be disposed of very carefully.

Most cities have hazardous materials disposal programs. These programs were set up to keep toxins out of the wastewater stream and out of surface water and groundwater. Because it is so important that our waters remain free of toxins, these programs are free of charge. Old paints, stains, varnishes, solvents, oily rags, pesticides, herbicides, medicines, motor oil, oil filters, fluorescent bulbs, mercury thermometers, sawdust and scraps from treated lumber, and other dangerous or hazardous chemicals can be brought to the hazardous waste site and handed over to the technicians, who will send them to the proper disposal site.

Many hazardous waste facilities have materials exchange programs where cans of paint and stain can be dropped off, checked out by technicians, then given to other residents who need them. Giving unused paint to people who can use it is far preferable to letting excess cans of paint harden and rust in the basement. But before those cans of paint completely solidify, they make dandy fire accelerators.

LET THE PROFESSIONALS DEAL WITH THESE

Paints, stains, paint thinner and solvents, art and
    hobby materials
Aerosol cans
Pool and spa chemicals
Pesticides and poisons
Motor oil, antifreeze, starter fluid
Batteries
Household cleaners and disinfectants
Prescription pills and other medications, hypodermic
    needles and lancets

Read the Label, Then You Won't Need to Weep

Some products are extremely dangerous when combined with other substances: Some mixtures will burst into flame while others produce toxic gases.

It can be quite difficult to comprehend the ingredients on the labels of most synthetic products. (Some chemists have told me that they can't really tell what is in some products because manufacturers often use different names for the same chemicals, possibly in an attempt to prevent the public from knowing what is in their products.) Since we are dealing with the incomprehensible, it is very important that we read and heed the label warnings. Never mix products together unless they are specifically designed to be used together in teams such as detergent and fabric softener, shampoo and cream rinse, or two-part epoxy, for instance.

Household products that contain chlorine bleach should never be mixed with anything at all. Highly toxic chloramine gas is released when chlorinated products are mixed with products containing ammonia, such as window cleaner or dish liquid. When chlorinated products are mixed with strongly acidic products, such as rust removers or toilet bowl cleaners, deadly chlorine gas is released.

The most common household products that contain chlorine are chlorine laundry bleach, mildew stain removers, automatic dishwasher detergents, some powdered bathroom cleansers, and

> ~🦋 Michigan Lawsuit Abuse Watch (M-LAW) holds a yearly contest to find the most idiotic warning label. The first prize winner for 2004 was the label on a bottle of drain cleaner, which says "If you do not understand or cannot read all directions, cautions and warnings, do not use this product."
>
> It is a ridiculous warning, and I'm sure it doesn't help the two-year-old children or pets who accidentally encounter carelessly stored drain cleaner. But I have been talking to people about dangerous chemicals for more than twenty years now, and I am fairly certain that most people never read the warnings on products. If they did, they would probably be too nervous to use these products at all.

some toilet cleaners. The most common household products that contain ammonia are glass cleaners, metal cleaners, and dishwashing liquids. These are such everyday products that it is easy to use them carelessly. For example, you can produce chloramine gas simply by scrubbing the bathroom sink with a bleach-containing cleanser, then cleaning the mirror with an ammonia-based window cleaner.

Anything with chlorine in it is potentially dangerous and should be avoided if at all possible. If two products do the same job and one contains chlorine while the other doesn't, choose the chlorine-free product.

Age-Induced Instability

Chemicals tend to degrade over time and either lose their potency or become less stable. Packaging also degrades over time. Some elderly products degenerate into unstable chemicals precariously housed in crumbling containers. If neighboring chemicals leak and fraternize, completely unpredictable reactions may occur.

A child could discover a disintegrating box of pesticide and spill poison all over himself. Any chemicals that are more than a couple of years old should be taken to the local hazardous waste facility.

If you come across an unlabeled chemical, don't touch it; don't smell it; don't taste it. Bring it to a household hazardous waste facility, and let the professionals figure it out.

Household hazardous waste workers regularly have to contend with nearly full gallon jugs of DDT, which was banned more than three decades ago. Doubtless, the householders who purchased these enormous quantities of pesticide thought they were saving money by buying the large economy size. Even if DDT hadn't been banned, it is highly unlikely that the typical householder could have used that much DDT in a lifetime.

Buy only as much product as you need; better yet, buy safe alternatives to dangerous chemicals.

Divide and Conquer

Tim Lundell, a household hazardous waste technician at the Western Lake Superior Sanitary District in Duluth, Minnesota, said it's important to keep products in their original containers whenever possible. If the package is disintegrating and you must transfer the product to a new container, label the new container carefully—if possible, tape the original label to the new container. Hazardous waste technicians do not appreciate mystery materials. If you have questions about how dangerous your waste is, call your local hazardous waste disposal facility, tell them what you have, and ask them how to transport it.

A Rolling Fire Drill

Mr. Lundell told me that a few fires have erupted in vehicles that were being driven to the hazardous waste facility because incompatible chemicals had been poured into a single container for transport to the facility. It takes a while for enough heat to build up, but eventually, *poof!*

Mixing a very strong acid with a very strong base can easily generate enough heat to start a fire, and it's a lot easier than it sounds: Just pour (acidic) toilet bowl cleaner and (alkaline) drain cleaner into the same container. If you're really unlucky, you will produce toxic gases as well as a fire.

Repacking for the Trip

If a container is failing, put the whole thing into an intact plastic five-gallon bucket, close the lid, and seal it with duct tape. These buckets are made of plastic that is compatible with most chemicals. Use a separate bucket for each hazardous material and label each new container accurately.

When a completely unknown chemical comes in, the hazardous waste facility tests it in a small lab to determine whether it's an oxidizer (likely to catch fire), an acid, or a pesticide.

❧ BURN BARRELS: WASTE REDUCTION FROM HELL; OR DO-IT-YOURSELF HAZARDOUS WASTE PRODUCTION

Most hazardous materials are manufactured in factories. The major exception to this rule is the dioxins that are formed when plastics are burned at low temperatures. Though municipal trash incinerators are highly efficient and reach temperatures that are high enough to destroy dioxins, home burn barrels are inefficient and cannot reach high temperatures. Burning trash in open barrels spews more dioxins into our air than any other source.

A single exposure to dioxin can cause eye, nose, throat, skin, and lung irritation; stomach and intestinal upsets; and headache and memory loss. Long-term exposure to dioxins can cause asthma, birth defects, learning disorders, infertility, immune system disorders, cancer, and leukemia.

Burning trash is definitely not an environmentally friendly activity! Open burning of trash is illegal in many states. Even if trash burning is legal in your state, remove all traces of plastic from your trash before putting it in the barrel. This is more easily said than done, however, since almost all food packaging contains plastic: waxed cartons, such as milk cartons and some cracker packaging, is no longer waxed, it is plastic-coated; the cereal bags inside cereal boxes used to be waxed paper, but now they are plastic; the interiors of many tin cans are coated with plastic; candy wrappers and drinking straws, which used to be paper, are now plastic; the insides of bottle caps, which used to be made of cork, are now plastic; and many shipping cartons, which used to be wax-coated, are now plastic-coated. Asphalt, rubber products, treated wood, and petroleum products are also unsafe to burn.

What to Wear

The technicians who receive hazardous materials are nattily attired in plastic aprons, goggles, Solvex gloves (which are resistant to most chemicals), and respirators. What are you planning to wear for this solemn disposal occasion? If you have to deal with a leaking chemical, wear plastic gloves (acid can eat through latex), and don't forget your splash goggles! A plastic apron may also be a good idea.

When to Call for Help

Most people don't own respirators, or if they do, their respirators are not sophisticated enough to deal with highly toxic chemical fumes. If you think gases or fumes are being produced by household or garden chemicals, you may need to call the fire department to help you out.

If you have inherited a shed or basement that contains a chemical arsenal, it may be necessary to call your fire department's nonemergency number to ask advice on how to proceed. If the chemicals are very old, some of them may have crystallized and become unstable enough to combust or explode if disturbed. Old fireworks and highway flares can also be quite unstable. In some parts of the country, it is possible to inherit old explosives that were used in farming or mining.

Better safe than sorry. *Ask for help.*

Fire Safety

During infrequent sleepless nights, I generally attempt to solve global problems single-handedly, as well as protect my family against all imaginable hazards. As I fret about the possibility of our house burning down, my worrying is generally confined to the problem of evacuating family members from second story bedrooms. This is a very narrow-scope worry, which I really should try to expand.

If burning a single barrel of household trash produces more dioxin than does a municipal incinerator, imagine what happens when the whole house burns.

🐝 REST ASSURED, THERE WILL BE NO FIRE RUNNING IN OUR VEINS . . .

Though the fear of fire may make the idea of fire retardant chemicals appealing, some fire retardant chemicals have been found to be quite toxic and hazardous. Polybrominated diphenyl ethers (PDBE), which have been used for thirty years to treat everything from children's sleepwear to mattresses to computers, have been flowing in ever increasing amounts in streams and rivers, sewage sludge, human bloodstreams, and mothers' milk. Nowhere on earth is uncontaminated: PBDEs have even been found in remote Arctic lakes.

Ronald A. Hites of Indiana University in Bloomington, surveyed studies of PBDE concentrations in people and presented his findings at an Environmental Protection Agency conference in Chicago in August 2003. Professor Hites found that PBDE concentrations in North Americans are ten to twenty times higher than they are in Europeans. Tests of stored breast milk have shown that human concentrations of PBDEs have been doubling every four to five years since the 1970s.

Researchers at Indiana University also analyzed PBDE concentrations in the umbilical cord blood of newborn infants and in their mothers' blood. In 2003, Linda S. Birnbaum, the EPA's director of experimental toxicology in Research Triangle Park, North Carolina, told *Science News* that these concentrations of PBDEs may leave "no margin of safety" for humans.

Per Eriksson and his colleagues at Uppsala University in Sweden exposed ten-day-old mice to PBDE and managed to produce hyperactive, memory impaired animals that had trouble learning mazes.

PBDEs are persistent organic pollutants (POPs). The European Union banned two of the three most common PDBEs starting in 2004, and other countries and some manufacturers are phasing them out. European law requires proof of safety before a new chemical can be used in manufacturing and released into the environment; U.S. law requires that a chemical be proven dangerous before it is removed from the marketplace.

The latest news from the American chemical industry is that PBDEs will be gradually phased out because better, more environmentally safe alternatives have been found. I remain skeptical. "Better living through chemistry" has often proven otherwise. The chemical prevention of naturally destructive processes such as combustion or decay seems to be a never-ending cycle of invention, marketing, scientific alarm and recall of the chemical, then invention of a new chemical. We've had asbestos, PCBs, and PBDEs to prevent fire; we've had pentachloride, arsenic compounds, coal-tars, chromium compounds, and chlorinated compounds to prevent rot. Chemicals come and go like fashion fads.

The uncontrolled combustion that occurs during a house fire releases a horrifying amount of extremely toxic materials, a quantity so large that the environmental damage cannot be balanced by an entire lifetime of careful avoidance of synthetic pesticides, herbicides, solvents, and cleaners.

Therefore, domestic fire prevention is one of the most basic pollution control techniques available to us. The value of preventing house fires is probably the only subject on the planet on which everyone agrees.

Arise! Awake!

Thanks to PBDEs, American blood may be ten to twenty times more fire resistant than European blood, but that hasn't prevented us from having one of the highest rates of fire fatalities in the industrial world. More Americans die in fires each year than in all other natural disasters combined. Fire is the third leading cause of death for young children in the United States, right after traffic accidents and drowning.

Fire 101

Fire is a chemical reaction that requires oxygen, fuel, and heat, which are the three components of what is often referred to as the fire triangle. If any of the three sides of the fire triangle are missing, a fire cannot start; if a piece of the fire triangle is removed, a fire will go out.

When a flammable material chemically combines with oxygen, producing heat, the chemical reaction is called combustion. Combustion can be either very fast, as when a match is held to a piece of newspaper, or slow, like iron gradually rusting, or a damp bale of hay gradually heating up. When the heat from slow oxidation is allowed to build up, spontaneous combustion sometimes occurs.

Keeping fuel and ignition sources separated is the basic principle of fire safety. Though it has but a single principle, fire safety encompasses a lot of details . . .

From Small Sparks, Huge Fires Grow

The United States Fire Administration tells us that it can take only half a minute for a tiny flame to grow into a major fire. A house can fill with thick black smoke or be engulfed in flames in minutes.

The Grand Prize Fire Starter

Careless smoking is the leading cause of fire deaths in the United States; this particular irresponsibility causes 30 percent of all fire fatalities each year. In 1998, smoking caused nearly $7 billion worth of property damage.

Arguing the case against smoking feels almost like shooting fish in a barrel; there really is no rational case for smoking and such a plethora of reasons not to smoke. But since this book is about nontoxic housekeeping, I will simply point out that a potent poison like nicotine does not belong in a nontoxic household.

In 2000, epidemiologists from the University of California, Davis began adding up the costs of smoking-related fires. The data showed that smoking is a leading cause of fires all over the world. In addition, the researchers estimated that worldwide, one million fires are started each year by small children playing with cigarette lighters and matches.

The first rule of fire safety is prevention. If you are truly concerned about your family's safety, *don't allow smoking in your house!*

Cooking Up an Ounce of Prevention

The National Fire Protection Association says that cooking is the leading cause of home fires, as well as domestic fire injuries in the United States. Most cooking fires are caused by human error rather than by mechanical failure. Here are some recommendations for reducing dangerous kitchen mistakes:

1. Wear proper attire. The charred look is definitely out. A well-dressed cook avoids loose or trailing clothing and long or loose sleeves that might brush against burners. Avoid synthetic cloth-

ing; it can melt when exposed to high temperatures. If you have long hair, tie it back to prevent it from brushing against a burner.

A note to outdoor cooks: Wool clothing will actually protect you from heat, flame, and sparks, and it really is the best thing to wear around campfires. Synthetics melt.

2. Purchase a fire extinguisher that is approved for trash, wood, and paper fires; liquid and grease fires; and electrical fires. Keep the extinguisher just outside the kitchen where you can reach it easily in an emergency.

Once a month, read the dial to make sure that the extinguisher is still charged; when it loses pressure, it must be either recharged or replaced. Extinguishers with metal heads hold a charge longer, are refillable, and are more durable than extinguishers with plastic heads.

3. Keep all things flammable away from the stovetop. Don't decorate your kitchen with billowing curtains, which at best get grimy from airborne grease and at worst can catch fire by blowing across the stove. And even if you think the stove is turned off, never leave flammable items such as cutting boards, wooden cooking spoons, pot holders, towels, napkins, plastic containers, plastic dinnerware, plastic bags, newspapers, or magazines on or near the stove. I have seen far too many cutting boards, pot holders, and cooking spoons with burner marks on them, and far too many melted plastic containers to believe that people really check before they put things down. Store plastic bags and pieces of paper where they can't blow across a hot stove and start a fire.

4. Use utensils wisely. Always turn pan handles toward the center of the stove where youngsters can't reach them and adults won't knock into them. If you have young children, use the back burners for large stock pots. A kettleful of boiling water can kill or maim a young child.

Never let the electrical cords of kitchen appliances dangle down where children can reach them. One tug on the cord attached to a deep fat fryer could be fatal to a youngster.

Don't forget to turn off the teakettle. If the water boils dry, the bottom of a teakettle can actually melt out. Maybe this is why teakettles have whistles!

5. Don't put a hot pot or pan down on a countertop made of Formica, Corian, acrylic, cultured stone, or other synthetic materials; these petroleum-based materials are flammable and will melt. Use a trivet or put the pan on a fireproof surface such as stone, ceramic, or metal.

6. Purchase pot holders that are made of natural materials such as cotton or wool; synthetic fabrics and filling can melt when exposed to flame or high heat. And use those pot holders! If you attempt to manipulate a hot skillet bare-handed, you may end up dropping it on the stove and starting a grease fire.

7. Prevent grease fires. Overheated cooking oil will ignite, so never leave a frying pan unattended. If you are frying something and have to answer the phone, tend to a child, or go to the door, *turn off the burner*! It's very easy to get distracted and forget that you left something on the stove.

   When I was a child, one of our neighbors burned her kitchen down twice by leaving a frying pan of oil on the stove. The woman was an artist—and her oil paints were obviously calling louder than her cooking oil.

   Pools of grease in a stove's burner pans or reflector bowls are fire hazards. Wipe grease up as soon as it cools.

8. Extinguish grease fires. The best, cleanest, and easiest way to put out a grease fire in a frying pan is to turn off the burner and put a tight-fitting lid on the pan. (Immediately turn off the exhaust fan too. If the fan is going, it can suck the fire into the ductwork.) The lid will cut off all the oxygen and the fire will extinguish without any further ado. Even a five-gallon pot of oil will stop burning if a lid is put on it. I like to have a large pot lid on the counter next to the stove when I am frying, just in case.

   If you have a grease fire, you want it to stay confined to your skillet and not spread to flammable items near the fire. Never try to carry a pan of burning grease outside or put it in the sink. You are likely to blaze your trail with flaming grease. Extinguish the cooking fire where it is.

Don't ever pour water on a grease fire. Water can splash the grease around and actually spread the fire. Spraying a grease fire with a fire extinguisher may also spread burning grease around. If you don't have a lid handy, throw baking soda on the fire.

Keep a clearly labeled container of baking soda near the stove. You can pour baking soda on a grease fire to extinguish it. However, note that baking soda and corn starch are often sold in very similar boxes. Be very careful not to throw corn starch on a grease fire, since the corn starch will immediately burst into flame.

Apparently, many people try extinguishing grease fires by throwing flour or sugar on the flames. This is like throwing sawdust on a campfire. Any flammable material that is ground into very fine particles will burn explosively when exposed to heat or a source of flame. (This is what causes dust explosions in grain silos.) If you throw flour on a fire, a column of flame will shoot up the flour as it's being poured.

Sand is an excellent fire extinguisher. A bucket of sand in the kitchen can be a useful firefighting tool.

9. *Never* use a cupboard or shelf above the stove to store candy, cookies, toys, or anything else that might be attractive to a child. A child who climbs on top of a stove is in mortal danger.

10. Prevent oven fires by cleaning the oven and broiler pan and keeping them free of grease and food debris. (See chapter two, "The Kitchen," page 88.) When you are baking pies, sweet potatoes, or other gooey items, put a cookie sheet under them so they don't leave flammable bits of themselves on the oven floor. When you are preparing potatoes for baking, remember to stab the potatoes repeatedly and deeply with a fork so steam can escape and the potatoes won't explode.

11. Refrain from storing flammable items in the oven or broiler, even if you have a double oven. You may have a perfect memory and never make a mistake about which oven to use, but unless you are a hermit, other people may occasionally enter your home and

might not understand that the top oven is where you store the gummy worms. If these visitors start preheating the storage oven in the mistaken belief that it's a good place to roast a Thanksgiving turkey, burned gummy worms, melted plastic wrap, and chaos will ensue.

It is a good idea to check inside both the oven and the broiler before using either one. If you don't live alone or if your memory is bad, you never really know what you might find.

This incident occurred on February 17, 2004, in Howard, Wisconsin:

A couple returned from vacation, and the wife turned on the oven to start dinner. Suddenly they were dodging bullets and were forced to seek shelter behind the refrigerator.

Before they left for their vacation, the husband had hidden three handguns and ammunition in the oven. Naively, the wife had neglected to do a weapons check before making dinner.

Miraculously, no one was injured.

12. If you do have an oven fire, turn off the oven, leave the oven door closed, and let the fire burn itself out. Opening the door will replenish the oxygen and encourage the fire.

13. Before you use a new kitchen appliance, read the instruction booklet and follow the directions. Many modern gadgets are dangerous if used improperly. Electrical appliances and water do not mix well, and many appliances can be damaged by improper cleaning.

14. Antique pressure cookers are infamous for their fickle and dangerous natures. Projectile pressure valve caps, steam burns, and food stuck to the ceiling were all rather common occurrences in our grandmothers' kitchens.

That being said, canning in pressure cookers is the only recommended way to process low-acid foods (almost everything that isn't a jam, jelly, or pickle) so the resultant canned fruits and vegetables will be free of botulism and safe to eat (see page 101). Your community garden program or county extension agent will have plenty of information on safe canning techniques. Some communities even have community canning equipment and canning classes.

If you want to can low-acid fruits or vegetables, invest in a brand-new, high-quality pressure cooker and follow the manufacturer's directions. Do not attempt to save money by buying a pressure cooker for $10 at a garage sale; new pressure cookers have safety features that the older models are lacking. Your mother's or grandmother's antique pressure cooker is a stovetop bomb; I recommend you either throw it out or plant petunias in it.

Microwave Fire Prevention

Microwaves are notorious for causing fires when the wrong materials are put into them. Read the instruction manual and learn about the recommended operating procedures before using a new microwave oven. Heed the safety precautions.

- Use only cookware and dishes that are labeled microwave safe. Turn over your glass or ceramic plates, bowls, and cups, and peruse their bottoms before you nuke them.
- Metals can cause electrical arcing and sparking inside a microwave, and may start a fire. Never put metal flatware or aluminum foil in the microwave; metallic glazes and decorations on ceramic dishes and glassware can also cause problems. The seals under the lids of many bottles and jars are made of metal foil. (My husband once tried warming up a bottle of maple syrup in the microwave, and the tiny bit of aluminum seal left on the mouth of the bottle arced and partially melted the glass!)
- Putting paper in a microwave may not be a good idea. Greasy paper can heat up and ignite. Newspapers, recycled paper products, and colored paper towels may contain inks that absorb microwaves, heat up, and ignite. So it is best to avoid putting paper products in the microwave unless they are specifically labeled as microwave safe.
- Follow the instructions on the labels of microwaveable foods. Some packaged foods are not microwave safe, and will be labeled as such. Stand by when you're microwaving popcorn. Popcorn can scorch

and begin to burn in just two minutes, so set the microwave's timer for the minimum recommended popping time.

- If something ignites in your microwave, turn the power off in order to stop the fan. Leave the power off and the door closed, and the fire will suffocate. After the fire is out, wait at least an hour before opening the oven door.

Microwave Burn Prevention

Foods that are heated in a microwave oven can behave in very unusual ways. A little bit of prevention can avert a lot of suffering.

Sticky Explosions

- Refrain from using tight lids and plastic wrap in the microwave. Tightly sealed foods can get superheated and explode violently when the microwave door is opened.
- Many foods carry their skintight packaging around with them. Poke holes in potato skins, hot dog casings, and eggshells before microwaving.
- Foods should be loosely covered in the microwave in order to prevent spattering. Putting the food on a microwave-safe glass or ceramic plate and covering it with a microwave-safe bowl is a safe, easy way to keep your oven clean.
- Some very sticky foods may self-seal when heated in the microwave and pose an explosion hazard if overheated. If you insist on reheating your tapioca pudding in the microwave, let it sit and cool off for several minutes before you open the oven door.
- Many of the stickier varieties of babyfood are hazardous when microwaved; their labels include warnings. No jar of baby food should ever be heated with its lid on because the whole jar may explode when the microwave door is opened.

Liquid Explosions

Microwaves can superheat liquids past the boiling point and turn a cup of water into a booby trap. Superheating occurs when a liquid heats up to the boiling point, but no bubbles form to carry heat out of the liquid. Superheating can only occur in a very smooth container that is so slippery that there is nothing for bubbles to cling to. (Yet another instance when imperfect housekeeping is safer housekeeping. If you keep using and reusing your coffee mug, it will acquire a lovely patina that will hold bubbles.) Movement also encourages bubble formation. Most teakettles jiggle as they heat on a stove, thus preventing superheating.

If a cupful of water is superheated in a microwave, the water can suddenly and violently boil up and out as soon as the cup is moved. Adding a dry substance such as tea, sugar, or coffee to superheated water can also cause an explosion. The boiling geyser effect can be prevented by reducing the heating time and letting the water cool in the oven for a minute after the power turns off.

Steam Explosions

Be careful when removing the covers from microwaved food. Use hotpads to tip the lid away from yourself so the escaping steam doesn't burn you. Microwaved food can be deceptively hot.

Barbeque

After we've finished all our chores, there's nothing quite as much fun as a barbeque. Here in the frozen north many people barbeque year-round, and barbequed turkey is a Thanksgiving favorite.

Health

The barbeque is our link to our meat-burning ancestors. Though many studies have shown that burned or barbequed meat forms carcinogenic compounds called heterocyclic amines (HCAs) and polycyclic aromatic hydrocarbons (PAHs), who wants to forgo barbequed chicken and ribs? Life is too short.

In 2005, the American Institute for Cancer Research announced that marinating meat before grilling can reduce HCA formation by up to 99 percent, while reducing the amount of fat that drips onto the coals helps prevent the formation of PAHs.

You can make barbequing less toxic by marinating your meat before grilling it; by choosing smaller, leaner cuts of meat that cook quickly and drip less fat; and by pushing the hot coals to the edges of the barbeque so that meat cooking in the middle of the grill won't drip onto hot coals.

You can make barbequing even less toxic by trading in your can of lighter fluid for a barbeque chimney starter, which is a metal cylinder with ventilation holes at the bottom, a metal grid partway down, and a sturdy handle on the side. Crumpled newspaper is used to light the briquettes.

A chimney starter can be purchased at most hardware stores for less than $20, and it will last indefinitely. Using a chimney starter is safer, healthier, and cheaper than using lighter fluid, and it produces far less air pollution. Your food will taste better, too: Essence of lighter fluid is not a positive addition to the taste of grilled corn, hot dogs, or chicken.

BBQ Cleaning

Remove the crusty residue from your barbeque tongs and grill racks by soaking them overnight in hot water and baking soda. The loosened crust will be easy to remove in the morning.

BBQ Safety

The point of barbequing is to add a delicious smoky flavor to your food, not to char your home or garage.

- Locate your barbeque grill well away from siding, deck railings, eaves, and overhanging branches.
- Do not allow grease or fat to build up in the trays below the grill. Fat is extremely combustible.
- Never use a propane or charcoal grill indoors. They are not designed for safe indoor use and may start a fire or cause asphyxiation.
- Store unused charcoal in a cool dry place inside a waterproof metal container with a tight-fitting lid. Damp charcoal can spontaneously combust.

Deep-Fried Turkey

In November 2003, in an attempt to avert further tragedies, the National Fire Protection Association issued a warning against the use of turkey fryers, appliances which have caused numerous fires and injuries. Underwriters Laboratories has refused to certify any turkey fryers, deeming them too dangerous. It seems that boiling three or more gallons of oil in a long-legged vessel over an open flame is just not a good idea. Who would have thunk it?

The Next Biggest Fire Thing

And the second runner-up in the death-by-fire competition, right after careless smoking, is home heating. This problem is, of course, exacerbated in very cold weather when people start using supplemental heaters.

Preventing Heating Related Mishaps

1. Have your furnace professionally cleaned and checked before the start of each heating season.
2. If you burn wood, have your chimney inspected and cleaned yearly. Even if you only burn wood occasionally, your chimney still needs to be inspected and cleaned annually to prevent the build-up of flammable creosote, which fuels chimney fires. Note that the chimney should be equipped with a metal spark arrester to prevent sparks from landing on the roof.
3. Fireplaces should have tightly fitted glass doors that prevent all sparks from jumping out of the fireplace, rather than metal screens, which can allow some sparks to escape. Make sure the fire in your fireplace is out before you go to bed.
4. *Never* close the damper when the fire is burning or hot ashes are in the fireplace. A closed damper will allow carbon monoxide to build up in your home.
5. Ashes should be placed in a tightly covered metal container and stored outside, well away from buildings. Never assume the ashes are safe and cold until they have been sitting for at least a week.
6. Never use an unvented fuel-burning (nonelectric) appliance for space heating. *All* nonelectric heaters, whether they burn kerosene, propane, charcoal, or other fuel, must be vented outside.

  Even in a heating emergency, you should not try to use your

cooking oven or stove burners to heat your home. Gas ovens may not burn fuel efficiently with their doors open, thus creating deadly carbon monoxide. Leaving the oven door open may also make the pilot light blow out, allowing unburned gas to leak into your home. Stove burners and electric ovens are simply not designed for space heating; you will waste a lot of energy and gain almost no heat.

7. Be very careful with portable electric heaters. Whenever possible, plug them directly into wall outlets and try to avoid using extension cords. If you must use an extension cord, be sure it is a heavy-duty one that is rated for more current than your heater will draw.

8. Read the instruction booklets that come with all your heating equipment and heed the warnings. Combustible household items, such as furniture, bedding, clothing, curtains, toys, cooking oil, newspapers, and magazines, must be kept more than three feet away from heaters. If at all possible, store paints and solvents outside the house; if paints must be stored in the house, they should *not* be kept in the same room as heaters or furnaces. Gasoline, kerosene, diesel fuel, and sawdust should never be stored in the house, and should be kept far away from heat- and spark-producing equipment, such as power tools and engines.

9. Keep the area near the furnace, room heaters, water heater, stove, and portable heaters free of clutter. Clutter is a fire hazard as well as a navigational hazard. Walkways should be kept completely clear so passersby don't trip and burn themselves on a heating appliance.

10. If you have young children, keeping combustibles away from furnaces and heaters includes preventing your progeny from dropping small plastic toys through the heat registers or grating . . .

A few years ago, a friend kept complaining about a noxious smell in her house. Her husband repeatedly told her, "It's nothing, honey." Eventually the stench grew so strong that he could no longer ignore it. He ended up having to cut a piece out of their furnace so he could remove the plastic zebra that had fused to its inside wall.

Carbon Monoxide

Even vented appliances can cause trouble if they are not running properly. Malfunctioning gas appliances such as furnaces, stoves, water heaters, and clothes dryers can produce deadly amounts of carbon monoxide (CO), an odorless yet deadly gas that is produced by all types of combustion. Carbon monoxide displaces oxygen in the blood, causing disorientation that may prevent victims from escaping and—if they don't manage to escape—bright red corpses.

Unvented fuel-burning heaters can cause a lethal amount of carbon monoxide to build up. Heating temporary shelters such as mobile homes, tents, and ice fishing houses with unvented fuel-burning heaters can make you both red and dead.

You should, of course, have a detector, which will alert you to a buildup of CO. But here are other signs that a fuel-burning appliance is malfunctioning:

- Early symptoms of CO poisoning are fatigue, drowsiness, and headache.
- Gas flames should be blue. Yellow or orange flames, pilot lights that blow out frequently, or black soot stains around the appliance are all signs warning you to call a repair person immediately.

If your appliance isn't getting enough oxygen, it won't be long before you won't, either. In order to encourage healthy respiration, make sure the appliance's vents, grilles, flues, and air intakes are unobstructed.

Very tight, energy-efficient houses are more likely to build up dangerous levels of carbon monoxide than are draftier, less efficient houses.

An estimated three hundred people die of carbon monoxide poisoning each year in the United States. Malfunctioning appliances are unlikely to produce smoke, so smoke alarms cannot alert householders to a buildup of carbon monoxide due to gas appliances. You can protect your family by installing carbon monoxide detectors on each level of your home, especially near heating units and bedrooms. If the alarm sounds, leave the building immediately while your mind is still functioning.

Don't forget to test your CO detectors monthly.

Electrical Fires

According to the National Fire Protection Association (NFPA), electrical fires are one of the leading causes of fire deaths in the United States; each year electricity kills hundreds of people, either by electrocution or in electrical fires.

Easy Does It

Many residential fires are caused by overloaded electrical outlets and circuits. The overloading creates heat that can eventually start a fire. Appliances that draw 1,000 or more watts—such as refrigerators, hot plates, microwave ovens, deep fryers, dishwashers, air conditioners, and space heaters—should not share the same outlet or circuit.

If you are not sure which outlets are on the same circuit, try looking inside your fuse box. Many electricians label the fuses inside the box so you can tell which outlets and major appliances are on which circuit. If your fuses are unlabeled, here's how to figure them out yourself: Plug an extension cord into an outlet, then plug a portable trouble light into the extension cord. Carry the lit trouble light over to your fuse box. Turn off the fuses one at a time until the light turns off. Write down the location of the outlet next to its appropriate fuse. Check to see whether any appliances have turned off. Repeat with each remaining fuse.

While you are checking the label, make sure that your appliance is UL (Underwriters Laboratory) listed. Underwriters Laboratory is an independent, nonprofit organization that tests electrical components and equipment. An UL listing means that the device met UL safety standards for shock and fire hazard.

Some homeowners' insurance policies have clauses that limit the company's liability for damage caused by the failure of non-UL-listed appliances or electrical equipment.

When I think about electrical safety, I am irresistibly reminded of cartoon cats with frizzed out fur, enormous bottle-brush tails, and wild, pop eyes. The following suggestions will help you keep your dander down:

Socket Safety

- Do not overload outlets. High-wattage appliances, such as refrigerators and microwaves, should never share a single outlet.

- Don't plug more than one extension cord into an outlet.
- Don't use extension cords that allow you to plug more than one appliance into a single socket.
- Outlets with ground fault circuit interrupters should be installed in the bathroom, kitchen, laundry room, and other rooms that contain faucets or are very damp. Ground fault interrupters shut off the current within a tenth of a second if a short occurs.
- If a socket feels warm, turn it off at the fuse box and call an electrician.
- Use plastic safety covers on unused electrical outlets to prevent young children from trying to plug objects into the sockets.

Cord Safety

Malfunctioning electrical cords start many electrical fires each year. Overloaded electrical cords can heat up and cause fires. Damaged insulation can expose live wires that spark on contact; exposed wires are fire and electrocution hazards.

- Stop using any appliance that has a damaged, frayed, or loose cord, or that has a plug with damaged or loose prongs. Replace either the damaged cord or the appliance.
- Protect the insulation on electrical cords by keeping the cords away from hot surfaces. If you accidentally melt your iron's cord, immediately turn off the iron and unplug it. The cord is now damaged, see above.
- Outdoor appliances should be plugged only into outlets that have ground fault circuit interrupters. If you are using a corded electric lawn mower, hedge trimmer, or other bladed tool, be very careful to keep the cord behind you, well away from the blades. If you are mowing or trimming and find that you are losing your concentration, stop and take a break; losing your concentration may be a shocking experience.
- Pets and electrical wires can be a deadly combination. If your dog chomps on an electrical wire or cord, you will be lucky if he is the only member of your family who dies. A dead dog or rabbit with its

teeth stuck in a live wire is a fire hazard as well as an electrocution hazard. If you have a pet that might chew on electrical wires, block all its access to live wires.

Electrical Extension Cords: Do Not Fold, Spindle, or Mutilate, or You and Yours May Incinerate . . .

Your main objective when using an extension cord should be to protect the integrity of the cord's insulation, wires, and plug, and to prevent it from building up heat.

Shock and Short Prevention

- Avoid stapling extension cords to walls or ceilings; staples can damage the insulation and cause a short circuit.
- Do not hang extension cords over nails.
- When using outdoor appliances, use only approved exterior extension cords, not the household type normally used indoors. Household cords are not weather- and waterproof.
- Replace damaged plugs and frayed or worn cords immediately.
- Never run wires across doorways where people may walk on or trip over them, nor under rugs or carpets, where they can be damaged as people walk across the rug.

Keep It Cool

- Extension cords are designed for temporary use only. If you must use extension cords, do not overload them with several appliances or use too many cords in one socket. Do not string multiple extension cords together. Use the largest possible gauge of extension cord for any given job.
- Coiling, kinking, knotting, or bending an extension cord increases its resistance to the passage of electric current; greater resistance produces more heat. Make sure you use the proper gauge extension cord for the appliance you are operating.
- Leave electrical cords uncovered and out in the open where heat

can dissipate. Avoid trapping cords against walls where heat can build up. Replace any cords that heat up while in use.

Appliance Safety

Most electrical appliances are not designed to be used near water. Keep appliance cords dry and away from showers, sinks, faucets, and tubs.

If you are not sure whether an appliance is safe to use near water, read its safety manual and label. A water-safe appliance is only safe as long as its cord and case are intact; never use a damaged appliance of any kind near water.

Unplug your appliances by pulling the plug, not by pulling on the wire.

Never throw water on an electrical fire; you might electrocute yourself. Use a multipurpose, dry-powder fire extinguisher.

This'll Curl Your Hair

Small appliances such as irons, curling irons, and hair dryers may seem innocuous, but they can be treacherous. Never leave the room without turning off and unplugging small appliances that contain heating elements.

Never let the hot surfaces of appliances touch combustible items. Remember that most "marble" tops on bathroom vanities are actually made of plastic; if you leave a hot appliance such as a hair curler on the bathroom counter, the counter will melt and eventually ignite.

Safely Unplugged

You should always read and follow the directions before using or cleaning an appliance. Always unplug an appliance before trying to clean it. For example, if your toast is stuck, unplug the toaster before trying to pry out the toast with a wooden chopstick or bamboo skewer. *Never* put a metal object in a toaster, or you could be toast!

Don't even think about trying to repair or work on an appliance without first reading its label and instruction manual. Many modern appliances—microwaves and television sets, for instance—can hold a charge even after they are unplugged. If the label on your appliance says Caution, Shock Hazard, removing the back panel of that appliance may be the last thing you ever do. Let a professional fix it.

Electric Wolves in Sheep's Clothing

Electric blankets and heating pads are essentially rows of electric wires laid in fabric. Basic extension-cord safety rules also apply to them.

According to the United States Consumer Product Safety Commission,

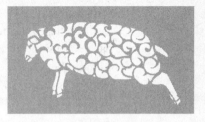

electric blankets started four hundred fires in 1996; the fires killed ten people, injured thirty, and caused $6.6 million in property damage.

Though electric blankets and heating pads seem comforting and homey, they are a bit tricky to use safely. You should read the label before using an electric blanket or heating pad, but here are some of the safety basics:

1. Buy an Underwriters Laboratory (UL) tested blanket or heating pad. Never buy a used electric blanket or heating pad; it is impossible to tell whether internal wires have been damaged.

2. Electric blankets are nothing like regular blankets. Otherwise perfectly normal bed making, sleeping, and laundering habits become fire hazards when practiced on electric blankets and heating pads. Here are some basic safety tips:

   a. Turn off your electric blanket before you fall asleep. Many electric blankets don't have sensors that will shut the blanket off when it gets too hot.

   b. Turn your heating pad off after half an hour; if the heating pad runs longer than that, enough heat can build up to burn skin.

   c. Never put anything on top of an electric blanket while it is energized; enough heat can build up between the item and the blanket to cause a fire. This means no pillows, no coverlets, no bedspreads, no clothing, no dolls, no toys, no pets, no small children . . . Even the most sedate cat or dog can literally become a ball of fire if he naps on top of a heated electric blanket.

   d. Never sit upon, lean against, or lie down on an electric blanket or on an electric heating pad, whether or not it is turned on; the internal heating coils are delicate and easily damaged. Damaged heating coils can start fires.

e. Never "tuck in" an electric blanket. The bending may damage the heating coils, and if the blanket is activated while it is tucked in, heat will build up under the mattress and may ignite the blanket, your sheets, or your mattress.

f. Never tightly fold or roll up an electric blanket, lest you damage those delicate coils. Unplug the blanket when it is not in use and store it flat.

g. While it is activated, the blanket should be kept flat on the bed; excess heat will build up in a crumpled blanket.

h. Never wash an electric blanket. The blanket will be dangerously damaged by the washing machine's action.

i. Heating pads can burn or damage skin, and should never be used on infants, small children, or medically delicate adults.

I have never owned an electric blanket because I know that I am not conscientious enough, nor a quiet enough sleeper to use an electric blanket safely. Even if the blanket wasn't turned on while I slept, my impressively athletic sleeping style would eventually damage its wiring.

Lighting Safety

Lightbulbs

- Incandescent lightbulbs can get hot enough to start fires. When you replace a lightbulb, read the label inside your lamp and make sure you don't use a bulb with too high a wattage.
- Never let anything touch a lit lightbulb. Though draping a light with a pretty cotton cloth might seem romantic, I'm not sure that many firefighters end up falling in love with people they rescue from burning buildings.
- Beware: Halogen lights aren't called torches for nothing. They get incredibly hot. Never let a halogen lamp touch anything at all.

Mood Lighting

Candles are wonderful for setting a mood, but they are open flames and need to be treated with respect. House fires were much more common before the advent of electric lights. Here are some tips for keeping your candles' flames where they belong.

- Candles are very untrustworthy and should never be allowed to burn without adult supervision. Extinguish all candles before leaving the house or going to bed.
- Keep burning candles a minimum of one foot away from combustible items.
- Candleholders should be stable, sturdy, and nonflammable. Though glass is not flammable, thermal shock from the candle flame can shatter a glass candle holder. You may want to set your glass candle holder in a large dish of sand, just in case.
- If your electricity goes out, *do not use candles for light*. Use flashlights. Candles are far too dangerous to carry around the house.

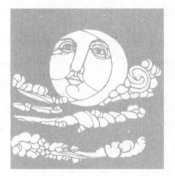

We live in a rural area that is subject to frequent power outages. Here, moonless nights are truly as dark as the inside of a cow. When the power goes out at night, one is liable to fall down the stairs unless an alternate source of light is found immediately. After our first experience with total darkness, we bought wonderful rechargeable flashlights that turn on automatically when the power goes out. We have these marvels plugged into an outlet on each floor of the house as well as in each bedroom. Now when the power goes out, we can immediately locate our fully charged flashlights.

Molotov Cat Tails

Cats and candles are a very bad combination; many house fires have been started by cats that have brushed their tails against burning candles, then fled, setting fires as they ran.

The location of a burning candle is at least as important as its color or scent.

Spontaneity Is Not Always a Good Thing . . .

Though most fires are ignited by sparks, open flames, or very high heat, a few fires are self-starters. Spontaneous combustion can occur when combustible materials heat up enough to ignite without being exposed to an external source of heat or flame.

Rags that have been soaked with a flammable liquid such as paint, wood stain, solvent, kerosene, or gasoline are fires-in-waiting. Though it is obvious that one shouldn't expose these soaked rags to a source of open flame or heat, it is less obvious that, given enough time, they will set themselves on fire.

A heap of paint, solvent, or oil-soaked cleaning rags will heat up as the flammable liquid combines with oxygen. Slowly, gradually, the heat builds up until *poof*! We have ignition. Solvent-soiled rags should be stored in clearly labeled, airtight metal containers. Pour enough water into the container to completely cover the rags. Bring the submerged rags to a hazardous household waste facility for disposal.

Astonishingly, steel wool that has been soaked in a flammable liquid is also subject to spontaneous combustion. Remember that combustion occurs when a material combines with oxygen; rust is steel or iron combined with oxygen. Very tiny pieces of combustible materials burn much more easily and quickly than larger pieces of the same material. So, if you combine steel wool with a flammable liquid and let it sit around long enough, eventually you will have a fire. Put that solvent-soaked steel wool in water in an airtight metal container, and take it to a hazardous waste facility.

Moral of the story: Clean up your cleanup materials!

Hay, Hay!

Spontaneous combustion can also occur without flammable liquids: Decomposition also produces heat. If that heat is not allowed to dissipate, eventually the decomposing material will become hot enough to ignite. Very large decomposing piles of damp organic material such as municipal compost piles, industrial sawdust piles, or even haystacks sometimes build up enough heat to catch fire.

Red Hot Laundry

Most of us don't have to worry about our compost piles catching fire, but we shouldn't feel left out—there's still something we can worry about! Spontaneous combustion caused by decomposition doesn't necessarily require a large amount of material; all that is necessary is a sufficient build up of heat.

Several years ago, a custodian told me a wonderful little story: Once upon a time, the custodian's partner mopped the floor, put the damp mop in its bucket, then put them in the utility closet and locked the door. The mop sat, rotting and moldering happily away in its tiny closet for about a week, getting warmer and warmer until, finally, the other custodian opened the closet door, admitting fresh air to the hot, stuffy closet and, *poof!* The mop caught fire. Moral of the story: Wring out your mop and hang it up to dry.

Also, don't allow heaps of damp laundry to congregate in your basement or laundry room; you know how incendiary those unwashed types can be. And if you must store every newspaper and magazine you've ever bought in your lifetime, remember that the piles must not only be kept away from heat, sparks, flame, electrical extension cords, and flammable liquids, they must also be kept dry, or you may end up with a flaming pile of composting paper.

Special Holiday Fire Section

If you conduct a survey of a dozen people, the odds are good that at least a few of them have had personal experience with a flaming Christmas tree.

Ideally, Christmas should be a heartwarming holiday, not a blistering, searing experience. But unfortunately, a rapidly desiccating Christmas tree can provide fuel for an explosive fire. Here are some safety tips that a few of my friends have learned the hard way:

TREE CARE

- Cut your tree as late in the season as possible. If you are buying a precut tree, bend some needles to test them for flexibility. Fresh needles bend. Dry needles break.

- Dry evergreens are extremely flammable. Keep your tree as lively and green as possible by using a Christmas tree stand with a water well in the bottom. Make sure the well is filled at all times.
- Locate your tree at least a yard away from all sources of heat and combustion, and close enough to an electrical outlet so extension cords are not necessary.
- Keep the tree upright by tethering it to the wall or ceiling with a strong cord or cable.
- When the needles begin to fall, the tree is dry and should be taken down.
- Under no circumstances should a defunct Christmas tree be burned in the fireplace or woodstove. Evergreens are full of extremely flammable resins.
- Many municipalities offer Christmas tree recycling. The old Christmas trees are ground up and used for mulch.

CHRISTMAS LIGHTS

- Avoid plugging several sets of Christmas lights into one another. The extra resistance may create enough heat to set the tree on fire. Small lights create less heat than large ones.
- Do not leave the lights turned on when the family is asleep or when no one is home.
- Using real candles on a Christmas tree may seem like a romantic idea until they set the tree alight. Refrain.

What Firefighters Want You to Know

Back in the days when houses and their furnishings were made mostly of wood and other natural materials, the first breath of smoke from a house fire made people drowsy as carbon monoxide displaced the oxygen in their bloodstream; after a few more breaths, they would drop to their knees before they passed out. But flaming modern building materials are so astonishingly

🐝 PROTECTING FIREFIGHTERS

A statistical study, published in the *American Journal of Industrial Medicine* in 2003, showed that male firefighters were four times more likely to develop testicular cancer than were men in the general population. This study by Dr. Andreas Stang of the University Hospital of Essen, Germany, echoed the results of a 2001 study in New Zealand showing that firefighters were three times more likely to develop testicular cancer. Though the reasons for the increased cancer risk to firefighters are unclear, Dr. Stang pointed out that firefighters are exposed to many toxic "combustion products" created by burning synthetic materials.

toxic that one good lungful of synthetic smoke can make you lose consciousness.

Eighty years ago, firefighters used no self-contained air when they entered a burning building; they just held their breath and went in. They proudly referred to themselves as "leather lungs." It was considered normal and admirable to vomit after fighting a fire (though it certainly wasn't healthy).

Unfortunately, hydrocarbon-based materials—such as the foam padding in furniture, mattresses, plastic toys, PVC plumbing, synthetic carpeting, and polyester fabrics—burn faster and at higher temperatures than the natural materials they have largely replaced. These burning hydrocarbon-based materials also release toxic and flammable gases that increase the danger for firefighters. Nowadays, far more people die of the toxic smoke and fumes produced by house fires than of burns. The air in modern burning buildings is so toxic that firefighters must carry their own oxygen supply with them, or they will die. And they must be very careful about removing their breathing apparatus because many toxic gases—for example the cyanide gases emitted by burning PVC pipes and electrical insulation—are invisible. That is why, especially in airtight homes, a very small fire can generate enough toxic gases to kill people. Even a very slowly smoldering short circuit, such as one caused by accidentally driving a nail through an electrical wire, can release enough toxic byproducts to kill you even though the amount of smoke being released is not detectable to humans. (Don't procrastinate! Go buy a carbon monoxide detector!)

The Firefighters' "Perfect" Dream Home

If you are contemplating building your dream house, remodeling, or simply redecorating, remember that natural fibers and materials make your home a much less toxic and far less flammable place.

If firefighters had their druthers, all residences would contain only natural materials from floor to ceiling:

Fire Safe Floors

Nonflammable floors made of stone, brick, concrete, or ceramic tile are safest in the event of a fire. The safest floors that are not hard as a rock are those that are made of natural materials such as wood, bamboo, cork, and linoleum, which are flammable but do not produce toxic smoke.

Vinyl flooring, like other polyvinyl chloride (PVC) products, produces deadly hydrogen chloride gas and dioxin when it burns. Firefighters are not fond of vinyl floors, nor are they fond of PVC plumbing.

Carpeting

Synthetic carpets and rugs, whether nylon, olefin, polyester, or acrylic, are just fuzzy species of petroleum and, as one would expect, they burn toxically and melt easily.

Natural carpeting will tend to be less dangerous than synthetics in the event of a fire, simply because the smoke is less toxic. Carpets made of coir, sisal, seagrass, jute, hemp, and cotton are all easily available, but will burn fairly easily. The true fire safety champion is the wool rug because wool is naturally fire retardant.

Petro-Fabrics

Anyone who has ever worn synthetic outerwear near a campfire can tell you that these materials melt when a spark lands on them. If you must wear synthetic materials near a flame, emulate Forest Service firefighters, who wear a layer of cotton or wool between their skin and the synthetic material. That way, if the synthetic melts, it will not stick to the skin. Many safety experts recommend that travelers avoid wearing any synthetic clothing in airplanes because synthetics are so dangerous during fires.

Petro-fabrics include nylon, polyester, polypropylene, polyethylene, Capilene, Polartec, Thinsulate, acrylic, modacrylic, olefin, vinyon, Saran, and spandex.

Natural Fabrics

Whenever possible, choose clothing, carpeting, decorating fabric, and stuffing made from natural materials such as cotton, linen, ramie, hemp, bark cloth, wool, cashmere, camel hair, alpaca, qiviut, angora, silk, or leather.

The following stuffing materials are also animal- or plant-based: down, eider down, feathers, wool, horsehair, kapok, cotton, cattail fuzz, milkweed silk, and latex rubber.

Naturally Fire Resistant

Leather and wool are the most flame-resistant materials available for home decorating.

Man-Made Fibers Made From Rearranged Natural Materials

The following are materials synthesized from natural materials. They are synthetic materials but are not petroleum-based, and they are nontoxic: rayon, viscose rayon, high wet modulus (HWM) tayon, Modaltm, polynosic rayon, acetate, triacetate, lyocell, Tencel, and foam and fiberfill made from polylactic acid (PLA).

When Prevention Fails

Accidents happen. Prevention cannot avert all fires. If a fire occurs, fire safety systems can greatly improve our odds of survival.

Let's begin with the cheapest component of a fire safety system, the smoke alarm . . .

The Care and Feeding of Your Smoke Alarm

According to R. David Paulison, head of the U.S. Fire Administration: "The majority of the children who die in fires die in those homes that don't have working smoke alarms. People don't realize how quickly a fire spreads through a house . . ."

Smoke alarms can give you and your family enough time to safely escape a fire. Though smoke alarms have become commonplace, *working* smoke alarms are still a bit unusual: About a third of all smoke alarms are nonfunctional. The most common reason for smoke alarm failure is that the batteries are dead, missing, or disconnected.

- Install smoke detectors on every level of your home. Smoke rises, so smoke alarms should be installed six or eight inches below the ceiling. Many fire departments will recommend specific smoke detectors. Some fire departments give away smoke detectors or sell them at cost. (Remember, if you pass out from fumes, firefighters will endanger their lives while trying to save yours. Do them a favor and keep your smoke detectors in working order.)
- Change the batteries at least once a year. Changing the smoke detector batteries is a good New Year's chore.
- If a smoke detector is chirping, its batteries need to be replaced. But if its batteries are dead or missing, it will not chirp. Test smoke detector batteries monthly: Pushing the button should cause an ear-splitting squeal.
- All appliances eventually wear out; replace your smoke detectors every ten years. Write the replacement date on the smoke detector with a permanent marker: "Replace detector in January 2014."
- Vacuum the smoke detector regularly to keep it working properly.
- Let the detector do its job. If it goes off because you have burned the toast, don't pull out its batteries; ventilate the room and wave a vinegar-soaked kitchen towel in front of the detector to clear the air.

A Quenching Shower

According to the National Fire Protection Association (NFPA), in 2002, fire departments responded to a fire somewhere in the United States every nineteen seconds. This adds up to a total of 1,687,500 fires in which 3,380 civilians died and 18,425 were injured. Seventy-nine percent of the civilian fire deaths occurred in homes. Many cities require new commercial buildings to have fire sprinklers so, ironically, we are in far less danger from fire in most theaters than we are in our own homes.

The odds are even worse for rural residents. There is a morbid saying that volunteer fire departments save basements and foundations. This is not because the volunteer fire departments aren't hard working or dedicated. Country homes are often quite far from the fire station and synthetic materials burn so hot and so quickly that houses actually burn faster than they did eighty years ago. Unless a fire department arrives within five minutes of the start of a fire, they won't be able to save the building.

I have never coveted anything as much in my life as I now covet a fire sprinkler system. Fire sprinklers knock fires down very quickly, preventing the formation of toxic gases. A fire sprinkler system nips a fire in the bud; a fire department fights a fire that's already in full bloom.

According to Captain Marcus Hardin of the Duluth, Minnesota, fire department, "If every house had fire sprinklers, my job would be much easier, and we'd lose fewer lives. I love my job. I love going into a burning building and saving people. But I don't like having to go in and bring out a dead body."

Flashover Times

Patrick Coughlin, director of Operation Life Safety, a public/private partnership whose goal is to reduce residential fire deaths and injuries through the use of fire sprinklers and smoke alarms, was quoted in an article in *Plumbing and Mechanical Engineer* (*PM Engineer*): "Residential fire sprinklers operate quickly enough to stop a fire before flashover occurs. In fact, they operate quickly enough to keep the room of origin tenable to life. Without them, the room becomes untenable to life about halfway to flashover." Flashover is what happens when the combustible materials in an area reach a temperature high enough to burst into flame. Rooms that contain synthetic materials reach the flashover point in about five minutes.

If my math has not failed me entirely, Mr. Coughlin is saying that residents in homes without fire sprinklers have two and a half minutes to safely exit their homes during a fire.

Cheaper than Carpeting

The average cost of installing a residential fire sprinkler system is between $1 and $2 per square foot in urban areas, and about $3 per square foot in rural areas. But as sprinklers become more common, the price will drop. After Scottsdale, Arizona, mandated residential fire sprinklers, the cost of sprinkler installation dropped from an average of $1.14 to 59 cents per square foot. For comparison, I called a national carpeting company and was informed that installation of the least expensive carpeting costs about $2.50 per square foot.

Water, Mother Nature's Fire Control

Now we are getting to the crux of the issue:

While testifying in front of the Iowa City Board of Appeals, which was debating a proposal to require automatic fire sprinklers in fraternity and sorority houses, Dominick Kass of the National Fire Sprinkler Association stated that smoke detectors can warn you that you are about to die, but fire sprinklers can actually prevent your death.

Fire sprinklers have been in use in the United States since 1874. In all that time, there have been no recorded instances of more than two civilians being killed by fire in a fully sprinklered building. The National Fire Protection Association states that the fatalities in sprinkler-equipped buildings have generally occurred when the victims were in direct contact with the fire before the sprinkler was triggered. In other words, unless you have been playing with explosives, a sprinkler system will probably save your life in a fire.

Most fires are not acts of god; they are caused by careless acts of man. As Heracles said to the wagon driver who was stuck in the mud: "The gods help those who help themselves."

Money Makes the World Go Around

The residential fires that inflict so much human suffering are also expensive: In 2002, residential fires in the United States caused $6.1 billion worth of damage, so insurance companies are quite interested in fire prevention.

According to the *Scottsdale Report*, which was released in 1997, there have been no fire deaths in Scottsdale in homes with sprinklers since the fire sprinkler ordinance went into effect in 1986.

Though many of us have seen movies in which all the fire sprinklers in a building go off randomly and simultaneously, ruining everything beneath them, this is fiction. Fire sprinkler heads are activated by heat, not by smoke.

When the most common type of residential fire sprinkler reaches a temperature of about 150° Fahrenheit, a metal disk in the sprinkler head melts, and water flows out of the sprinkler. In most cases, only the sprinkler nearest the fire goes off. The authors of the *Scottsdale Report* noted that in addition to saving lives, the fire sprinkler ordinance has also reduced property damage. Part of this reduction is no doubt due to the fact that a residential fire sprinkler sprays an average of 341 gallons of water to extinguish a fire, while firefighters use an average of 2,935 gallons. Not surprisingly, many insurance companies give a 10 to 15 percent discount to homeowners whose homes have sprinkler systems. Encouraging homeowners to install sprinkler systems is in the insurance companies' best interests, since fire sprinklers reduce property losses by one-half to two-thirds.

Despite what script writers would have us believe, the accidental triggering of fire sprinklers is quite rare, usually involving a homeowner who knocks into a sprinkler head with a ladder; a student who hangs clothing from them; or a child who sets off the sprinkler while playing with a cigarette lighter. If your children are playing with cigarette lighters, a sprinkler head going off is the least of your worries.

Home Maintenance

Paint, stain, and varnish function as a building's protective skin, helping prolong the life and looks of the siding.

Paint Purchasing

Buy enough paint to finish the job, but do not try to store large amounts of paint for touch ups. Paint does not store well for prolonged periods of time, and solvent-based paints are extremely flammable. Rather than storing bulky cans or jars, keep a file of color swatches from the paint store. These handy pieces of paper not only accurately reproduce paint colors, they also include the formula used to mix the color. Label the swatch with the date of purchase and when and where you used that color. Then if you need to do a little bit of touching up, you can buy a small can of lump- and rust-free, perfectly matched paint.

If you just want to keep a small amount of paint, put it in a glass jar that is just big enough to hold it. The less air in the jar, the longer the paint will be usable.

The new style of plastic paint can, with a screw top and a built-in spout, is a big improvement over the standard metal paint can. Plastic is not only more airtight, it will not rust and ruin the paint.

Help prevent paint from slopping over the sides of metal paint cans by poking drip holes in the rim: First remove the lid, then use a small nail and a hammer to poke a few holes at the bottom of the rim. The drip holes will allow paint that spills into the rim to drip back down into the can. When you put the lid back on the can, it will cover the rim and the holes, so the closed can will still be airtight.

No matter what type of container your paint is in, the lid should be tightly closed whenever the paint is not in use. Tightly sealed paint will last longer and will release fewer pollutants.

Aerosol Paints

Aerosol paints are *not* environmentally friendly: Aerosol propellants are both flammable and toxic, and the fine mist of paint produced by spray cans is easily inhaled. Do your lungs a favor and avoid spray paint.

Watch Out for That Can!

Aerosol cans become bombs at temperatures above 120° Fahrenheit, giving new meaning to the term "Aerosol can propellant." Therefore, they should never be burned or incinerated, and they should be stored in cool, dark places far away from sunlight and sources of heat such as radiators, furnaces, and stoves. During warm weather, closed motor vehicles can easily get hot enough to explode aerosol cans.

Never use an aerosol product near any source of ignition, such as a pilot

---

Aerosols are often used to dispense paints, enamels, adhesives, lubricants, lacquers, rust preventives, and insecticides. These materials are all quite toxic, and a fine aerosol mist is an ideal method for delivering a large dose of airborne toxins directly to the lungs. Aerosol products should only be used in very well-ventilated areas (preferably outdoors).

Many aerosol propellants are also extremely toxic, inducing intoxication if inhaled in small amounts, and death if inhaled in large amounts.

The sixteenth-century Renaissance physician Paracelsus wrote: "All things are poison and nothing is without poison. It is the dose that makes the thing a poison."

It is not just the dose that makes the poison, it is also the method of delivery. (If milk is injected intravenously, for example, it is more deadly than heroin because the proteins in the milk induce a fatal inflammatory reaction.) It is illegal to sell spray paint to minors; consequently, some underage "huffers" try to get high by inhaling other types of aerosols, often with disastrous results. For instance, aerosol cooking oil, if inhaled, can completely seal off the lungs and cause death by suffocation.

light, lit stove, or candle. If the spray reaches a flame or a spark, it will ignite, and flame will flash back to the can, which, you may remember, you are holding in your hand.

Whenever possible, choose nonaerosol products. Pump-spray dispensers work perfectly well for many purposes. Some spray cans use safe propellants like compressed carbon dioxide or compressed air and nitrogen.

Safe Cleanup

Read the product label and follow the manufacturer's directions for disposing of rags, towels, masking tape, steel wool, paint scrapings, and other materials that are moistened or saturated with oil paints, oil-based finishes and stains, paint thinner, solvents, gasoline, or other flammable liquids. Combustible materials that are soaked with flammable liquids may spontaneously combust if not disposed of properly (see page 330). A rag used to apply boiled linseed oil can catch fire in less than an hour.

Paint Pollution

There is no such thing as the Perfect Solution to most problems. Take cleaning up after painting, for instance: Cleaning latex paint out of paintbrushes and roller pans contaminates large amounts of water, which must then be disposed of; and cleaning oil paint out of paintbrushes requires the use of volatile, petroleum-based solvents. In order to reuse paintbrushes, they must be cleaned between jobs.

Paintbrush Maintenance

Using paintbrushes for just one job then disposing of them creates far less pollution than cleaning the brushes. Prevent your paintbrushes from stiffening by keeping them continually damp until the entire job is finished, then throw them away.

When you take a break from your painting chores, store the paint-filled brush in a plastic bread bag to keep it from drying out. If you will be taking a prolonged break, put the brush in its bread bag in a freezer bag, and seal it tightly. Store the brush in the freezer until you are ready to paint again.

Disposable paint trays are flimsy and precarious to use, but cleaning the latex paint out of a reusable roller tray consumes a lot of water. Here's a happy compromise: Line your sturdy metal roller tray with a plastic bag before you pour in the paint. When you are done painting for the day, lift out the liner and throw it away.

Paint Stripper

The main ingredient in most commercial paint strippers is methylene chloride, which has been classified by the EPA as a probable human carcinogen. Methylene chloride is extremely volatile and evaporates rapidly, releasing large quantities of toxic fumes. This type of paint stripper can be very dangerous unless used with extreme caution (and perhaps while wearing a hazmat suit and a respirator).

If you need to strip paint, use a heat gun and scraper, or choose paint strippers that contain natural citrus-based solvents. (Homeowners should *not* attempt to strip lead-based paint.) Always wear rubber gloves and safety goggles when stripping paint.

In my opinion, the most effective way to strip paint from portable objects such as furniture or window shutters is to bring the object to a refinishing shop and have it stripped professionally. The professionals dip the objects into large vats of paint remover that is used and reused. Professional paint stripping costs a bit more, but the paint is removed more efficiently, the residue is properly disposed of, and you will save enormous amounts of time and energy.

Removing Old Wallpaper

To remove old wallpaper, wet it with full-strength distilled white vinegar, wait until the vinegar has soaked through the paper, then wet it again and wait five minutes. Use a metal spatula or scraper to lift the wallpaper off the wall. Start by removing a horizontal strip across the middle of the wall and shred strips of paper off from the starting strip.

After the paper is stripped, scrape the walls with a putty knife, then scrub the rest of the residue off with a wet sponge.

My friend Jean, whose house was liberally covered with hideous wallpaper when she and her husband moved in, suggests that removing wallpaper may not be worth doing because it requires large amounts of time, patience, sweat, and muscle power, and initiates numerous arguments, much discouragement, and many trips to the hardware store.

If the wallpaper has been applied directly to wallboard, it is impossible to remove the wallpaper without damaging the wallboard. If you remove the wallpaper anyway, you will need to use a wallboard-joint compound to skimcoat the damaged surface, *or* put on a new layer of wallpaper over the old, *or* paint primer over the old wallpaper, then paint it.

If the wallpaper has been applied over lead-based paint, your best option is probably to make sure that it is securely glued to the wall—and wherever it isn't, glue it back down—then prime and paint over the wallpaper.

Cleaning Wooden Decks

Use baking soda to clean mold, mildew, and dirt from a wooden deck:

1. Hose down the deck.
2. Sprinkle baking soda over the entire surface.
3. Use a long-handled scrub brush to scrub the surface.
4. Wait ten to fifteen minutes, then rinse off the baking soda.

Killing Moss on Wooden Shingles

Though moss is very pretty, it will eventually damage wooden shakes and shingles.

- If your roof is growing moss, sprinkle it with baking soda. The soda will kill the moss. (Moss on asphalt shingle roofs may be a signal that it is time to reroof.)
- A strip of copper nailed to the ridge of the roof will leach miniscule amounts of copper every time it rains. That tiny amount of copper is enough to prevent moss from growing.

Digging Outside

Call all utility companies before you dig in your yard. The utilities will be happy to send crews out to mark the locations of electrical, gas, water, and phone lines for you. Better safe than sorry (or dead!).

A friend of mine once dug down six inches while planting a lilac and broke a gas line next to her driveway. She was shocked that the gas line was so close to the surface. The gas company told her that due to frost heaving and erosion, gas lines in cold climates often end up near the surface.

Ice and Snow

- Use sand, grit, clean kitty litter, or calcium chloride (CaCl) to make your walkways less slippery. These substances are all easier on the environment and less likely to damage your plants than regular salt (NaCl). Calcium chloride is sold in hardware stores as an ice melter.
- Wax your snow shovel with a candle stub to prevent snow from sticking.

It is surprising how many wives and daughters have stories about watching their menfolk fall off roofs while shoveling snow or snowblowing. Walking or standing on a snowy, icy, sloped roof is generally not a good idea. It is safer to stand on the ground or on a ladder and use a long-handled roof rake.

The Nuts and Bolts of Rust Removal

Remove rust or mineral deposits from nuts and bolts by soaking them in vinegar.

If a bolt is too rusty to move, wrap it with a vinegar-soaked rag and cover it with a plastic bag secured with a rubber band. Wait a day, then try to move the bolt. Repeat until the bolt loosens.

Soft drinks are quite acidic. If you want to impress your children, use a favorite soft drink as a rust remover. It should work more rapidly than vinegar. Casually mention that if you borrowed a baby tooth from the tooth fairy and soaked it overnight in a soft drink, the tooth would be completely dissolved by morning.

Automotive Care

Some people spend so much time driving that their vehicles begin to resemble tiny, cluttered offices and snack bars. Clutter is no more functional in a car than it is in a home.

Cleaning

- Clean squashed bugs and scuff marks from the paint, headlights, chrome, and windshield of your car by scrubbing them off with a paste made of baking soda and water. The paste will not scratch the car's finish.
- Remove tar from your car's paint by applying olive oil to the spots. Let the tar soften, then rub it off with a soft cloth dipped in olive oil. After the tar is gone, use a clean, soft cloth to wipe off the olive oil.
- Your clothes will stay cleaner if your seat belts and upholstery are clean. Use a light spray of vinegar and a clean rag to wipe down the car seats and seat belts. Vinegar will not leave a dirt-attracting residue.
- Dry dirt and dust are abrasive and can scratch a car's finish. Wash your car clean; do not attempt to wipe the dust and dirt off a dry car.
- Polish the chrome on your car with a crumpled sheet of newspaper.

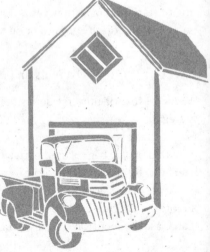

Automotive Clutter-Busting

- Strap an automotive trash bag behind each front seat.
- Store your important automotive documents in a tightly

closed tin in the glove compartment; insects, moisture, and nesting rodents will not be able to touch them.
• Set up a file folder for each vehicle. It should contain the car's registration, sales receipt, owner's manual, tire receipts, repair records, service records, etc. When you eventually sell the car, you can give the file to the new owner.

Pollution Prevention

The environmentally savvy way to wash a car is to take it to a commercial car wash: The businesses are required to install filter systems that catch dirt and pollutants, and must use environmentally friendly soaps, detergents, and waxes. The water pressure is high at car washes, so less water is used per vehicle. The runoff from home-washed cars is much more likely to pollute groundwater.

If you must wash your car at home, park it on the lawn so the grass can absorb the dirty water and prevent it from running directly onto the street, into the storm sewer, or into surface water. Use cleaners or detergents that are labeled Nontoxic and Biodegradable. Conserve water by turning the hose off when you are not rinsing the car. When you are done washing the car, pour the soapy water down the toilet, not down a storm sewer or on the street.

Motor Oil

The world's worst oil-based accident occurred in 1989 when the *Exxon Valdez* ran aground off the coast of Alaska and spilled 11 million gallons of oil. The environmental devastation was heartbreaking.

The United States Environmental Protection Agency estimates that every year, American do-it-yourselfers illegally dump or burn about 180 million gallons of used motor oil. Each of these illegal acts can cause enormous damage: One gallon of waste oil is sufficient to pollute a million gallons of fresh water, rendering it unsuitable for aquatic life and useless as a source of drinking water. (Coincidentally, one gallon of oil is the volume of one oil change.)

It is against federal and state laws to dump used motor oil on the ground, pour it down a storm sewer or drain, or flush it down the toilet. It is also illegal for private individuals to throw used motor oil in the trash, take it to a landfill, or burn or incinerate it. The only legal way to dispose of used motor oil is to take it to an oil collection site.

Quick lube businesses recycle all their used motor oil and oil filters. Taking your car in for an oil change is quick, efficient, easy on the wardrobe, and relatively inexpensive. You can also be sure that the used oil will be recycled properly. Motor oil never breaks down; it merely gets dirty. Used oil can be recycled, re-refined, and used again.

If you do your own oil changes, you need to bring the used oil in to a dealer, mechanic's garage, or hazardous waste facility for recycling. *Never* pour motor oil down a drain, on the ground, or down a storm sewer.

A clean plastic milk jug is a recommended container for transporting used oil to the collection facility. Do not pour used oil into a container that has held other petroleum products such as gasoline, antifreeze, paint, solvents, or kerosene, or the oil will not be recyclable.

Antifreeze

Standard antifreeze contains ethylene glycol, a highly toxic chemical with a sweet smell and taste that can be fatally attractive to dogs, cats, wildlife, and young children. A teaspoon of ethylene glycol is enough to kill a cat; two ounces can kill a dog.

Any liquid that is both sweet and poisonous poses a grave danger to pets and children. But even though the mechanic of the household may refrain from tasting the antifreeze, he or she may still suffer from its toxic effects: Ethylene glycol is easily absorbed through the skin, and chronic exposure, no matter how it enters the body, can cause kidney and brain damage and severe skin allergies; prenatal exposure can induce birth defects.

There is a safer alternative: Propylene glycol antifreeze, which is advertised as green, safer, or environmentally friendly antifreeze, is available at most auto stores. Propylene glycol is considered relatively nontoxic, though drinking large amounts (more than 100 milliliters) may cause gastrointestinal upset.

All antifreeze becomes polluted with heavy metals during use. This means that all used antifreeze is considered hazardous waste and must be recycled properly. Have your antifreeze changed at a garage that recycles antifreeze, and demand propylene glycol antifreeze for your refill.

The following companies make propylene glycol antifreeze. If you cannot buy their products locally, you can order them online:

Amsoil: www.amsoil.com
Neo Synthetics: www.neosyntheticoil.com
Sierra Antifreeze/Coolant: www.sierraantifreeze.com

Transmission and Brake Fluid

These may be recyclable in some communities, but whether they are recycled or not they must be brought to a proper disposal facility.

Never mix chemicals: Put them in separate clean plastic jugs and bring them to a hazardous waste facility or to a garage that recycles automotive fluids.

Handling Grease

Avoid degreasers that contain methylene chloride, which is a suspected human carcinogen. Use water-based detergents or citrus-based degreasers. Better yet, steam clean your engine at a car wash that features steam cleaning equipment. Never use gasoline to clean auto parts.

Protect your health by working in a well-ventilated area and wearing rubber gloves when working with gasoline, motor oil, and other petroleum products.

Cleaning Up Spills

Never use a flammable material such as sawdust or cornmeal to soak up flammable liquids. Use clay-based kitty litter to absorb grease and oil spills on concrete surfaces; clay is not flammable.

Recycling Solid Parts

• Used auto batteries can contain large quantities of dangerous chemicals and heavy metals; it is illegal to throw car batteries in the trash or send them to a landfill. Many automotive dealers, auto parts stores, and battery stores will accept used batteries for recycling. (When you buy a new battery, ask the retailer whether you can leave your old one at the store for proper disposal.)

- When you buy new tires, leave the old ones with the dealer, who will dispose of them properly.

Saving Transportation Energy

- Walk, bicycle, and take mass transit whenever possible.
- Carpool when you can. The fuel efficiency per person rises with the number of people riding in a vehicle: Twice as many people equals approximately twice the fuel efficiency.
- Plan ahead. Plot your route when you are doing errands so you get as much done as possible in a single trip and don't have to backtrack.
- Keep a local phonebook in your car. Being able to look up addresses and phone numbers will help keep you on track.
- Keep your car tuned-up and well maintained for maximum efficiency. A tune-up can improve your gas mileage by 4 percent.
- Synthetic oil is a bit more expensive, but it lasts longer and works more efficiently than regular oil. It will increase your car's fuel efficiency.
- Check your tire pressure at least once a month. According to the EPA, a tire that is under-inflated by only 2 PSI can increase fuel consumption by 1 percent. (If your vehicle normally gets 30 miles per gallon and your tank holds 15 gallons, the wasted gas is enough to power your car for 4.5 miles.)
- Choose a fuel efficient car.
- Remove roof racks and other rooftop carriers when you are not using them. They cause extra wind resistance that reduces fuel efficiency.
- Do not "top off" the gas tank when you are filling your car. The gas pump stops automatically when your tank is full. When you top off you are risking a fuel spill.
- The fuller the gas tank, the less room there is for evaporation: Keep your gas tank as full as possible and save gas.
- The higher the temperature, the more rapidly gasoline evaporates: Park your car in the shade during hot weather.
- Unless you are driving a large diesel-powered coach bus or semi-truck, there is no good reason to keep your motor idling while you run into the store or the post office or talk to a friend. If the weather

is very cold or very hot and you are waiting for someone, turn the engine off and go wait inside a building.

- If your engine is overheating, turn off the air conditioning. (Air conditioning uses a lot of energy, creates a lot of heat, and puts a strain on the engine.) Then turn on the heat. The heater will pull heat away from the engine and send it into the passenger compartment. You will overheat, but with any luck your engine won't catch fire. (I killed one of our cars one fine, hot August day because I reck-

---

VEHICULAR SAFETY

Many people think that large, heavy, tank-like vehicles are the safest because they could win a ramming contest against smaller vehicles. This is a false assumption: The safest cars are those that are the most maneuverable, whose drivers can avoid obstacles and prevent accidents.

Several months ago there was a photo on the front page of our local newspaper that showed the aftermath of a car accident. A small sedan had gone out of control in an intersection, and broadsided a large SUV that was stopped at the light. The sedan was barely dented and its occupants were fine, but the SUV had flipped over and its occupants sustained injuries. So much for the ramming contest.

Sometimes truth is stranger than fiction: Just as I was writing this, there was an accident not a hundred yards from our front door. A young woman was driving to work in her Ford Explorer, going about 25 miles an hour on a straight section of road. She hit a patch of ice and the next thing she knew, she was upside down in our ditch.

When it comes to vehicles, big is not beautiful; big is inefficient, cumbersome, top-heavy, and dangerous. The National Highway Traffic Safety Administration (NHTSA) conducted rollover tests on the 2004 models of vehicles (www.safercar.gov), and here is a quick summary of the results: The lowest rollover likelihood of any SUV was 13 percent; the highest was 34 percent. The lowest rollover likelihood for a pickup truck was 15 percent; the highest was 28 percent. The lowest rollover likelihood for a van was 12 percent; the highest was 15 percent. The lowest rollover likelihood for a car was 7 percent; the highest was 16 percent. A quarter of all SUVs tipped up on two wheels during the testing; about a quarter of the trucks tipped during the testing; none of the vans and none of the cars tipped during testing.

Check the Consumers Reports before buying a car: The safest cars are those that are rated high in maneuverability, stability, and crash test safety.

lessly and foolishly turned the heat off when the outside temperature topped 90 degrees. I had driven about ten miles with the heater off when smoke began shooting out of the front end of the car. My husband had neglected to tell me that the car had been overheating and he'd been running it with the heater on to keep the engine cool.)

No Fires, No Floods, No Explosions— and They Lived Happily Ever After

We may be able to teach our four-year-olds to clean up their rooms, our eight-year-olds to do the laundry, and our ten-year-olds to do all the routine household chores, but ridding our homes of hazards will always be a job for adults.

CHAPTER 9

In and Around the Garden

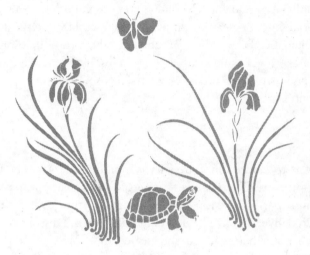

This chapter deals with gardening, home and garden pest control, and how to make your homestead safe and healthy for your children and pets.

Gardening is an expansive subject that cannot be completely dealt with in a single chapter. Although I have been landscaping professionally for a couple of decades and have written two books about gardening, I have still barely scratched the surface of gardening knowledge. There are many fine books on the market that go into more detail about all aspects of gardening.

Whether you are a backyard potato farmer or a couch potato, you can choose to make your yard or garden environmentally friendly.

The water that runs off your property can contain enough contaminants to degrade the quality of nearby surface water. Microorganisms are the main building blocks of all ecosystems. Any contaminant that kills or weakens microorganisms or upsets the balance between organisms can ruin an ecosystem.

You can reduce the toxicity of the water sloshing across your property by using only biodegradable, chlorine- and phosphate-free soaps and detergents for your outdoor cleaning projects. Antimicrobial detergents are especially problematic because they can immediately disturb the ecology of any body of water. Avoid using synthetic pesticides, herbicides, and fungicides, and don't pour petroleum products, paints, solvents, or other toxic products on the ground.

Home Treatment

Another way to reduce runoff toxicity is to minimize the amount of runoff from your property. The trick is to divert as much water as possible away from storm-sewer systems and paved surfaces. Storm water that travels quickly can deliver a heavy load of contaminants and dissolved silt. If that same storm water had stopped and tarried in a low spot, it would have dropped its load of silt, perhaps encountered a few chemical-eating microorganisms, and soaked slowly into the ground. Water that has been absorbed slowly into the ground is less likely to flood; groundwater is released slowly and gradually into waterways, and it is more likely to keep streams, creeks, and springs running year-round.

Wetlands can be thought of as Mother Nature's kidneys, where contaminants are broken down and removed from circulation. This cleansing is accomplished by wetland plants, animals, and microorganisms. It is so efficient that artificial wetlands are being used to treat the raw sewage from small communities; the effluent from livestock production; contaminated agricultural and urban runoff; and industrial wastewater. Treatment in artificial wetlands has been found effective at reducing levels of toxic pesticides, herbicides, fertilizers, and microbial pathogens, and also in removing heavy metals from waste water.

Rain gardens are shallow depressions that act as tiny wetlands. They host a variety of wetland plants and are designed to catch storm water and allow it to percolate slowly into the earth. Rain gardens are capable of absorbing about 30 percent more water than comparable areas of lawn.

Building a Rain Garden

Rain gardens should be situated where they can collect runoff from roofs, lawns, driveways, and other paved areas, and where they will catch water before it runs onto the street or sidewalk.

It is not a good idea to encourage runoff to sink into the ground next to a building: Use a drain pipe or dig a swale or depression to carry water away from a downspout to the rain garden. Native flowering plants and shrubs that tolerate "damp feet" are good choices for rain gardens, and they will make the rain garden an attractive oasis for birds, wildlife, and beneficial insects. Contact your state's Department of Wildlife or agriculture department for information on which plants are most suitable for rain gardens in your area.

A rain garden does not need to be deep. A level depression that aver-

---

🌿 NATIVE VS. NATURALIZED

Native plants are not the same as naturalized plants. Naturalized plants are plants that have been imported from another region. Often, naturalized plants thrive too well and become weedy problems. The list of naturalized plants that have become rampant ecosystem-suffocating pests includes water hyacinth, iceplant, purple loosestrife, tamarisk, and kudzu—all of which were introduced as ornamentals. Don't plant premixed wild garden or naturalizing wildflower seed mixes, which are often full of potential problems. Avoid planting anything that is labeled an invasive species by state or federal agencies, and heed the warnings of neighbors about overly aggressive plants.

Native plants are those that are endemic to a particular area and are thus perfectly adapted to local conditions. Natural landscaping provides habitat for native birds, butterflies, and beneficial insects. Contact your local Department of Natural Resources, University Extension Service, Department of Agriculture, or Audubon Society for information about native plants and natural landscaping in your area.

ages 3 or 4 inches lower than the surrounding ground, with a slightly lower area in the middle, is adequate. You are merely trying to encourage rainwater to tarry on your property long enough to soak into the ground rather than roll down the road: A puddle will do, a pond is not necessary. If you want to plant bog plants that require standing water, such as cranberries, papyrus, bog rosemary, or wild rice, dig a deeper depression for your rain garden, and incorporate clay into the soil in the depression so that the water will seep down more slowly.

A naturally low area where water tends to collect can be turned into a rain garden if you dig up and remove the sod or turf, then plant the area with native flowers and shrubs.

Many municipalities sponsor workshops in order to encourage residents to plant rain gardens. Contact your agricultural extension agency or Department of Natural Resources for more information.

Rain Barrels: Saving for a Dry Day

Set up rain barrels to catch runoff from roofs. Capturing rainwater before it hits the ground reduces the amount of runoff that reaches waterways, and the stored rainwater is wonderful for watering gardens during dry spells. If you get your water from a well that occasionally runs dry, rain barrels are an exceptionally good idea.

These are the components of an efficient rain collection system:

1. Roof gutters to collect rain from the roof of the building.
2. Downspouts to funnel water into the rain barrels.
3. Barrels with closed tops.
   a. A hole is cut into the barrel lid to accommodate a downspout. Mosquitoes cannot lay eggs in closed barrels.
   b. A hose-adapted spigot is installed near the bottom of the barrel.
   c. Multibarrel systems are connected by tubes installed near the top of the barrels. As the first barrel fills up, water begins to flow into the next barrel through the connecting tube.

Rain barrels are available through garden stores and catalogues; many municipalities offer workshops to teach residents how to fabricate their own rain barrels.

Permeable Pavement

Permeable paving surfaces, such as gravel, wood chips, or bricks or paving stones laid in sand, reduce runoff by allowing water to percolate down into the ground. These surfaces are more than adequate for most domestic purposes.

Lightly used parking areas or driveways can be paved by setting decorative, perforated concrete blocks into the ground, filling in and around them with sandy loam, then planting the area with grass and tough ground cover. The blocks make a pretty pattern and prevent ruts from developing in the grass. In areas with cold winters, the blocks will need to be set into a bed of sand, just as bricks are, in order to prevent frost-heaving.

These green parking areas are environmentally and aesthetically preferable to solid expanses of concrete or asphalt: They reduce water runoff, reduce heat build up in the summer, and produce oxygen. What more could you ask of a parking area?

Maintaining a green parking area is simple: Because the tops of the concrete blocks are at ground level, you simply mow as you would any other bit of lawn.

Contaminated Soil

Sometimes, through no fault of our own, we find ourselves dealing with contaminated soil. Dirt that has been contaminated by old lead paint is common in many cities, for instance. Garden soil that has been subjected to large doses of pesticides is also common. If you are concerned about the purity of your soil, contact your county agriculture agent and inquire about how to have your soil tested for contaminants.

The solution to both lead and pesticide contamination is to cover the contaminated area with large amounts of composted manure or sewage sludge, and leave it covered. (Fully composted materials have no smell.) Studies have shown that biologically active compost locks up toxic metals—

such as lead, cadmium, and zinc—making them less toxic and less likely to be absorbed by people, animals, and plants. Compost also helps speed up the breakdown of synthetic chemical compounds. Call a local nursery to ask about sources for composted manure.

Once you have buried the problem, however, you must make sure that it stays buried. Compost will gradually break down, exposing the original layers of contaminated dirt. You must add compost liberally and regularly, or the lead will once again be exposed.

Many cities offer lead-abatement programs to help homeowners cope with lead-contaminated soil. These Lead Safe Yards programs do free lead testing and offer education, information, grants, and loans to help home-owners make their yards safe for young children. Contact your local health department and ask for lead-abatement information.

Compost

Every bit of material that was once part of a plant or an animal will eventually biodegrade if it is exposed to air, warmth, and moisture. A compost pile can be as simple as a bunch of autumn leaves left to its own devices in a far corner of the garden for a few years; or as complex as a multiple bin system that is layered, watered, turned, and nurtured as tenderly as if it were a potted orchid.

Efficient composting requires a combination of brown (dry plant material) and green (fresh plant material). Brown materials are rich in carbon; green materials are rich in nitrogen. Composting experts agree that a compost pile should be constructed of alternating brown and green layers, using three times as much brown material as green material. Experts disagree about the amount of watering, turning and fussing required after that. The truth of the matter is that composting is an art. Some people are good at it, and others are not. I am not. Many years ago I learned to add red wriggler composting worms to my compost pile each spring. The worms made the difference between a pile that took several years to break down, and a pile that turned to compost in one season.

Though all organic material is biodegradeable, some materials are unsuitable for home compost piles. These include construction materials, which may contain hazardous substances; sawdust or shavings from treated wood; painted items; paper and newspaper; anything that has been contaminated with petrochemicals, pesticides, or heavy metals; human waste or droppings from carnivorous animals (this includes cats and dogs); and meat (unless your compost pile is completely fenced in or in a building that is inaccessible to vermin). Acceptable materials for a domestic outdoor compost pile include grass clippings, dry leaves, weeds, garden waste, worn-out cotton clothing, and small diameter hedge clippings. Food waste may attract varmints to an outdoor pile. If you want to compost food waste, you might consider starting an indoor vermicomposting bin.

In his book *All I Really Need to Know I Learned in Kindergarten*, Robert Fulghum wrote about a shoemaker who, after declaring a pair of Mr. Fulgum's shoes beyond repair, put the shoes into a paper bag along with two cookies and the following note: "Anything not worth doing is worth not doing well. Think about it . . ."

I have thought about it, long and hard, and I have come to the conclusion that the truly wonderful thing about composting is that anything organic that is too worn out to be reused or recycled can be composted. If those worn-out Bass loafers had been members of our shoe family, I would have composted them and felt great about it. It's not so hard to give things up if you know they will break down into beautiful compost in your pile.

Anything not worth doing is worth not doing well. I can't think of a better way to put it: If it can't be used in its present form, transform it! Composting is the opposite of fixing; it is unfixing. This is, of course, one of the best reasons to buy natural products: Their end-of-life-solution is so satisfying.

Vermicomposting

Apartment dwellers, folks whose yards are tiny or nonexistent, people who live in intemperate climates or where there is an abundant varmint population may need to forgo traditional outdoor composting. Luckily, vermicomposting (worm composting) is an easy alternative. This amusing indoor activity requires a minimum of equipment, space, and effort, and it yields extremely high-quality fertilizer. Organic materials ranging from unbleached paper towels to eggshells to cellulose sponges to apple cores can be vermicomposted. Red wriggler composting worms are available through many gardening catalogues, and I have written a useful little booklet on vermi-composting, called "Laverme's Handbook of Indoor Worm-composting," which is available through www.greenmercantile.com.

Mulch

The well-dressed yard wears a nice layer of mulch. Mulched soil retains moisture longer; mulched plants are more drought resistant; and a mulched garden grows fewer weeds. The difference between compost and mulch is that compost is made up of organic material that has partially biodegraded and is ready to become part of the soil. Ideally, mulch sits on top of the soil and biodegrades slowly, or not at all.

Ornamental Mulches

Mulch is any loose material that sits on top of the soil, though some mulches are considerably more attractive than others: A layer of windblown grocery bags covering a vacant lot could technically be considered a mulch; the layer of shredded leaves in a well-tended rose garden is also a mulch.

Here is a short list of mulches that are suitable for a nontoxic garden: bark; undyed, untreated wood chips; leaves; wine-grape pomace; rice hulls; licorice root; and pine needles. The most attractive biodegradable mulches are dark in color. The larger the particles, the more slowly the mulch will break down, but all plant-based mulches will need to be renewed on a regular basis.

Cocoa bean hulls are a popular and attractive mulch, but they may pose a toxic hazard to dogs. If your dog has a tendency to eat dirt, avoid using cocoa bean hulls in your garden.

Stones and gravel make a permanent mulch, but they do not suppress weeds as completely as does a thick organic mulch.

Functional Mulches

The following homely mulches are suitable for vegetable gardens or other utilitarian locations: plain uncoated cardboard and worn-out carpeting made of natural materials such as wool, cotton, seagrass, or jute.

Though these mulches will eventually break down, they generally prevent weed growth for at least one season, after which you will need to add another layer of mulch.

The Value of Trees

Controlling Global Warming

Everything we humans do, from eating and breathing to burning fuel to using aerosol cans, tends to dirty the air, raise the temperature, and use up oxygen. The more active we are, the more desperately we need help from trees.

As plants photosynthesize, they remove carbon dioxide (a greenhouse gas that contributes to global warming) from the atmosphere and release pure oxygen. Wood is a more durable, long-term storage system for carbon than are more ephemeral plant products such as blades of grass, leaves, and flowers. One of the best ways to reduce global warming is to plant more trees and to do one's best to keep them healthy.

Most tree species are heavily dependent on mycorrhizal fungi (thread-like fungi), which live in and on their roots and deliver nutrients to the tree in exchange for sugar. These fungi are an essential component of healthy soil. Chemical fertilizers, fungicides, and deep tilling can damage or kill them. You can nurture the fungi by using organic fertilizers, adding compost, and avoiding the use of synthetic pesticides, herbicides, and fungicides.

Mycorrhizal fungi are being grown commercially, and inoculant (fungal starter) is available online through various companies. If you tend your

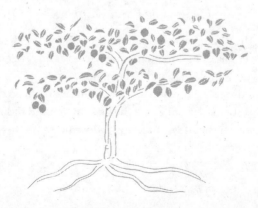

≈ FLOOD AND EROSION CONTROL

In May 2004, Tropical Storm Jeanne swept over the island of Hispaniola, killing 11 people in the Dominican Republic and 2,665 people in Haiti. The greater loss of life in Haiti was not directly related to the force of the storm, which actually hit the Dominican Republic harder, but rather to the fact that Haiti has been almost totally deforested. Haiti's denuded mountains were incapable of absorbing the heavy rainfall. The subsequent river flooding and mud flows caused the huge loss of life.

About 80 percent of Hispaniola is mountainous. In 1959, about 25 percent of Haiti was forest-covered; by 2004, only about 1.4 percent of Haiti had tree cover. Much of the Dominican Republic is still forested: Its soils can still absorb water, are relatively fertile, and can be cultivated. The estimated amount of forest cover in the Dominican Republic ranges from 22 to 40 percent, depending on the definition of "forested."

According to the Central Intelligence Agency's "World Fact Book," the per capita gross domestic product (GDP) in the Dominican Republic is the U.S. equivalent of $6,000; the per capita GDP in Haiti is $1,600.

The economic differences between the two sides of the island are almost entirely due to the nearly total destruction of Haiti's forests and the consequent erosion, loss of soil fertility, and lowered water table.

---

soil lovingly and gently, it should need inoculation only once. Here are a few online sources for these fungi:

Fungi Perfecti: www.fungi.com
Horticultural Alliance, Inc.: www.hortsorb.com
Bio Organics: www.bio-organics.com

Controlling Local Warming

Large trees actually change the climate in their immediate vicinity, making the air cooler and moister and reducing the "heat island" effect caused by the sun beating down on buildings and pavement.

Planting deciduous trees where they will throw shade on the south sides of buildings helps shade the buildings in the summer and reduces heat build up. In the winter, the leafless branches allow most of the available sun through to help warm the building.

A comprehensive regional plant book is the most essential piece of landscaping equipment. Do your research before choosing and planting trees: You do not want a tree that will drop branches on the roof of your house, crack its foundation, or invade the water or sewer lines. Look up the trees' size at maturity so you can plant them an appropriate distance away from the house. Avoid planting trees with invasive root systems near water and sewer lines. Trees described as "brittle" or "messy" should not be planted near buildings, roads, paths, or paved areas. (The "mess" from some trees, eucalyptus, for example, can be up to twenty feet long and eight inches in diameter.)

It is easiest and most efficient to plant smallish trees, up to a five-gallon pot size, because they are easy to transport and sustain less shock when they are planted, rather than to try to plant large specimens that often languish for years after they are planted.

After seeing the wretched aftermath of many a professional planting, I think it best that trees are planted by people who love them. If you don't already know how to plant, perhaps you will be lucky and someone who loves trees will teach you how. In the meantime, read up on the subject. If you want to hire a professional, try calling a local tree service that employs ISA (International Society of Arboriculture) certified arborists, and ask them to recommend a gardener or landscaper who knows how to plant trees properly. Arborists love trees, and day after day they make valiant attempts to save trees that have been damaged by improper planting; they will know which of your local gardeners and landscapers are competent.

Lawns

Maintaining the All-American Lawn is often an exercise in futility. The common suburban lawn is meant to emulate the lush, rolling, sheep-grazed grounds of an archetypal manor house in Merrie Olde rural England. England has a uniquely wet, mild climate that is perfect for growing large expanses of grass; nowhere in the United States is there a similar climate.

The lawn lost something essential in its translation from English to American: British green swards were composed of grass, clover, and other flowering plants, while the classic American lawn in the post–World War II era is a monoculture consisting of just grass.

Unfortunately, monocultures are fragile and difficult to maintain; great quantities of toxic chemicals are necessary to keep the Great American Lawn lush, green, and weed- and pest-free. We may be able to force our lawns into synthetic lushness by pouring large amounts of money, time, water, and chemicals into them, but they will never fit easily or healthily into this continent's ecosystem.

Bags of Weed and Feed (lawn fertilizer with herbicide) are almost as common as bags of dirt in our great country. In fact, the average American lawn is blasted with three to six times more pesticide per square inch than is the average field of corn or soybeans.

The weed component of Weed and Feed is 2,4-D, an herbicide that was known as Agent Orange when it was used as a defoliant during the Vietnam War. After many years of denial, the U.S. government finally admitted that many Vietnam veterans and their offspring had been made seriously ill by Agent Orange, and the Veterans Administration began paying for veterans' treatment for the following diseases that were found to be caused by exposure to Agent Orange: soft-cell sarcoma, non-Hodgkin's lymphoma, Hodgkin's disease, chronic lymphocytic leukemia, and chloracne (a serious skin disorder). The government also admitted there was a direct link between service-related exposure to Agent Orange and the incidence of acute myelogenous leukemia in the children of Vietnam veterans. Other diseases that have been linked to Agent Orange exposure are diabetes, prostate cancer, respiratory cancer, and the birth defect spina bifida.

I cannot count the number of times in the past twenty years that my friends, acquaintances, and readers have told me that their neighbor—whose child had just been diagnosed with cancer or had just returned from the hospital after receiving treatment for leukemia—was still using a lawn service. The connection between childhood leukemia and pesticide exposure has been known or suspected since the late 1960s.

I will not comment on the subject of chemical lawn services versus children with leukemia lest I run afoul of obscenity laws.

*   *   *

There are corn-based organic substitutes for Weed and Feed, which are designed to be spread on a lawn in exactly the same way as their chemical competitors. One of these organic lawn fertilizer/preemergent herbicides, called WOW!, is manufactured by Gardens Alive! The website is www.gardensalive.com.

Lawn Alternatives

There is no ecologically sound way to maintain a monocultural lawn. A much safer approach to lawn tending is to plant several different types and species of grasses, clovers, creeping groundcovers, and low-growing herbs. This melange is called a flowering lawn, and it is much hardier, easier to care for, and drought-tolerant than an all-grass lawn. I recommend a mix of tough lawn grasses, low-growing White Dutch clover (*Trifolium repens*), and low-growing groundcovers such as chamomile (*Anthemis nobilis*), creeping thyme (*Thymus* species), English Daisy (*Bellis perennis*), Irish and Scotch moss (*Sagina subulata*), and creeping speedwell (*Veronica repens*). (*Note:* If someone in your household is allergic to bee stings, you will have to forgo the clover and thyme, which attract bees.)

No matter what plant species inhabit your lawn, the following rules will make your lawn healthier and more drought and pest resistant.

- Set your lawn mower blades as high as possible. The longer the grass, the harder it is for weed seeds to reach the ground and germinate. Longer grass also shades the ground and helps conserve moisture in the soil.
- Leave the grass clippings on the lawn to decompose and nourish the soil. (But if your grass clippings are more than an inch long, they can kill the grass under them. Rake these haylike clippings up and throw them in the compost pile.)
- Don't give weeds an opening: When you find a bare spot in the lawn or create one by pulling a weed, sprinkle grass and clover seeds into the breach, then cover the seeds with a thin layer of dry grass clippings, compost, or straw.

- Water seldom but deeply; a lawn needs a minimum depth of an inch of water per watering. (If you use a sprinkler, set out a container where it will catch water from the sprinkler. When there is an inch of water in the container, turn off the sprinkler.) Shallow watering encourages shallow root growth. Shallow roots are easily damaged by foot traffic, heat, and drought.
- The more heavily you feed your lawn, the more quickly it will grow and the more often you will have to mow.

Do yourself and the environment a favor by fertilizing lightly, infrequently, and organically. Chemical fertilizers have a nasty tendency to migrate to waterways during rainstorms. Compost and other natural fertilizers are released slowly over the course of a whole season, and they are less likely to wash off during heavy rains.

Chemicals kill the microorganisms in the soil, cause soil compaction, and make the grass dependent on a chemical fix. Organic material encourages soil microorganisms; the result is livelier, healthier soil. Chemically fed plants are weaker and more likely to attract insect pests than are plants that have been nourished with slower-acting natural fertilizers and compost.

How to Feed

Sprinkle an inch of well-aged composted manure, fine-grained garden compost, or a natural fertilizer on the lawn, then comb the area with a leaf rake until the grass blades pop up above the layer of compost. Repeat every spring and fall.

Natural or organic fertilizers can contain a variety of ingredients, which may include worm castings; cricket droppings; bat guano; composted cattle, sheep, or chicken manure; seaweed; bacterial and fungal inoculants; enzymes; blood meal; bone meal; fishmeal; and feather meal. Natural fertilizers are available at garden centers, in the garden department of many hardware stores, and at farm and feed stores. In addition, here are a few good online fertilizer sources:

Gardens Alive!: www.gardensalive.com
Peaceful Valley Farm & Garden Supply: www.groworganic.com

Planet Natural: www.planetnatural.com
Arbico Organics: store.arbico-organics.com
Worm's Way: www.wormsway.com

Mowing

Consider using a manual push mower if your lawn is small. If you have a large expanse of lawn and it is not the home field of a ball club, you might consider reducing your expanse of mowed grass. If your lawn is still too big for a push mower, a quiet, exhaust-free, rechargeable electric mower is prefer-able to a smelly, noisy, gas mower. (If your gas-powered lawn mower was built in the twentieth century, you should replace it. The emissions standards for small engines were tightened in 1999. An older gas mower produces almost as much air pollution in an hour as a new car does in two days.)

Solar-powered, self-guided, robotic lawn mowers have been on the market for several years. These robotic replace-ments for grazing sheep are more expen-sive than either a manual mower or an electric mower, but they make (short) hay while the sun shines.

> ⚒ Other gas-powered garden equipment is similarly dirty:
>
> ◆ Using a gas-powered hedge trimmer for an hour creates as much pollution as driving a 1995 model car more than 650 miles.
> ◆ Using a two-stroke gas powered chainsaw for one hour produces as much pollution as driving 1,250 miles in a 1995 model car.
> ◆ A gas-powered leaf blower pro-duces twice as much pollution as the average car. Use a broom or a rake; the exercise will do you good, and your neighbors will be happy to listen to the sounds of silence.

Safe Garden Hoses

If your water is clean but the delivery system is contaminated, the end prod-uct will be dirty.

Choose hoses that are labeled Drinking Water Safe. Even if you never drink from a hose, your vegetables, pets, or children probably do.

Many cheap hoses are made of polyvinyl chloride (PVC), a compound that degrades easily in sunlight unless it is stabilized. Unfortunately, lead is one of the most common PVC stabilizers. *Consumer Reports* found very high levels of lead in many PVC hoses, and also in the water coming out of them.

Weed Control

Evicting Itchy and Scratchy

Poison oak, ivy, and sumac, and thorny brambles can be a challenge to eradicate. But there is no reason to panic and resort to chemical warfare; there are perfectly usable, nontoxic solutions to these problems.

Some lucky locales have Rent-a-Goat businesses, which hire out herds of goats for weed eradication. When a homeowner with a pernicious weed problem or a utility company with overgrown powerline right-of-ways contracts with the Rent-a-Goat company, the goats are transported to the job location and confined within a strong fence. Then under the watchful eye of a knowledgeable goatherd, the animals are allowed to decimate all the scrubby brush, weed trees, poison oak or ivy, brambles, or other noxious weeds within the confines of the fence. After all the target vegetation within the enclosure has been destroyed, the fence is moved so the goats can browse the next sector.

If the Rent-a-Goat option is not available and you don't want to brave the rashes or scratches yourself, you might consider hiring a brawny, rash-resistant teenager to attack your problem plants.

Having eradicated plenty of blackberry brambles myself, I can offer the following advice to do-it-yourselfers:

1. Bramble eradication is a cool-weather job: An all-encompassing layer of protective clothing is essential, and you don't want to overheat.
2. Wear heavy jeans, work boots, a heavy work shirt, heavy leather gloves with long gauntlets, a stiff, large-brimmed work hat, and mesh-front safety goggles.
3. You will need heavy-duty pruning loppers, a pick-mattock (this tool resembles a huge, pointy hammer-head on a long stout handle), and a pointed shovel.
4. Stand at the near end of the bramble patch, and begin lopping off the brambles and putting them in a pile. Lop off the long ends, then cut the main cane, leaving about two feet sticking up from the ground to use as a handle when you dig out the roots.
5. Continue lopping and piling until you have created a forest of two-foot-high bramble canes and a big pile of thorny debris.
6. Use the shovel and the mattock end of the pick-mattock to dig out the roots.
7. After the roots have been dug out and the pile has been removed, water the area thoroughly and cover it with black sheet plastic.
8. Weigh down the edges with dirt and stones. Let it sit for a summer and cook in the sun. The following year, remove the plastic, add compost, and plant the garden.
9. Brambles can be composted, burned, or bundled up and set out with the trash. Their final disposal depends upon your inclination and your local laws.

The technique for eradicating poison oak, ivy, or sumac is similar to the technique for brambles, with the following additions:

1. If you are sensitive to the toxins from these plants, delegate the job to someone who is less sensitive.
2. If possible, wear old but intact clothing that can be thrown out with the plant debris when the job is done.
3. Wear disposable rubber or plastic gloves over your work gloves. Dispose of them along with the plant debris.
4. Pour boiling water on the root cavities after digging out the poisonous roots.
5. After the job is done, seal the poison oak and ivy stems, leaves, and roots inside plastic garbage bags. Double-bag the debris, and try to avoid contaminating the outside of the second bag. Put the bags out with the trash.

    Warning: Never burn poison oak, ivy, or sumac! Burning does not destroy the irritating oils, so the smoke from these plants is extremely dangerous.

6. Clean your tools and work boots with a nontoxic degreaser such as Simple Green.
7. When you go indoors, avoid contaminating household surfaces with the irritating plant oils. Nondisposable contaminated clothes must be laundered in very hot water.

Pickled Weeds

United States Department of Agriculture (USDA) scientists tested the herbicidal properties of vinegar and found that a spray of common household vinegar (5 percent acetic acid concentration) killed weed seedlings. Older weeds succumbed when sprayed with pickling vinegar (9 percent acetic acid concentration). Even Canada thistle, one of the world's toughest weeds, did not survive a vinegar drenching.

Fill a spray bottle with full-strength vinegar and spray the weeds thoroughly. The vinegar will burn the leaves and kill the plants. This treatment works best on hot, sunny days.

Note: Vinegar will damage all plants, not just weeds. Avoid getting vinegar on plants that you want to keep.

Boiled Weeds

Kill weeds by pouring boiling water on them. This method works exceptionally well for cleaning weeds out of the cracks in pavement.

Poisonous Plants

There are few weeds that are as hazardous to children and pets as many of our common garden plants.

It is tempting to assume that all chemicals are bad or dangerous and all natural substances are good; unfortunately, nothing could be further from the truth. Not everything organic is safe or beneficial: Salt is inorganic, for example, and is relatively benign; cyanide is organic, extremely poisonous, and found in apple seeds and apricot, cherry, nectarine, peach, and plum pits.

It is often difficult for adults to accurately identify poisonous plants. Rather than attempt to teach young children to identify dangerous plants, begin by teaching them never to lick, chew, kiss, and—above all—swallow any plant parts.

If you have young children, try to avoid landscaping with poisonous plants. Here is a heavily abridged list of dangerous plants:

Warm Climate or Houseplants

Oleander, *Nerium oleander*: Deadly. This one is far too poisonous to ever be used as a houseplant. Adults have died after using oleander twigs to roast hot dogs.

Poinsettia, *Euphorbia pulcherrima*: Mildly toxic.

Decorative

Mistletoe, *Phoradendron flavescens*: The berries of this symbolic plant can be deadly to children and pets.

Precatory bean (rosary pea, crab's eye, jequirity), *Abrus precatorius*: The shiny red seeds, which are used for beadwork and rosaries, are extremely toxic. If chewed thoroughly then swallowed, one of these seeds will kill a human being.

Outside

Trees

Black locust, *Robinia Pseudo-acacia*: The bark, shoots, and leaves are poisonous.

Buckthorn, *Rhamnus cathartica*: The bark, leaves, and berries are purgative and will violently clean out your system.

Cherry, *Prunus* species: The leaves develop extremely toxic hydrocyanic acid when they wilt.

Horsechestnut (buckeye), *Aesculus* species: The leaves and nutlike seeds are poisonous.

Shrubs and Bushes

Box (boxtree), *Buxus sempervirens*: The leaves and stems are poisonous.

Burning bush, *Euonymus* species: The leaves and fruits are poisonous.

Daphne, *Daphne* species: The bark, leaves, and fruits are poisonous. The bright red and, in some species, orange berries have killed a number of children.

Datura (Angel's Trumpet), *Brugmansia* species: All parts are deadly.

Holly, *Ilex* species: The berries of all species are reported to be poisonous.

Privet, *Ligustrum vulgare*: Horses have been poisoned by browsing the leaves of privet hedges, and children have been poisoned by eating the berries.

Mescal bean and Japanese Pagoda Tree, *Sophora* species: The seeds are poisonous.

Yew, *Taxus* species: The wood, bark, leaves, stems, and seeds are all deadly, but the flesh of the berry is not. (This may cause some confusion, since a child will survive if she sucks the flesh off the seed then spits out the seed without chewing it, while a child who swallows the entire yewberry—flesh, seed, and all—may die.) British children have died of yew poisoning.

Elderberries

Black elderberry, *Sambucus canadensis*: The berries are used in jams and pies, but the fresh leaves, flowers, bark, young buds, and roots are poisonous. Children have been poisoned by chewing or sucking the bark, or by using hollow tubes of elder bark to make pea shooters or flutes.

Red elderberry, *Sambucus racemosa*: The berries are poisonous.

Vines

Bittersweet, *Celastrus scandens*: The berries and leaves are poisonous.

Ivy, *Hedera helix*: The whole plant is poisonous. Children have been poisoned by eating the berries. Animals have been poisoned by browsing the leaves or feeding on clippings. Contact with ivy leaves can cause severe dermatitis.

Perennials

Rhubarb, *Rheum cultorum*: Rhubarb stems, as many northern cooks know, are excellent in pies, jams, and sauces, but the leaves are poi-

> ### ❧ INSECTICIDAL RHUBARB SPRAY
>
> Remove the rhubarb stems and make them into a pie. Put the leaves in a stockpot and cover them with water. Bring the pot to a boil. Turn off the heat and let the pot sit and cool for an hour. Strain the leaves out of the cooled liquid. Use a spray bottle to apply the rhubarb tea to infested plants.

sonous and should never be ingested. In fact, rhubarb leaves can be used to make an excellent insecticidal spray for plants.

Aconite Family: All parts of all the plants in this family are poisonous, including:
- Monkshood, Aconite, *Aconitum* species
- Larkspur, *Consolida ajacis*
- Delphinium, *Delphinium* species
- Baneberry, *Actaea* species
- Blue cohosh, *Caulophyllum thalictroides*

Bulbs

The bulbs and foliage of most ornamental bulbs are poisonous. Children and pets should be kept away from all flowering bulbs, including the following:

AMARYLLIS FAMILY

Amaryllis *belladonna*
Crinum species
Hymenocallis species

LILY FAMILY

Lily, *Lilium* species
Narcissus, Daffodil, and Jonquil, *Narcissus* species
Meadow saffron, *Colchicum autumnale*
Tulip, *Tulipa* species
Lily of the Valley, *Convallaria majalis*

Miscellaneous
Jack-in-the-pulpit, *Arisaema* species

Bean Family, Leguminosae
This family encompasses all the familiar edible legumes, which include green beans, lima beans, dried beans, and lentils. Unfortunately, many of the other members of the bean family produce highly poisonous seeds, all of which resemble their edible cousins. It is safest to presume that any bean-like seed is poisonous until proven otherwise.

PERENNIAL LEGUMES

Lupine species: The seeds, pods, and leaves of many lupine species are poisonous.

Canary bird bush and wild pea, *Crotalaria* species: All parts of these species are poisonous.

Crown vetch, *Coronilla varia*: The seeds are poisonous.

ANNUAL LEGUMES

Castor bean, *Ricinus communis*: A tropical-looking ornamental. The entire plant is appallingly poisonous, especially the beans.

Weeds

DEADLY NIGHTSHADE FAMILY

Nightshade, *Solanum* species: The poisonous red, purple, or black berries look like tiny tomatoes and are very attractive to children. The leaves of all the plants in this family—which includes potatoes, tomatoes, eggplant, and peppers—are poisonous.

It would be nice to assume that once one's children have reached the age of reason, poisonous plants no longer pose a threat; unfortunately, that may not be the case. Our son, when he was old enough to drive, shave, and attend college, once made an amusing, but potentially sickening, mistake: I asked him to harvest some basil in the vegetable garden, and he returned with a beautiful bouquet of healthy green leaves. I thanked him, began chopping them up, and gradually realized that I wasn't smelling anything. Our brilliant son, who has no sense of smell, had harvested green pepper leaves. Luckily I caught the mistake before the pepper leaves were added to our dinner.

Umbelliferae Family

Poison hemlock (*Conium maculatum*), Fool's parsley (*Aethusa cynapium*), and Water hemlock (*Cicuta maculata*) are all dangerously toxic and strongly resemble their edible relatives: carrots, dill, fennel, caraway, angelica, and anise. It is easy to make a mistake with this family.

Garden Pest Control: Of Mice and Men

Pests are notoriously tough. Any poison that is toxic enough to kill a nuisance organism is strong enough to harm a human being. Though we like to think we are very different from the pests that annoy us, we all live on the same planet and share much of the same genetic material.

Genetic sequencing techniques have revealed that about 99 percent of the genetic material in mice and men is identical. (This may give new poignancy to the old insult, "Are you a man or a mouse?") These genetic similarities allow humans to use animals as our stand-ins when we are testing the safety of drugs, chemicals, and medical procedures and apparatus.

It is a rare poison or toxin that is toxic to rodents and not to humans.

We are All Siblings Under the Skin, Exoskeleton, or Bark

Forty-four percent of mammals' and insects' genetic material is identical; and 18 percent of our genome is identical to that found in plants. The most ancient, basic functions that are essential to most organisms—such as the chemical signals that govern embryonic development and those that control the immune response and the hormonal system—are the most likely to be identical.

Researchers at the University of Wisconsin are studying fruit flies in an attempt to figure out the genetic causes of some types of human deafness and blindness. This research is only possible because many of the genes that govern embryonic development in flies perform the same functions in human beings.

The nerves of insects and humans are similar enough that grasshoppers and cockroaches are commonly used as laboratory animals when scientists need to test the effects of new drugs and chemicals on the nervous system.

These genetic similarities mean that any synthetic poison that attacks an insect's nervous system, embryonic development, resistance to infection, or hormonal signaling system may pose an acute danger to humans as well. Herbicides that kill weeds by making them grow themselves to death, such as 2,4-D, may also damage our own ability to stop uncontrolled cell growth (this phenomenon is called cancer when it affects humans and other animals).

A Clean Safe Kill

Since most of the poisons that work on pests also work on us, it behooves us to think hard before resorting to chemical warfare against unwanted organisms in our homes and gardens.

The first question we should ask is "What are we trying to protect?"

The second question is "How important is my objective?"

My first objective is always to protect the health and happiness of my family; any lesser objective does not merit the use of dangerous chemicals. For example, life- or health-saving drugs can be quite toxic, but I am willing to use them to save a human life; chemical dandelion-killers are also quite toxic, and I am unwilling to use them to save a lawn.

There is, I believe, a design flaw in our world, to wit: Only the good die young. Though disease-causing bacteria eventually develop immunity to all antibiotics, we will always be able to depend on those antibiotics to decimate the normal, necessary intestinal bacteria that our health depends on;

and if you use a pesticide to kill a garden pest, you can bet that eventually the pest will acquire a taste for the poison, but the poison will remain remarkably efficient at killing helpful creatures such as toads, frogs, bats, honeybees, and ladybugs.

Insects have been on the planet far longer than we have, and there is little doubt that they will outlive us. The harder we try to poison them, the more quickly they adapt.

The best defense against plant-eating pests is to plant a diverse garden and keep it healthy. Insects are just as lazy as everybody else: When they have to choose between journeying long distances between their favorite food plants, or hopping conveniently from plant to plant, they will choose convenience. Diversify, and most of those pests will pass you by.

Destructive insects such as cinch bugs, tent caterpillars, thrips, and Colorado potato beetles thrive on the monotony of a monoculture, while beneficial insects such as assassin bugs, ambush bugs, ladybugs, parasitic wasps, and praying mantises crave variety. Diverse plantings that bloom over a long season will encourage beneficial insects and discourage pests.

Don't Judge by Appearances

The most important pest control tool is a well-illustrated arthropod (insect and spider) identification book. There is no point in going into emergency alert mode over a harmless or beneficial insect or spider. Some of the least attractive arthropods are beneficial.

A simple rule of thumb: Predatory creatures are generally faster than their herbivorous prey. An insect scuttling along at a fast clip is probably on the hunt.

Insect Control with Backbone

Birds, bats, frogs, snakes, shrews, and moles eat destructive insects, slugs, and snails. If you improve the habitat in your yard by including a variety of plants, a few cozy, brushy hiding places, a little available drinking water in the form of a pan of water or small pond, and you refrain from using garden chemicals, these grateful creatures will happily tackle your pest problem.

Pickled Slugs and Snails

For more than sixty years, the only slug and snail baits available in the United States contained metaldehyde. The U.S. Environmental Protection Agency has classified metaldehyde as a "slightly toxic compound that may be fatal to dogs or other pets if eaten."

It seems rather odd that a compound that "may be fatal . . . if eaten" could be considered "slightly toxic." When I was a child, my friend's poodle ate snail bait and ended up more than "slightly dead." These dangerous products—which bear names such as Slug-Tox, Cory's Slug and Snail Death, and Deadline— might just as well have been named "Pug and Poodle Death" or "Deadfeline."

Finally, after all those toxic years, a different type of snail bait was developed in Europe; it was approved for sale in the United States in 1997. Its active ingredient is iron phosphate, which is fatal to land mollusks but relatively nontoxic to humans and pets.

These iron phosphate–based snail baits are available at many garden centers, and they bear such names as Escar-Go!, Sluggo, and Worry Free.

If you would rather not use poisons of any sort in your garden, try the following homely remedies against marauding mollusks:

- A saucer of beer set into the ground in the garden will attract slugs and snails, many of which will become inebriated enough to drown.
- Slugs and snails like to hide under things. You will find many potential victims if you set habitat traps for them: Put wooden boards on the ground, and turn the boards over every morning.
- If you want to put all the mollusks to good use, acquire a pet duck. Ducks adore dining on escargot and will happily follow you as you make your gardening rounds.

• Young gardeners who thrill to the excitement of the hunt may want to play a more active role by executing the mollusks with a spray of straight vinegar. The killing ground should be either bare or paved so your cherished garden plants will not be damaged by the spray. Compost the slippery corpses.

Garbage Can Security

If you compost your food wastes, animals will not be attracted to your garbage can. Waste that cannot be composted, such as meat, bones, and fat, should be stored in the freezer until just before the estimated arrival time of the garbage collector.

Indoor/Outdoor Pests

Ants, cockroaches, and mice are all very well in their own place, but not in mine. Though some indoor pests are actually dangerous (cone bugs, black widow spiders, and rats, for instance) the presence of a few small, uninvited guests is an inadequate justification for poisoning one's family.

According to toxicologist William Pease of the University of California, Berkeley School of Public Health: *"Indoor air use of pesticide products in the home is the main source of exposure for children."* Pease worries particularly about moth balls, no-pest strips, foggers, and other products that are designed to release pesticide continuously. Studies have shown that children who live in households where these pesticides are used have an increased risk of leukemia and brain cancer. These products are even more dangerous when used where they can contaminate food and kitchen surfaces.

There are many safe, nontoxic ways to evict pests from your home; better yet, prevent them from entering your abode in the first place. The most basic piece of domestic insect-control equipment is the humble window screen. All windows should be equipped with screens to keep out flies, mosquitoes, wasps, and other insect pests.

If you don't have window screens, all your other pest control efforts are likely to prove futile.

Being Chased by the Furies

Fear and panic can induce people to take inappropriate action. Dr. Merlin Tuttle, the world's foremost authority on bats, once told me that many people jump out of second or third story windows when they think there's a bat in their house. Often the bat is actually a bird; occasionally it is a butterfly. But even if one were bitten by a bat that was rabid, being vaccinated against rabies requires only a few small pokes in the arm. I took the series so I could work with wild bats; the needles were so small that I didn't even feel them. Jumping out a second or third story window would undoubtedly be a lot more painful than being vaccinated!

My husband and I once did a bat exclusion (eviction) job for a retired couple who had poured an entire jug of insecticide in their attic in a vain attempt to kill the resident bats. (Using pesticides to kill bats is strictly prohibited by federal law, by the way.) Luckily for the bats, the insecticide was heavy and didn't affect those that were hanging from the attic ceiling. Unfortunately for the humans, the pesticide was heavy, and it filtered down from the attic into their living room.

Ants Indoors

Ants are most likely to invade a house when there is a drought or a shortage of food outdoors. Follow the line of ants to discover where they are getting into the house, and if possible, caulk the openings.

If the ants are searching for water in your house, try putting pie pans of water outdoors near their trails. They may prefer drinking outdoors.

Sprinkle peppermint leaves, red pepper, or paprika across ant trails to divert them from the house.

Either don't leave pet food out all day, or make an ant moat by putting the pet food bowl in a slightly larger bowl that has an inch of soapy water in it. Ants are not good swimmers.

Try dusting boric acid or borax into cracks

that cannot be caulked. This can be accomplished by pouring a small amount of the powder near the crack then brushing it into the crack with a soft dust brush or paintbrush.

On a lighter note, one Thanksgiving when my father was in his late eighties, we were planning to prepare the meal at his apartment. While the turkey was thawing on his counter, he phoned and said that there were ants all over his floor, and he'd had to spray Raid. I was not happy with this news, thinking we were going to have to buy a new turkey. We rushed over and asked him to show us the can of Raid. He showed us an aerosol can of cooking oil. (My dad had macular degeneration, and his eyesight was really bad.) The ants were indeed defunct; they'd been gooped to death. Several hours later, we feasted on a delicious and nontoxic turkey.

Ant Bait

The type of bait one puts out for ants depends upon their dining habits. If the ants are lining up to get to your unwashed frying pans, they are grease ants, which dine on fats and proteins; if they are carrying off bits of grape jelly, they are sugar ants.

1. Make a bait for grease ants by mixing a teaspoon of boric acid with a quarter cup of bacon grease or butter. Kill sugar ants by mixing 1½ teaspoons boric acid with ⅓ cup sugar and 1 cup water. Soak some cotton balls in the boric acid solution.

2. Put a few of the wet cotton balls or a dollop of the greasy bait in a small bottle with a screw-on lid, poke ant-size holes in the lid, then screw the lid back on. Lay the bottle on its side in a location

where pets and children cannot reach it, such as behind the refrigerator or under the sink.

Ants Outdoors

Indigenous ants are an essential part of the ecosystem. They protect their territory, attack termites, and eat flea eggs, so unless they are coming indoors or are pasturing their dairy aphids on your favorite apple seedling, you should probably leave them alone. (Aphids exude a sweet secretion that is called honeydew. Some ant species keep herds of domesticated aphids that they milk for their honeydew.) You can distract ants from their domesticated aphids by putting containers of honey beneath aphid-afflicted plants. The aphids will languish without the gentle ministrations of the ants.

Ants and pine trees go together like peanut butter and jelly. If you live in a pine forest, there will always be anthills in your yard. No matter how many ants you kill, more will take their place within a few days.

Inconveniently located anthills can be destroyed by opening them up with a shovel, then drowning them with boiling water. This delicate operation should be performed at night, when the ants are inactive. Be aware that killing off an entire colony of harmless ants will leave their habitat vacant, and a less desirable species may move in.

Cockroaches

Indoor cockroach control is similar to that for ants, except that roaches are nocturnal. All the roach-preventive cleaning must be done before dark.

- Keep the kitchen clean and the food put away.
- Don't leave water sitting in pots, pans, glasses, or plant saucers.
- Do not leave pet food out overnight.
- Apply a very thin dusting of boric acid or borax in dark places where roaches like to hide, such as under the refrigerator, under the stove,

and in cracks in walls and floors. Roaches will avoid piles of boric acid, so the layer must be very thin.

- Make a cockroach bait by mixing 4 tablespoons boric acid powder or borax, 2 tablespoons sugar, and 1 tablespoon cocoa. Put the bait in jar lids and place them under the refrigerator, in the cabinet beneath the kitchen sink, behind the stove, and in other areas that are inaccessible to pets and children.

    Caveat: If you live in a large, cockroach-infested apartment building, cockroaches that live in neighboring apartments will continue to visit. Cockroach eradication in multifamily buildings can only be accomplished as a group project.

- Research conducted at Iowa State University showed that catnip oil repels cockroaches. If you don't own cats, strew catnip on your kitchen shelves. Catnip has a pleasant, minty smell.

Infested Food

Flour and grain moths, beetles, and weevils can infest and ruin stored grain, flour, pasta, dried beans, nuts, dried fruit, and other food. Strong smelling spices will repel or kill these pests. Put a couple of peppercorns, a cinnamon stick, or a bay leaf into a small cloth bag and drop it into your flour tin to ward off pests. The spices will not affect the taste or smell of these dry foods.

Mice, Rats, and Squirrels

The first step in rodent control is to seal off entry points to buildings. Check for cracks in walls, and inspect the entry points for pipes and wires and the places where the roof and the walls intersect. If you can fit a dime in a hole, a mouse can squeeze through. Rats can slip through nickel-size openings, gray squirrels can squeeze through quarter-size holes; both are capable of enlarging inadequate entry holes by gnawing. Rats are even capable of chewing through porous, low-quality concrete blocks.

Signs that an opening is being used by varmints include grease-darkened edges and a few droppings. If you cannot locate the rodents' access points, try dusting the area near suspected entry points with fine white flour. The next morning, check the flour for the footprints of tiny intruders.

Use rodent-proof material such as 26 gauge galvanized sheet metal, galvanized hardware cloth (metal mesh), or cement mortar to seal any openings in the building.

Habitat Control

You can sharply reduce the rodent population by reducing the available food supply and nesting areas:

- Do not stack junk or firewood in the yard close to the house. Rats love to live in piles. Stack fire wood away from buildings and at least eighteen inches off the ground.
- Birdhouses and feeders should be elevated on rat- and squirrel-proof metal poles or hung from metal cables.
- Store pet food and birdseed in metal containers with tight lids. Do not leave pet food out overnight.
- Collect fallen fruit and vegetables in the garden and orchard and put them in the compost pile. Bury them under several inches of dirt or finished compost.
- Metal garbage cans are rat-resistant; plastic ones are not.
- Store dry goods in the kitchen in airtight metal or glass containers, not in plastic bags, cardboard boxes, or plastic containers.
- Rats and mice are primarily nocturnal. Clean up the kitchen, put food in rodent-proof containers or in the refrigerator, clean up crumbs, take out the trash or compost, and wash the dishes before you go to bed.
- Peppermint repels mice. Plant peppermint next to your foundation (along with catnip, if you also have a termite problem). Strew peppermint leaves on kitchen shelves or dab peppermint oil on shelf edges.

Eradication

Poisoning rodents is never a good idea. Even if you have a successful kill with no collateral casualties among your pets and juvenile humans, when a poisoned mouse dies inside a wall and begins to stink, how does one remove it?

Rats and mice skulk along the edges of rooms: They keep in contact with the walls and navigate by feel. Rat and mouse traps should be set close to walls. Snap traps, which kill instantly, are considered more humane than sticky traps. Use peanut butter as bait; it is more attractive to rodents and lasts longer than cheese. Rats are extremely fond of Froot Loops; putting a single Froot Loop on top of the peanut butter bait in a trap may make the bait completely irresistible.

To dispose of a dead rodent, put it in a plastic bag, seal the bag tightly, and place it in a tightly covered garbage can.

Live Trapping

Do not attempt to live trap a rat and set it free to live out its life in blissful harmony with nature. Rats are dangerous. No one wants or deserves your relocated rat.

Trapping live mice is futile: The word that best describes a relocated mouse is "lunch."

Flies

The best way to deal with flies is to deny them access to food and breeding areas.

Indoor Fly Control
- Make sure your window and door screens are intact and properly closed.
- Keep the kitchen cleaned up, the food put away, and the garbage cans covered.
- Sticky flypaper strips catch and kill flies effectively without using poisons. These long coils of shiny, sticky paper look rather festive when they are first pulled down from their small cardboard cylinders, but they quickly lose their decorative value as they become dotted with the corpses of flies.

  Hang the flypaper from the ceiling in a location where no one will walk into it. It is exceedingly unpleasant to get flypaper stuck in one's hair.

Outdoor Fly Control

- Cover the compost pile with black sheet plastic, clean dirt, or finished compost.
- Don't allow fallen fruit to rot under trees; pick it up and bury it in the compost pile.
- Clean up animal droppings and dispose of them properly by flushing them down the toilet, burying them, or putting them in a closed container in the trash.

Two different species of tiny parasitic nematodes attack and kill immature flies as well as the larvae of other soil-dwelling pests. These nematodes, *Steinernema carpocapsae* and *Heterorhabditis bacteriophora,* invade the bodies of insect larvae, reproduce, and kill their hosts.

Laboratory-grown parasitic nematodes, which can be mixed with water and sprayed on the lawn or garden, are available online and through gardening catalogues. Nematodes are tiny delicate creatures, so follow the application directions carefully. One application will kill insect larvae for a full year.

Nematodes prey on the young of the following pests:

Flies: Walnut husk fly, fungus gnats, Onion maggot

Caterpillars: cutworms, army worms, sod webworms, artichoke plume moth

Beetles: cucumber beetles, Colorado beetle, Japanese beetles, June beetles

Ticks

Fleas

Termites

Here are a couple of sources for parasitic nematodes:

Peaceful Valley Farm & Garden Supply: www.groworganic.com
Gardens Alive!: www.gardensalive.com

Termites are colonial insects that feed on dead wood. These decomposers play a necessary and valuable role in the larger scheme of things, but unfortunately, termites cannot distinguish between a fallen log and a wooden house. Some of the subtle signs that your home has been invaded by termites include grooves in the wood; little piles of sawdustlike termite droppings; or long, thin mud tubes stretching from the ground, across the foundation, and up to the wooden siding of your home. Sagging floors or wooden columns may be evidence of a long-term, severe termite infestation.

There are three different types of termites: dampwood termites, which are most prevalent in the Northwest; drywood termites, which are most common in the South and in California; and subterranean termites, which are common across much of the continental United States and in Hawaii.

General Termite Control

Termites are attracted to dead wood. The wooden components of a house should never be allowed to come in contact with the soil, and neither lumber, nor firewood, nor dead or decaying wood should ever be stored next to or under the house.

Do not lean pieces of wood or lumber against the house where they can serve as termite bridges from the ground to your home's wooden siding.

Shield all wooden components of your house from direct contact with the soil, either by wrapping wooden posts in sheet metal or by building atop masonry foundations.

The same parasitic nematodes that were mentioned in the "Flies" section of this chapter (page 386) will also attack and kill termite larvae in the soil. They are effective against the soil-dwelling dampwood and subterranean termites but not against the drywood termites, which live exclusively in wood.

Specific Termite Control

Dampwood Termites. These west coast natives live in and eat damp wood. Because they are so specialized, they are the easiest termites to control: Keep your house dry by eliminating leaks and other sources of moisture, and replace damp, damaged wood. (See chapter seven, "Preventing Fungi, Mold, and

Mildew," page 290, for more detailed information on keeping your house dry.)

Drywood Termites. These warm-climate termites may be found in any part of the house. Experts recommend spot-treatment of infested areas using either a pyrethrin- (botanical) based pesticide or a high-voltage Electro-Gun. This job requires a pest-control professional who will also have the equipment to locate the colonies. (In some parts of the country, specially trained dogs are employed for sniffing out termite infestations.)

Subterranean Termites. These are the most rapidly destructive termites. They live in the soil and build mud tubes to reach their wooden food.

Sand barriers made of coarse, twelve grit sand have been proven effective against termites in Hawaii. Here's how to install a sand barrier: Remove all the dirt in a swathe several inches deep and a couple feet wide next to your foundation. Replace the dirt with coarse, twelve grit sand. Tamp the sand down firmly next to the foundation. Termites cannot build their access tubes in sand. Contact your local housing authority for more information on the use of sand barriers in your area.

Clothes Moths

The tiny larvae of clothes moths attack wool, silk, and fur. These larvae are too delicate to survive in clothing that is being worn; they can attack clothing only when it is not in use. To prevent moth damage, clean woolens before storing them; moth larvae are attracted to food stains, sweat, and body oils. Store woolens in tightly closed, airtight containers during the off season, and enclose pieces of aromatic cedar or a few sprigs of lavender or rosemary to repel moths.

Never bring used woolen clothing or furs into your home without treating it to kill moths.

1. Enclose your new acquisition in a clean, black plastic garbage bag and seal it tightly.
   a. If the weather is below freezing, leave your bag in an unheated outbuilding to freeze for a couple of weeks.
   b. If the weather is hot, put the black plastic bag outside in the sun to broil for a few days.

2. If the item can safely be tumbled in the dryer, do so. The tumbling action of the dryer will kill the larvae; no heat is necessary.

Bloodsuckers

In order to make informed, intelligent decisions, we need to have facts. In almost no realm are people less likely to make well-informed decisions than where human skin interacts with pest organisms. Many people are so terrified of insects that they willingly poison their homes, their gardens, and ultimately, themselves, their children, and their pets.

The Centers for Disease Control (CDC) reported that as of January 2005, all states in the United States except for Washington, Alaska, and Hawaii had reported cases of human, bird, or animal West Nile Virus infection: There were 2,470 human cases in 2004, and 88 people died. The West Nile Virus is transmitted by mosquitoes.

In 2001, the CDC reported 62,034 deaths from influenza and pneumonia (which is frequently associated with the flu). In an average year, 36,000 Americans die of the flu.

If you are really worried about your health, get a flu shot.

Mosquitoes

Female mosquitoes lay their eggs on standing water. The larvae take a couple of days to mature and escape from their watery nursery. Most mosquitoes are homebodies that travel less than two miles from their natal waters.

Eradicate Breeding Areas
- Empty out pet water dishes, birdbaths, plant saucers, and wading pools at least every other day to prevent mosquito larvae from maturing.
- Scout your property for trash that can hold water: Get rid of old tires and discarded containers. Clean out your roof gutters so they don't become elevated mosquito hatcheries. Drill drain holes in the bottom of your tire swings.

- Put covers or screens on rain barrels.
- Buy *Bacillus thuringiensis israelensis* (BTi) mosquito dunks or granules and put them in ponds, puddles, and other permanent or seasonal bodies of water. These products are available at feed stores and home improvement stores. (BTi is a bacteria that kills mosquito larvae but is harmless to other organisms.)
- A layer of oil on top of the water will suffocate mosquito larvae. Pour cooking oil into seasonal puddles.
- Keep your window and door screens in good working order.
- A little brown bat can eat seven hundred mosquitoes in a single night. Encourage these busy little insectivores by putting up bat houses, and refrain from using pesticides; bats are very easily poisoned. Contact your local Department of Natural Resources for accurate information about building and siting wildlife houses.
- Wear light-colored clothing during mosquito season: Mosquitoes are attracted to dark-colored clothing.

From the Counterproductive Department:
Mosquito Attractants

Sound Waves

Dr. Richard Gorham of the Arctic Health Research Laboratory in Fairbanks, Alaska, tested the effectiveness of an ultrasonic mosquito repeller during the height of mosquito season in the Alaskan wilderness. The machine emitted a high-pitched whine that the manufacturer claimed would drive mosquitoes away.

The first step in the experiment was to establish the baseline mosquito density: The intrepid Dr. Gorham accomplished this by exposing the back of his hand and counting the number of mosquitoes that landed on and bit his unprotected flesh. He estimated that if he'd been stripped naked and tied to a tree, he would have died from loss of blood within two and a half hours. Then he turned on the ultrasonic mosquito repeller machine and ran the experiment again. The density of mosquitoes increased.

Conclusion: High-pitched whines attract mosquitoes. Don't waste your money.

Black Light

Electronic bug zappers use ultraviolet light to lure flying insects to a spectacular, flashy death. Researchers from the American Entomological Society, who obviously have a lot of patience, studied the zapped remains of 13,789 insects. They found that only 31 of them were biting insects.

Another study showed that for every mosquito zapped, 250 mosquito predators were obliterated. Researchers have noted that mosquitoes are attracted by the pretty light, but don't fly into the trap. Once they're near the bug zapper, they veer off in search of fresh blood.

Did a mosquito invent this machine?

Beam Me Up, Scotty

Further evidence that bug zappers are counterproductive comes from Dr. James Urban and Dr. Alberto Broce of Kansas State University, who discovered exploded bits of insects six feet away from the bug zappers that killed them. Live bacteria and viruses were transported along with the insect parts.

Mosquito Repellents

DEET (N,N-diethyl-m-toluamide) is the active ingredient in many commercial insecticides and repellents. It has been on the market in the United States since 1957. Repellents that contain DEET are registered with the Environmental Protection Agency for direct application to human skin, clothing, pets, tents, bedrolls, and screens.

DEET is an effective mosquito repellent that has some unfortunate drawbacks, including skin irritation, painful blisters, permanent scarring, irritation of the mucous membranes, and numbness or burning sensations in the lips. The National Institute for Occupational Safety and Health (NIOSH) found that employees at Everglades National Park who were heavy users of DEET-based repellents were more likely to report problems with insomnia, mood disturbances, and impaired cognitive function than were their coworkers who used less of the repellent. One young man who applied DEET before taking a sauna developed acute manic psychosis.

Though the repellent can cause nasty symptoms in adult users, it is even worse for youngsters. DEET exposure has caused agitation, weakness, disorientation, ataxia, seizures, coma, and death in young children.

These Beat Deet

- A plant-based insect repellent called Bite Blocker, which contains soybean oil, geranium oil, and coconut oil, was developed in Europe, and it has been on the American market since 1997. Studies conducted at the University of Guelph in Ontario, Canada, showed that Bite Blocker was 97 percent effective at repelling insects for at least three and a half hours. A DEET-based spray was 86 percent effective over the same time period.
- Apparently, catnip attracts cats, but repels mosquitoes. Research conducted by Dr. Joel Coats of Iowa State University and Chris Peterson of the U.S. Forest Service showed that the essential oil in catnip is ten times more effective than DEET.

Ticks

Lyme disease is a much-feared bacterial disease that is transmitted by infected ticks. The disease was first described in Old Lyme, Connecticut, in 1975.

Three Lyme disease studies that were published in the New England Journal of Medicine in 2001 found the following:

1. Lyme disease is difficult to catch; just 3 percent of people who are bitten by infected ticks actually get the disease. Most of the people who contract Lyme disease make a complete recovery without antibiotics. (If you do come down with the classic bull's-eye rash and fever or aches, you should, of course, get medical attention.)
2. Many of the symptoms of chronic Lyme disease, such as fatigue, memory loss, and impaired thinking, do not respond to antibiotic treatment. These symptoms are quite common in the general public anyway. These facts have led many researchers to conclude that the symptoms of chronic Lyme disease are unrelated to Lyme disease infection.

   I know a woman who suffered from debilitating chronic Lyme disease for many years. She was short of breath, anxious, and in so much pain that she curtailed her activities. Doctors could do nothing to improve her quality of life. Her symptoms miraculously disappeared when she divorced her husband.

3. The potent antibiotics that have been used to treat chronic Lyme disease are dangerous and have caused side effects ranging from destruction of the bone marrow to fatal infections originating at the site of the drug catheters. (These are the only fatalities associated with Lyme disease.)

Dr. Leonard H. Sigal, a Lyme disease expert at the Robert Wood Johnson University Medical Group in New Brunswick, New Jersey, commented that "Lyme disease, although a problem, is not nearly as big a problem as most people think. The bigger epidemic is Lyme anxiety." (People don't usually die from Lyme disease, but they may die from the treatment for Lyme Neurosis.)

Tick Control

Over the years I have pulled thousands of ticks out of horses and dogs, and perhaps a dozen out of family members. Ticks are unquestionably disgusting, but when dealing with repugnant life forms, one must keep one's head. The mortality rate from Lyme disease is essentially zero, but many people die every year from acute pesticide poisoning and pesticide-induced diseases.

When you carefully pull a tick straight out with a blunt tweezers, it must keep its head. It must also keep all of its innards. Do not squeeze or compress the tick in any way. Embedded bits of tick may cause an infection.

Fleas

Many animals utilize aromatic plants for pest control. Dusky-footed wood rats (*Neotoma fuscipes*), which live on the west coast of Mexico and the United States, strew bay leaves in their sleeping chambers. Richard B. Hemmes of Vassar College in Poughkeepsie, New York, and his colleagues conducted laboratory tests and found that bay leaves can kill flea larvae. Apparently the rats already knew that.

Starlings and Blue Tits fumigate their nests with fresh aromatic leaves.

When researchers removed the herbs from the nests, the number of blood-sucking mites in the nests increased and the health of the chicks declined.

Flea-Free Fido
- Fresh leaves of aromatic herbs such as lavender, rosemary, yarrow, and bay can help keep pets' bedding flea-free. Pet beds that are stuffed with aromatic cedar chips also help repel fleas.
- Add brewer's yeast to your pets' food and apple cider vinegar to their water to make your animals less appetizing to fleas.

Flea-Free Home
After she has gorged on blood, a female flea dismounts from her itchy victim and lays between four and six eggs. The mother flea strews her nesting area with bits of dried blood that will nourish her offspring after they hatch.

After about ten days, the baby fleas emerge from their eggs and innocently begin to feed on their dried rations. The transformation from larvae to pupae to adult flea can take from two weeks to a year, depending on the weather and the season. Adult fleas can live for up to a year, but generally live for only two months.

The vacuum cleaner is one of the best defenses against fleas. Though adult fleas are notoriously agile and difficult to catch, juvenile fleas are less mobile and more vulnerable. If you vacuum daily, you will eventually disrupt and stop the infestation.

Kill fleas and flea eggs on carpets by sprinkling the carpet liberally with table salt or with borax. Wait several hours, then vacuum the carpet. If you use borax, you must keep pets and children away from the carpet until the borax has been vacuumed up.

If fleas are hatching from between your floorboards, dust the table salt or borax directly into the cracks, wait a few hours, then vacuum.

After you finish vacuuming, remove the vacuum bag and seal it tightly in a black plastic garbage bag. Put the bag in a sunny location, and let it bake in the sun for several days in order to kill any survivors.

Fleas are generally warm weather pests, but if by some odd chance your house acquired fleas during frigid weather, after you finish vacuuming, put the vacuum bag in a garbage bag, then set it outside to freeze for a few days. If a flea-infested carpet is portable, roll it up, take it outside, and let the fleas freeze.

Pet Care

Ear Mites

If your pet scratches repeatedly at his ear, he may have ear mites. Massage slightly warmed olive oil into the animal's ear canal; the oil will suffocate the ear mites.

Cleaning Up Pet Hair

- A tip for those who dislike lugging a vacuum cleaner around every day: a Dutch Rubber Broom (see page 67) works magnificently for raking pet hair off rugs.
- It's easier to remove loose hair from the pet than to remove the pet's hair from the carpeting and upholstery. Brush your animal frequently to remove loose hair; do the job outdoors whenever possible.
- After you bathe your dog, rinse him with a solution of one part white distilled vinegar to three parts water. The vinegar will restore his skin's acid mantle. Don't get the vinegar water in the dog's eyes.
- Cleaning the hair while it's still on the dog is easy when it's snowy: while you and Fido are out walking, find a nice, clean patch of snow and use it to snow-clean your companion. Dry, crystalline snow works best for snow cleaning because it won't clump up in the dog's coat.
  1. Grasp the dog firmly by the collar, and tell him he's a really good boy.
  2. Rub handfuls of snow into his fur, working methodically so you cover his whole body. Scrub his whole body with snow a couple of times. (Most dogs love snow and don't mind this procedure at all. Our dogs hate being

bathed with water, but they love being scrubbed with snow.)

3. Brush the snow off the dog with your mittened hands. Put your nose on top of his head and inhale deeply. There are few smells quite as lovely as the smell of a snowy-fresh dog.

Cat Litter Boxes

After you empty and wash the litter box, pour about half an inch of distilled white vinegar in the box, slosh the entire interior with vinegar, then let it sit. Wait half an hour, then pour out the vinegar and dry the box. The vinegar will neutralize the urine smell.

Pet Safety

These common foods are toxic to dogs and cats: alcoholic beverages, avocados, chocolate, coffee, fatty foods, macadamia nuts, moldy and spoiled foods, onions and onion powder, raisins and grapes, salt, and yeast dough.

Pet Birds

Reducing the amount of toxins in your home will help keep your pet bird healthy. Birds react badly to the following contaminants: aerosol sprays, nonstick cooking sprays, the fumes emitted by hot nonstick pans, cigarette smoke, incense, and pesticides. Maybe we should all keep pet birds! If the bird stays healthy, we're likely to stay healthy, too.

Baby-Proofing

The reality of baby-proofing must be a shock to those who have never lived with a baby before. Babies explore the world with their mouths open and their taste buds primed.

I have heard many parents say things like, "But of course a baby wouldn't drink _____. It tastes horrible!" The truth of the matter is that babies' taste buds are quite different from ours. A baby may drink anything. Babies have been known to drink gasoline. How could any adult hope to guess what liquid might taste too horrible for a baby to drink? Or eat? A friend of mine who was baby-sitting a one-and-a-half-year-old boy was shocked and horrified to discover him eating a soap-impregnated steel wool pad. Her own daughter was the same age, yet was far too ladylike to have dreamed of doing such a thing.

Protecting Children from Dangers in the House

- Lock up everything that is not safe for a child to eat or grab. Make no assumptions about what very young children will or will not do. Assume that if she can reach it, it will be either licked or put in her mouth.
- Beware poisonous substances that look similar to food. Children who cannot read may not be able to tell the difference between these lookalikes:
  - a can of Comet cleanser and a can of parmesan cheese
  - moth balls and lemon- or butter-ball candies
  - pine cleaner and apple juice
  - a 64-ounce Drano jug and a jug of orange juice
- Put socket protectors in all your empty electrical sockets. Probing holes with a stick seems to be an innate primate activity.

Scald Prevention

After running bath water for your child, turn the hot water off first, then turn off the cold. That way the spigot and the drips will be cold, not hot. (Please refer to page 134 for more information on water heaters and water temperature.)

Protecting the House from the Children

- Stain prevention: Don't give small children purple grape juice, dark-colored candies, or dark cough syrups. Dark food coloring stains terribly, and it is not broken down by digestive processes. Grape Kool-Aid can stain straight out of the cup as well as after it has been jostled around in a youngster's stomach.

- Don't gum up the works: Very young children should never be given chewing gum unless you are already planning to replace your rugs, drapes, books, paintings, paperwork, wall coverings, pets, and upholstery.

  If a child is young enough to need to have gum removed from her hair, she is too young to be given gum. However, if the child and the gum have already melded, pour a little olive oil on the gum and it will lose its grip on the child's hair.

  Put gum-embellished clothing in the freezer to ease the removal process. Leave the clothing in the freezer overnight. The frozen gum will be hard and brittle and easy to break off the clothing.

  For more gum-removal tips, see page 259.

- Scribble avoidance: Supervise your young children while they color, and never let them use indelible ink under any circumstances. Access to marking materials such as pens, pencils, markers, and crayons, as well as to stickers and tape, should be parentally controlled unless you want to replace wall coverings, paint, furniture, books, and toys regularly. Chalk can be an uncontrolled substance that can be used freely outside or on chalkboards indoors.

- Urp-prevention: Feed babies and young children one type of liquid at a time. Milk with a chaser of apple juice is a reliable way to produce an upset stomach.

Cleaning Tricks

- Clean hard-water deposits out of baby bottles by soaking them in vinegar.

- Most stuffed toys are not machine washable. Unless a stuffed toy's label specifically states that it is safe for machine washing, don't put it in the washing machine. Small bits of shredded foam are difficult to clean out of clothing, washing machines, and filters, and foam may catch fire in the clothes dryer.

- Clean stuffed toys by putting them in a larger paper bag with a generous amount of cornmeal. Shake the bag vigorously then brush off the cornmeal.

- Stuffed toys may also be snow-washed in dry, crystalline snow. (See page 251 for detailed information on snow washing.)

Lice

If your child comes home from school with a lice advisory letter from the school nurse clutched in her little hand, don't panic, and don't rush to buy poison. Smearing a licicide in your child's hair may harm the child yet leave the lice unscathed. Lice, like many other pests, are becoming resistant to the poisons used against them; unfortunately, our children are not.

Lice are loathsome, but they are small and easily smothered. This is a pest control technique that will never go out of style:

1. Wash the child's hair thoroughly with your regular shampoo. Rinse, repeat.
2. Heat a half cup olive oil to blood heat. (When you stick your finger in, a blood temperature liquid should feel neither hot nor cold.)
3. Apply a heavy coating of the warm olive oil to the child's hair and scalp.
4. Cover the child's oiled tresses with a plastic shower cap or produce bag. (If your child is very young, you will have to watch her closely to make sure she neither suffocates in the plastic bag or shower cap nor oils your furnishings with her head.) The lice will smother under the heavy layer of oil.
5. Wait an hour then shampoo the oil out of her hair. Removing the oil will require at least two rounds of shampooing.
6. Towel dry the child's hair.
7. To loosen the dead lice, soak a clean towel in distilled white vinegar then wrap the towel turban style around the child's head, carefully covering every strand of hair.
8. Wrap a dry towel around the wet towel, and let your child's hair marinate for an hour.
9. Unwrap the towels and use a nit comb to remove the loosened lice.

To avert a household infestation, assume that everyone in the household has been exposed to lice. Treat everyone's hair with olive oil and vinegar. In addition, the afflicted child's clothes and the whole family's current set of sheets and towels should be washed in hot water and machine-dried. Sprinkle the furniture and carpets with boric acid or borax, wait an hour, then vacuum thoroughly. Put unwashable stuffed toys in plastic garbage bags and set them outdoors for a couple of weeks to freeze in the winter or broil in the summer.

Sit your child down and explain that having lice is too much work, and in order to avoid getting them again, she's going to have to keep her hats, headbands, brushes, and combs to herself, and avoid using those of other children.

Closing the Circle

This book ends with children because they are the ultimate reason that we need to learn to run our households without poisoning ourselves. If we keep our children uppermost in our minds, we will be far less likely to go off on dangerous chemical tangents that will damage our family's health and harm the environment.

It is not uncommon for people who are terribly concerned about their exposure to chemicals to lose track of what they are doing in their own homes and yards. I have, in the course of my landscaping career, had people proudly show me their organic vegetable gardens, then tell me about the pesticides and herbicides they use to maintain the rest of the yard; I've also met dedicated vegetarians who only eat organic food yet regularly drench their pine-shaded lawns with diazinon in order to kill ants.

A home should be a tool for enhancing life, not the be-all and end-all of life itself. Brain research has shown that the simple act of concentrating changes the physical structure of the brain.

We are what we eat; what we drink; what we breathe; what we touch; and perhaps most of all, what we think. If we focus too long and hard on what we fear and hate, our brains and consequently our minds and bodies will change for the worst. Fear not! Concentrate on what you love.

Bibliography

Cleaning, Cooking, Decluttering, and Home Maintenance Books

Andrews, Cecile. *The Circle of Simplicity: Return to the Good Life.* New York: Harper-Collins, 1997. www.cecileandrews.com

Aslett, Don. *Clutter's Last Stand.* Cincinnati, Ohio: Writer's Digest Book, 1984.

Bacharach, Bert. *How to Do Almost Everything.* New York: Simon and Schuster, 1970.

Barrett, Patti. *Too Busy to Clean? Over 500 Tips and Techniques to Make Housecleaning Easier.* Pownal, Vermont: Storey Publishing, 1990.

Berthold-Bond, Annie. *Clean & Green.* Woodstock, New York: Ceres Press, 1990.

Bredenberg, Jeff, editor. *Clean It Fast, Clean It Right.* Emmaus, Pennsylvania: Rodale, 1998.

Campbell, Jeff. *Speed Cleaning.* New York: Dell Publishing, 1991.

Dadd, Debra Lynn. *Home Safe Home.* New York: Jeremy P. Tarcher, 2004. www.dld123.com

Eighner, Lars. *Travels with Lizbeth: Three Years on the Road and on the Streets.* New York: St. Martin's Press, 1993.

Mendelson, Cheryl. *Home Comforts: The Art and Science of Keeping House.* New York: Scribner, 1999.

Morgenstern, Julie. *Organizing from the Inside Out: The Foolproof System for Organizing Your Home, Your Office, and Your Life.* New York: Henry Holt, 1998

Schwartz, Barry. *The Paradox of Choice: Why More Is Less.* New York: Ecco, Harper-Collins, 2004.

Steinman, David. *Diet for a Poisoned Planet: How to Choose Safe Food for You and Your Family.* New York: Harmony Books, 1990.

Strasser, Susan. *Never Done: A History of American Housework.* New York: Pantheon Books, 1982.

Gardening and Animal Books

Bradley, F. M., and Anna Carr, editors. *Chemical-Free Yard & Garden*. Emmaus, Pennsylvania: Rodale Press, 1991.

Campbell, Stu. *Let It Rot!* Pownal, Vermont: Storey Publishing,1990.

Daar, Sheila, Helga Olkowski, and William Olkowski. *Common-Sense Pest Control*. Newtown, Connecticut: Taunton Books and Videos, Bio-Integral Resource Center, 1991.

Frazier, Anitra. *The New Natural Cat*. New York: Plume, 1990.

Hill, John W.,and Doris K. Kolb. *Chemistry for Changing Times*. Ninth Edition. Upper Saddle River, New Jersey: Prentice Hall, 1998, 2001.

An Illustrated Guide to Organic Gardening. Menlo Park, California: Sunset Publishing Corporation, 1991.

Klein, Hilary Dole, and Adrian M. Wenner. *Tiny Game Hunting*. New York: Bantam Books, 1991.

Lifton, Bernice. *Bug Busters: Getting Rid of Household Pests Without Dangerous Chemicals*. Minneapolis, Minnesota: McGraw-Hill, 1985.

Milne, Lorus, and Margery Milne. *National Audubon Society Field Guide to North American Insects and Spiders*. New York: Alfred A. Knopf, 1980.

Rodale, J. I. *How to Grow Vegetables and Fruits by the Organic Method*. Emmaus, Pennsylvania: Rodale Press, 1990.

Sandbeck, Ellen. *Eat More Dirt: Diverting and Instructive Tips for Growing and Tending an Organic Garden*. New York: Broadway Books, 2003.

———. *Laverme's Handbook of Indoor Worm-Composting*. Duluth, Minnesota: De la Terre Press, 1998.

———. *Slug Bread & Beheaded Thistles: Amusing and Useful Techniques for Nontoxic Housekeeping and Gardening*. New York: Broadway Books, 2000.

Wallace, Dan, editor. *The Natural Formula Book For Home and Yard*. Emmaus, Pennsylvania: Rodale, 1982.

Wolverton, B. C. *How to Grow Fresh Air: 50 Houseplants that Purify Your Home or Office*. New York: Penguin Books, 1997.

Magazine Articles

Anderson, Rosalind C., and Julius H. Anderson. "Acute Respiratory Effects of Diaper Emissions." *Archives of Environmental Health* (September 1999).

"Asthma, Allergies, Bronchitis and Cough Linked to Chlordane Homes." *Bulletin of Environmental Contamination Toxicology*, 39:903 (1987).

"Chewing Leaves to Fight Fleas." *Science Now* (August 3, 1998).

Curl, Cynthia L., Richard A. Fenske, and Kai Elgethun. "Organophosphorus Pesticide Exposure of Urban and Suburban Preschool Children with Organic and Conventional Diets." *Environmental Health Perspectives*, vol. 111, no. 3 (March 2003).

Edelson, Edward. "Vietnam Herbicide Connection Called 'Suggestive.' " *Health Scout Reporter* (April 20, 2001).

Epstein, David J. "Secret Ingredients 'Inert' Compounds May Be Chemically Active and Toxic." *Scientific American* (August 2003): 22.

"Farm Harm; Ag Chemicals May Cause Prostate Cancer." *Science News*, vol. 163 (May 10, 2003): 291.

"Genetic Link May Tie Together Pesticides, ADHD, Gulf War Syndrome and Other Disorders." *ScienceDaily Magazine* (2003–03–18).

Harder, Ben. "Composted Sewage Captures Dirt's Lead." *Science News*, vol. 163 (March 29, 2003): 205.

Heselbarth, Rob. "Hold Your Fire; Despite the myths surrounding them, fire sprinklers are gaining acceptance in the home." *The Healthy Home Supplement Contractor* (July 1998).

Holladay, Steven D., and Ralph J. Smialowicz. "Development of the Murine and Human Immune System: Differential Effects of Immunotoxicants Depend on Time of Exposure." *Environmental Health Perspectives*, vol. 108, supplement 3 (June 2000).

"Immune System Macrophages Paralyzed By Chlordane." *Agents & Actions Journal*, 37 (1992):140–46.

Marion, Robert. "The baby who stopped eating" (infant with botulism). *Discover* (August 1998).

Mazdai, Anita, Nathan Dodder, Mary Pell, G. Abernathy, Ronald A. Hites, and Robert M. Bigsby. "Polybrominated Diphenyl Ethers in Maternal and Fetal Blood Samples." *Environmental Health Perspectives*, vol. 111, no. 9 (July 2003).

"Neuroblastoma & Leukemia After Chlordane Exposure." *Teratogenesis, Carcinogenesis, and Mutagenesis*, 7 (1987): 527–40.

"Overweight—a Symptom of Chlordane Exposure." *Toxicology & Applied Pharmacology*, 126 (1994): 326–37.

Pickrell, John. "Cancer Causer? Researchers Zero in on Leukemia Risks." *Science News*, vol. 162 (September 21, 2002): 179.

Qiao, Dan, Frederic J. Seidler, Stephanie Padilla, and Theodore A. Slotkin. "Developmental Neurotoxicity of Chlorpyrifos: What is the Vulnerable Period?" *Environmental Health Perspectives*, vol. 110, no. 11 (November 2002).

Raloff, Janet. "Inhaling Your Food—and Its Cooking Fuel." *Science News*, vol. 165 (April 10, 2004).

———. "New PCBs?" *Science News*, vol. 164, no. 17 (October 25, 2003): 266.

———. "Spray Guards Chicks from Infections." *Science News* (March 28, 1998).

Schönfelder, G., W. Wittfoht, H. Hopp, C. E. Talsness, M. Paul, and I. Chahoud. "Parent Bisphenol A Accumulation in the Human Maternal-Fetal-Placental Unit." *Environmental Health Perspectives*, 110:(2002): A703-A707.

Selevan, Sherry G., Carole A. Kimmel, and Pauline Mendola. "Identifying Critical Windows of Exposure for Children's Health." *Environmental Health Perspectives*, vol. 108, supplement 3 (June 2000).

Thompson, Becky. "Drinking from Garden Hose Can Be Dangerous to Health." *Consumer Reports* (2003).

Weiss, Bernard. "Vulnerability of Children and the Developing Brain to Neurotoxic Hazards." *Environmental Health Perspectives*, vol. 108, supplement 3 (June 2000).

Newspaper Articles

Bracken, Amy. "Deadly Floods in Haiti Blamed on Deforestation, Poverty." Associated Press (September 24, 2004).

Hair, Marty. "Rain Garden Preserves Natural Water Cycle." Knight Ridder, Detroit (October 30, 2003).

Kolata, Gina. "Lyme Disease Is Hard to Catch and Easy to Halt, Study Finds." *The New York Times* (June 13, 2001).

O'Neil, John. "Hazards: The Dirty Business of Cleaning." *The New York Times* (November 4, 2003).

Robbins, John Charles. "Survey, Fertilizer on Lawns Still Problem for Watershed." Michigan: *Holland Sentinel* (September 28, 2003).

"U.S. Traffic Deaths Increase to Highest Point in 12 years." *USA Today* (July 17, 2003).

Press Releases

Brunetti, Kathy. "California Proposes Cancellation of DDVP Pest Strips." California Department of Pesticide Regulation (February 19, 1999).

"Cockroaches Beware! This House Has Been Treated with Catnip." American Chemical Society (August 27, 1999).

"Composted Biosolids Bind Lead in Soil, Reducing Danger of Poisoning." University of Washington (March 3, 2003).

"Do You Know What You're Eating? An Analysis of U.S. Government Data on Pesticide Residues in Foods." Consumers Union of United States, Inc. Public Service Projects Department Technical Division (February 1999).

"Highest Vehicle Death Rate Since 1990, Increase in SUV Rollover Deaths, Prompts Call for Passage of Safety Provisions." Consumers Union (April 28, 2004).

"U.C. Riverside Study Indicates Mosquito Coils May Cause Cancer." University of California, Riverside (2003-09-08).

Government and University Publications and Reports

"Backyard Burning Is a Health Hazard." U.S. Environmental Protection Agency (September 2003).

Barron, Thomas, Carol Berg, and Linda Bookman. "Janitorial Products Pollution Prevention Project." U.S. Enviromental Protection Aagency. State of California, Santa Clara County, the city of Richmond, and the Local Government Commission (June 1999).

Brunetti and Fabre, editors. "Source Book of Urban Pest Management." California Department of Food and Agriculture (1984).

"Building Deconstruction and Reuse." U.S. Environmental Protection Agency (September 2002).

Coats, Joel, and Chris Peterson. "Catnip Drives Cats Wild, But Drives Mosquitoes Away." Iowa State University, College of Agriculture (August 27, 2001).

"Cosmetics and Colors," fact sheet. U.S. Food and Drug Administration Center for Food Safety and Applied Nutrition (December 9, 1999).

Glowacki, Douglas. "Drought Response Home." State of Connecticut (2002–3).

Gouveia-Vigeant, Tami, Joel Tickner, and Richard Clapp. "Toxic Chemicals and Childhood Cancer: A Review of the Evidence." University of Massachusetts, The Lowell Center for Sustainable Production (May 2003).

Larson, Elaine. "Hygiene of the Skin: When Is Clean Too Clean?" Centers for Disease Control and Prevention vol. 7, no. 2 (March–April 2001).

Meer, Ralph, and Scottie Misner. "The Latest in Kitchen Sanitation." The University of Arizona College of Agriculture, Cooperative Extension, Tucson (December 1997).

"National Report on Human Exposure to Environmental Chemicals." The Centers for Disease Control (March 21, 2001).

"Pests of the Garden and Small Farm." University of California Cooperative Extension, Integrated Pest Management Project (1990).

"Public Health Statement for 1,4-Dichlorobenzene." Agency for Toxic Substances and Disease Registry (December 1998).

"Rain Gardens: A Household Way to Improve Water Quality in Your Community." The University of Wisconsin Extension and Wisconsin Department of Natural Resources (2002).

Reports and Fact Sheets

"1,4-Dichlorobenzene, CAS No.106–46–7: Reasonably Anticipated to be a Human Carcinogen." Tenth Report on Carcinogens. U.S. Department of Health and Human Services, Public Health Service, National Toxicology Program (December 2002); http://ehp.niehs.nih.gov/roc/tenth/profiles/s062dich.pdf.

1,4-Dichlorobenzene Chemical Backgrounder. National Safety Council; http://www.nsc.org/ehc/chemical/14-dichl.htm.

"All About Faucets." National Retail Hardware Association (2002).

Broce, A. B., and J. E. Urban. "Potential Microbial Health Hazards Associated with Operation of Bug Zappers." Annual Meeting of the American Society for Microbiology, abstracts (1998).

"Case Study: Nondisposable Diapers—A Cost Effective Change." State of Michigan Departments of Commerce and Natural Resources, Office of Waste Reduction Services (February 1992): #9201.

"Citizens Guide to Pesticides." Environmental Protection Agency #426X.

"Fire Loss in the U.S. and Fire in the United States 1987–1996," 11th ed. National Fire Protection Association (1998).

Goldberg, Rob. "The Big Picture, Life Cycle Analysis." Academy of Natural Sciences, Philadelphia (May 1992).

"Greenseal's Report: Carpet." Greenseal, Washington, D.C. (December 2001).

"Greenseal's Report: Floor Care Products: Finishes and Strippers," Greenseal, Washington, D.C. (June 2004).

Hall, John R. Jr. "Home Cooking Fire Patterns and Trends." National Fire Protection Association (October 2003).

Hazardous Substance Fact Sheet: 1,4-dichlorobenzene, revised. New Jersey Department of Health and Senior Services (June 1998); http://www.state.nj.us/health/eoh/rtkweb/0643.pdf.

"Health Hazards from Flea and Tick Products." Natural Resources Defense Council Report (November 2000).

Horton, Sydney. "In-Home Pesticide Exposure Increases Parkinson's Risk." American Academy of Neurology (2000–05–09).

Material Safety Data Sheet: p-dichlorobenzene. Mallinckrodt Baker, Inc. (November 2, 2001); http://www.jtbaker.com/msds/englishhtml/D2224.htm.

"National Primary Drinking Water Regulations: Consumer Fact Sheet on Para-Dichlorobenzene (p-DCB)," updated. U.S. Environmental Protection Agency, Office of Water, Ground Water and Drinking Water (April 12, 2001).

"Candle Safety." National Fire Protection Association.

"Ozone Generators that are Sold as Air Cleaners: An Assessment of Effectiveness and Health Consequences" updated. U.S. Environmental Protection Agency (July 2004).

"Risky Chemicals: A Guide for Retailers and Other Downstream Users." Friends of the Earth, London, England (July, 2002).

Smith, Joyce A. "Textiles and Clothing." Ohio State University Extension.

Thorton, Joe. "Environmental Impacts of Polyvinyl Building Materials." The Healthy Building Network, Washington, D.C. (2002).

ToxFAQs for 1,4-dichlorobenzene. Agency for Toxic Substances and Disease Registry (June 1999); http://www.atsdr.cdc.gov/tfacts10.html.

Useful Websites

RECYCLING INFORMATION
    Apple Computer
    Apple Recycles Program:
        www.apple.com/environment/recycling/nationalservices/us.html

    Carnegie Mellon Green Design Initiative
    Website contains information about electronics recycling:
        www.ce.cmu.edu/GreenDesign/index.html

COMPAQ
Computer asset recovery services: www.hp.com/hpinfo/globalcitizenship/
environment/recycle/hardwarerecycle.html

Dell Computer, Dell Recycling
Dell Computer offers free recycling of your old computer when you buy a new
Dell Computer, and it also offers a slight discount on a new Dell computer
when you recycle your old Dell Computer through them:
www1.us.dell.com/content/topics/segtopic.aspx/dell_recycling

Earth 911
This website helps consumers find information about local environmental
resources, including hazardous waste disposal programs: www.earth911.org

Empties For Cash
Ink jet cartridge recycling: www.empties4cash.com

The Funding Factory
To recycle old cell phones and ink jet cartridges: www.fundingfactory.com;
www.inkjetcartridges.com; www.c-rep.net

Hewlett-Packard
Hardware Recycling: www.hp.com/hpinfo/globalcitizenship/environment/
recycle/hardwarerecycle.html

IBM
Product End-of-Life Management (PELM) Service:
www.ibm.com/ibm/responsibility/world/environmental/products.shtml

International Association of Electronics Recyclers (IAER)
Comprehensive list of electronics recyclers: www.iaer.org/search

National Recycling Coalition
Website hosts a database of electronics recyclers, reuse organizations, and
municipal programs that accept old electronic equipment: www.
nrc-recycle.org/programs/electronics/search/getlisting.asp

Recycler's World
Website lists computer and telecommunications equipment recyclers and
refurbishers, and it hosts a worldwide electronics materials exchange:
www.recycle.net/computer

CARPET RECYCLING
Antron Carpet Company: www.infinitynylon.com
Los Angeles Fiber Company: www.lafiber.com/sys-tmpl/recycleprogram
Milliken & Company: www.earthsquare.com

Carpet Made of Recycled Fibers

Beaulieu of America: www.beaulieu-usa.com
Collins and Aikman Floorcoverings, modular carpet tiles:
   www.cafloorcoverings.com
Greenfloors: www.greenfloors.com
J&J Industries: www.jjindustries.com
Lees Carpets: www.leescarpets.com
Mannington Mills: www.mannington.com
Milliken Carpet Earth Squares: www.millikencarpet.com
Talisman Mills: www.talismanmills.com

Styrofoam Packing Peanuts Recycling Information

Plastic Loose Fill Council (go to website for nearest recycling facility):
   www.loosefillpackaging.com

Cleaning Equipment Sources

Cumberland General Store (old-fashioned housekeeping aids):
   www.cumberlandgeneral.com
Euroshine USA, Inc. (Dutch Rubber Brooms): www.euroshine.net
Lehman's (old-fashioned store caters to the Amish): www.lehmans.com
Vermont Country Store (old-fashioned housekeeping aids):
   www.vermontcountrystore.com

Environmentally Friendly Cleaning Products and Toiletries

Burt's Bees (natural toiletries and cosmetics): www.burtsbees.com
Dr. Bronner's Magic Soaps (vegetable oil–based soaps): www.drbronner.com
Ecover (detergents and dish liquids): www.ecover.com
Green Mercantile: www.greenmercantile.com
Planet Inc.: www.planetinc.com
Seventh Generation (dish detergents, dish liquids, laundry detergent, recycled
   papergoods): www.seventhgen.com
Tom's of Maine (natural grooming products): www.tomsofmaine.com

Supplies for Making Cleaning Products and Toiletries

www.fromnaturewithlove.com
www.snowdriftfarm.com

Biodegradable, Disposable Tableware

Nat-Ur, Inc. produces corn- and potato-based biodegradable garbage bags, food
   service containers, and compostable, disposable plates, bowls, cups,
   cutlery: www.cereplast.com

Floor Strippers

www.enviro-solution.com
www.fuller.com
www.green-solution.com

www.hillyard.com
www.johnsondiversey.com
www.mdstetson.com
www.orisonllc.com
www.pioneer-eclipse.com
www.rochestermidland.com

Paints and Finishes
The Real Milk Paint Company: www.realmilkpaint.com
William Zinsser & Co. (real shellac, made from lac beetles): www.zinsser.com

Insulating Paint
GBS Kwik Company: www.heatshield-r20.com
Hy-Tech Inc.: www.hytechsales.com
Pawnee Specialties: www.koolcoat.com

Self-Cleaning Glass Manufacturers
AFG Glass Radiance Ti tm: www.afgglass.com
Pilkington Activtm: www.activglass.com
PPG Industries SunCleantm: www.ppg.com

Energy Efficient Appliances
The American Council for an Energy Efficient Economy (Appliance efficiency ratings): www.aceee.org

Child-Labor Free Wool Carpets
RUGMARK Foundation: www.rugmark.org

Organic Gardening Supplies
Arbico Organics: store.arbico-organics.com
Ben Meadows Company (forestry and garden tools and clothing; safety equipment: goggles, hardhats, gloves): www.benmeadows.com
Bio Organics Mycorrhizae Products (mycorrhizal innoculant): www. bio-organics.com
Fungi Perfecti (mycorrihizal inoculant): www.fungi.com
Gardens Alive! (natural fertilizers, supplements, and pest control): www.gardensalive.com
Horticultural Alliance, Inc. (mycorrhizal innoculant): www.hortsorb.com
Peaceful Valley Farm Supply (garden tools and supplies): www.groworganic.com
Planet Natural: www.planetnatural.com
Worm's Way: www.wormsway.com

Environmental, Health, Safety, and Government Websites
Centers for Disease Control and Prevention: www.cdc.gov
Office of Energy Efficiency and Renewable Energy (EERE): www.eere.energy.gov
Environmental Protection Agency: www.epa.gov

Integrated Pest Management information from the University of California at
    Davis: www.ipm.ucdavis.edu/PMG/PESTNOTES
Internal Revenue Service (tax forms and information): www.irs.gov
National Cancer Institute: www.cancer.gov
National Environmental Health Association (NEHA): www.neha.org
National Fire Protection Association (NFPA): www.nfpa.org
National Highway Traffic Safety Administration (NHSTSA): www.nhtsa.dot.gov
National Institute for Occupational Safety and Health (NIOSH):
    www.cdc.gov/niosh
National Institutes of Health (NIH): www.nih.gov
National Kidney and Urologic Diseases Information Clearinghouse
    (NKUDIC), a service of the National Institute of Diabetes and Digestive
    and Kidney Diseases (NIDDK), NIH: kidney.niddk.nih.gov/index.htm
Occupational Safety & Health Administration: www.osha.gov
U.S. Consumer Product Safety Commission: www.cpsc.gov
U.S. Department of Energy: www.doe.gov
U.S. Fire Administration: www.usfa.fema.gov
U.S. Food and Drug Administration (USDA) link to Pathology Lab
    Guidebook: www.fsis.usda.gov

CONSUMERS' ORGANIZATIONS
The Consumers Union (nonprofit organization that tests consumer products
    and publishes the magazine *Consumer Reports*): www.consumerreports.org
    and GreenerChoices.org
Friends of the Earth: www.foe.org
Greenseal (product testing): www.greenseal.org
Organic Consumers Union: www.organicconsumers.org

HEALTH ISSUES
American Society for the Prevention of Cruelty to Animals: www.aspca.org
The Poison Control nationwide number: 1-800-222-1222

RADON MITIGATION
The American Lung Association: www.lungusa.org
National Environmental Health Association (NEHA): www.neha.org

ENVIRONMENTAL ORGANIZATIONS
Blue Vinyl (information about PVC): www.bluevinyl.com
Children's Health Environmental (CHEC): www.checnet.org
Natural Resources Defense Council: www.nrdc.org
Union of Concerned Scientists: www.ucsusa.org

MANUFACTURERS ASSOCIATION WEBSITES
American Fire Sprinkler Association: www.SprinklerNet.org
Association of Home Appliance Manufacturers: www.aham.org
Gas Appliance Manufacturer's Association: www.gamanet.org

Index

baking soda *(cont.)*
    kitchen cleaning uses, 76, 77, 78–79, 81,
        82, 94, 96, 122, 125
    in laundry and stain removal, 201, 212,
        255, 256, 258, 260
    for mold and mildew, 344
    in moss removal, 344
    to neutralize acids, 147
    for odor removal, 173–74
ball point pen ink, 202
bamboo flooring, 231, 238, 246, 247, 334
barbeque, fire safety, 318–20
bark cloth, 240
bathtubs
    choosing, 134–35, 243
    cleaning, 138–39, 145–56, 149–52, 154–55
    clog busting, 143–45
bats, 381, 391
batteries, 42–43, 336, 349
beans/legumes, poisonous, 375
beauty products, 157–63
bedbugs, 184
beeswax, 161
bifidobacteria, 113
bills, 24
biodegradable products, 45, 63–64
birds, pet, 397
birth defects, 128, 160
bisphenol A (BPA), 127–28
black fungus, 291
blankets
    duvet covers for, 168–69
    electric, 327–28
bleaches, 179, 186–87, 192–95, 212
blinds, window, 239, 270–71
blood stain removal, 174, 199, 256
bloodsuckers, 390
bluing, 196, 227
body grease, 267
Bon Ami cleanser, 64, 81, 148
bonnetting, 252–53
books, recycling, 28
borax
    bathroom cleaning uses, 150
    in homemade dishwasher detergent, 74
    kitchen cleaning uses, 68, 74, 91
    in laundry and stain removal, 187, 195,
        210, 212, 227, 258, 259
    for mildew removal, 152
    for odor removal, 173

for pest control, 381–82, 383–84, 395, 401
    wall cleaning uses, 267
botulism, 101–4
bovine spongiform encephalopathy (BSE),
    111
boxes
    cardboard-box organizing system, 17–18
    labeling storage, 20
    photo, 23
brake fluid, 349
brass food containers, 126
brick flooring, 233, 334
bulbs, poisonous, 374
bulk-buying, 41, 42
burn barrels, 307
burnt food, 77, 79, 89, 91, 317, 319
bushes, 345, 372–73

cabbage leaves, in cleaning pewter, 126
cadaverine, 108–9
calendars, 39–40
camel hair, 214, 240
camping, 226, 312
campylobacter jejuni bacteria, 105, 106, 112–13
cancer, 205, 318–19, 333
candles
    fire safety, 329–30, 332, 338
    lead-stiffened, 282–83
    odor and, 79
    particulate pollution, 282–83
    wax removal, 125–26, 260
carbon monoxide, 283–84, 289, 320–21, 322,
    333
car care and safety, 346–51
cardboard
    above kitchen cabinets, 62
    recycling, 17–18, 48
carpeting and rugs, 233–38
    bathroom, 131, 236
    chemical contamination, 238
    choosing, 235–36, 335
    cleaning, 250–60
    color choices, 242–43
    dusty, 234–35
    fiber types, 233–34, 238
    fire safety, 334, 335
    kitchen, 67, 236
    mold and mildew in, 291
    pest control, 395, 396
    reclaimed, 236–37